The Impact of the COVID-19 Pandemic on Child, Adolescent, and Adult Development

Nava R. Silton
Marymount Manhattan College, USA

A volume in the Advances in Psychology, Mental Health, and Behavioral Studies (APMHBS) Book Series

IGI Global
PUBLISHER of TIMELY KNOWLEDGE

Published in the United States of America by
IGI Global
Information Science Reference (an imprint of IGI Global)
701 E. Chocolate Avenue
Hershey PA, USA 17033
Tel: 717-533-8845
Fax: 717-533-8661
E-mail: cust@igi-global.com
Web site: http://www.igi-global.com

Library of Congress Cataloging-in-Publication Data

Names: Silton, Nava R., 1981- editor.
Title: The impact of the COVID-19 pandemic on child, adolescent, and adult development / Nava Silton, editor.
Description: Hershey, PA : Information Science Reference, [2022] | Includes bibliographical references and index. | Summary: "This book delves into how the COVID-19 pandemic impacted children's schooling, relationships, mental, physical and developmental health and how it particularly, adversely impacted those with disabilities, providing best practices for moving forward"-- Provided by publisher.
Identifiers: LCCN 2021044529 (print) | LCCN 2021044530 (ebook) | ISBN 9781668434840 (hardcover) | ISBN 9781668434857 (paperback) | ISBN 9781668434864 (ebook)
Subjects: LCSH: Child development. | Child psychology. | Developmental psychology. | Maturation (Psychology) | COVID-19 Pandemic--Psychological aspects.
Classification: LCC HQ767.9 .I55175 2022 (print) | LCC HQ767.9 (ebook) | DDC 305.231--dc23/eng/20211013
LC record available at https://lccn.loc.gov/2021044529
LC ebook record available at https://lccn.loc.gov/2021044530

This book is published in the IGI Global book series Advances in Psychology, Mental Health, and Behavioral Studies (APMHBS) (ISSN: 2475-6660; eISSN: 2475-6679)

British Cataloguing in Publication Data
A Cataloguing in Publication record for this book is available from the British Library.

For electronic access to this publication, please contact: eresources@igi-global.com.

Advances in Psychology, Mental Health, and Behavioral Studies (APMHBS) Book Series

ISSN:2475-6660
EISSN:2475-6679

Editor-in-Chief: Bryan Christiansen, Global Research Society, LLC, USA, Harish C. Chandan, Argosy University, USA

MISSION

The complexity of the human mind has puzzled researchers and physicians for centuries. While widely studied, the brain still remains largely misunderstood.

The **Advances in Psychology, Mental Health, and Behavioral Studies (APMHBS)** book series presents comprehensive research publications focusing on topics relating to the human psyche, cognition, psychiatric care, mental and developmental disorders, as well as human behavior and interaction. Featuring diverse and innovative research, publications within APMHBS are ideally designed for use by mental health professionals, academicians, researchers, and upper-level students.

COVERAGE

- Personality Disorders
- Eating Disorders
- Emotional Health
- Counseling & Therapy
- Trauma & Stress
- Developmental Disorders
- Anxiety
- Substance Abuse
- Treatment & Care
- Socialization

The Advances in Psychology, Mental Health, and Behavioral Studies (APMHBS) Book Series (ISSN 2475-6660) is published by IGI Global, 701 E. Chocolate Avenue, Hershey, PA 17033-1240, USA, www.igi-global.com. This series is composed of titles available for purchase individually; each title is edited to be contextually exclusive from any other title within the series. For pricing and ordering information please visit http://www.igi-global.com/book-series/advances-psychology-mental-health-behavioral/110200. Postmaster: Send all address changes to above address.

Titles in this Series

For a list of additional titles in this series, please visit:
http://www.igi-global.com/book-series/advances-psychology-mental-health-behavioral/110200

Stabilization Approaches in Mental Health Care
Peter Leslie King (Australian DBT Institute, Australia)
Medical Information Science Reference • © 2022 • 320pp • H/C (ISBN: 9781799882282) • US $325.00

Counseling Strategies for Children and Families Impacted by Incarceration
Kenya Johns (Duquesne University, USA)
Medical Information Science Reference • © 2022 • 320pp • H/C (ISBN: 9781799892090) • US $265.00

Handbook of Research on Neurocognitive Development of Executive Functions and Implications for Intervention
Francisco Alcantud-Marín (University of Valencia, Spain) María Fernanda López-Ramón (University of Valencia, Spain) Esperanza Navarro-Pardo (University of Valencia, Spain) Veronica Moreno-Campos (University of Valencia, Spain) and Yurena Alonso-Esteban (University of Valencia, Spain)
Medical Information Science Reference • © 2022 • 494pp • H/C (ISBN: 9781799890751) • US $345.00

Mental Health and Wellness in Healthcare Workers Identifying Risks, Prevention, and Treatment
Clint A. Bowers (University of Central Florida, USA) Deborah C. Beidel (University of Central Florida, USA) Madeline R. Marks (University of Maryland, USA) Kristin Horan (University of Central Florida, USA) and Janis Cannon-Bowers (Cannon-Bowers Consulting, USA)
Medical Information Science Reference • © 2022 • 393pp • H/C (ISBN: 9781799888130) • US $295.00

Provision of Psychosocial Support and Education of Vulnerable Children
Simon George Taukeni (University of Namibia, Namibia) Joyce Mathwasa (University of Fort Hare, South Africa) and Zoleka Ntshuntshe (University of Fort Hare, South Africa)
Information Science Reference • © 2022 • 335pp • H/C (ISBN: 9781799888963) • US $195.00

For an entire list of titles in this series, please visit:
http://www.igi-global.com/book-series/advances-psychology-mental-health-behavioral/110200

IGI Global
PUBLISHER of TIMELY KNOWLEDGE

701 East Chocolate Avenue, Hershey, PA 17033, USA
Tel: 717-533-8845 x100 • Fax: 717-533-8661
E-Mail: cust@igi-global.com • www.igi-global.com

Editorial Advisory Board

Table of Contents

Detailed Table of Contents

The chapter aims to examine the adaptation to the coronavirus disease-2019 (COVID-19) pandemic process of adults previously diagnosed with a chronic illness. Chronic illnesses negatively affect a person's psychosocial functioning as well as their physical health. When the COVID-19 pandemic entered people's lives, a higher risk was expected for individuals with chronic illnesses. Several studies were conducted to understand their COVID-19 adaptation process and psychosocial consequences. Studies revealed high levels of depressive and anxious symptoms as well as non-compliance, fear of COVID-19, isolation, and loneliness. From another viewpoint, individuals with chronic illnesses were also able to cope with COVID-19-related stressors and some of them experienced better well-being outcomes. Online and telehealth interventions were offered for people in need of psychosocial support. The pandemic experience helped people develop an understanding of the management of health threats and a multidimensional perspective toward health.

The COVID-19 outbreak began in December of 2019 and affected many worldwide. Research posited that those with ADHD might struggle more with the conditions of the COVID-19 pandemic than their neuro-typical counterparts. The objective of this chapter was to collect and synthesize much of the present research surrounding those with ADHD and to determine how they have been impacted by COVID-19 in hopes of providing ways to mitigate those impacts. The chapter evaluates the research suggesting that ADHD may be a potential risk factor for contracting COVID-19 and discusses how to reduce the possible increased risk of transmission in both children and adults with ADHD. The chapter also examines the effects of lockdowns and online schooling and working from home on children and adults with ADHD as well as best practices for mitigating these impacts.

In early 2020, the SARS-CoV-2 Virus made its appearance and has, since then, substantially impacted our lives. Those with mental health issues have been significantly impacted and are still adjusting. Multiple studies since then have been conducted to study its effects. This literature review aims to expand on the research conducted regarding the effects of COVID-19 on patients with obsessive-compulsive disorder (OCD). After briefly reviewing research articles, coping and management techniques were discussed. Lastly, future research suggestions are provided. Five research studies are reviewed, and all of the results reveal that the pandemic has worsened OCD severity. For example, results of the Khosravani et al. study, which included 270 participants, showed that stress reactions related to compulsive checking and contamination exacerbated patient's OCD. A study by Tanir et al., which included 61 participants, discovered that contamination obsessions and cleaning or washing compulsions increased during the pandemic. Additionally, a study by David et al. with 30 participants found that contamination symptoms, particularly along with remitters, showed a worsening of OCD when compared to pre-COVID levels. Regarding coping mechanisms, patients with OCD used instrumental support, religion, denial, and self-blame when dealing with changes to their disorder. Researchers have advised therapists to monitor patients' screen time, since that's one of the ways that OCD levels of those with contamination, hygiene, and cleanliness obsessions tends to worsen. As for future directions, researchers should aim for longitudinal studies, which would fully measure the effects of the pandemic on OCD. The chapter concludes by elaborating on suggestions, since a vaccine is now available.

Foreword

As a physician in a Pediatric Intensive Care Unit, the Coronavirus Disease 19 (COVID-19) pandemic affected me and my patients in a very significant way. Though children were generally spared, there were some who experienced substantial illness. Numerous children ended up on ventilators and various forms of life support. Fortunately, the large majority of them survived, but the effect on the others should not be understated. Furthermore, the unknown nature of COVID-19 made caring for these children all the more difficult. We were faced with questions that we simply didn't have answers to: Will this treatment work? How long will my child need to be in the hospital? Will my child survive? Although we often deal with the unknown in medicine, these types of questions became exponentially more difficult during the pandemic. Thankfully, we know a lot more today than we did in the beginning of 2020, but there is still much to be learned about this elusive disease.

In the beginning of the pandemic, society, understandably, was focused on the physical health of those affected by COVID-19. The hard work of health care workers was vital. However, as we move past the acute phase of this horrid disease, the long-term effects of COVID-19 have arguably become more important. *The Impact of the COVID-19 Pandemic on Child, Adolescent, and Adult Development* has been written at the perfect moment. Society now needs to understand what we can expect from COVID-19 as we continue to move forward and Silton's text does just that.

The Impact of the COVID-19 Pandemic on Child, Adolescent, and Adult Development touches on numerous sensitive issues that, until now, have received little attention in the literature. The impact on people's physical health should not be understated, but it is equally important for us to understand the psychological effects of COVID-19. There are those with a history of mental illness who were severely impacted by this virus and those who developed a new mental illness as a result of it; vulnerable populations such as children, the elderly, and those with physical impairments, were impacted by COVID-19 in ways that might not be overt; underdeveloped countries did not have the proper infrastructure and resources to properly handle the pandemic. These are just some of the key topics covered in

Silton's text. Each of the chapters in the text can function as a valuable resource to healthcare and mental health professionals, teachers, and parents.

The hope is that this text eventually serves as a historical perspective of a dark time in our lives and that society never needs to deal with these atrocities again. But as we know, those who do not learn from history are doomed to repeat it. Let's not make that mistake. We should heed the lessons taught in this text and prepare for the future of COVID-19 or perhaps the next plague that wreaks havoc on the world.

Ariel Brandwein
NYP-Brooklyn Methodist Hospital, USA

Preface

The astute authors of the fascinating studies in this compendium investigate a topic so new and devastating that it has "jumped the tracks" as most pandemics do. Nimble, mutating and perilous COVID-19 has wreaked havoc on adults, children and especially on vulnerable populations. It has disrupted and continues to disrupt our lives and has spawned an ever-changing global reality.

"How lucky we are," we originally thought. Zoom was just waiting in the wings to help us. How fortunate that the children's studies could continue seamlessly and that their parents, in great part, could conduct business virtually, in their pajamas. Once churches, synagogues and mosques realized they could conduct religious services and offer comfort, they hurried to do so through the good services of Zoom. How opportune that telemedicine could serve patients who lacked medical services in underserved or rural areas. Now without one-on-one personal contact, patients and their medical providers could speak on the telephone and often use face-time to meet their needs.

Of course, the initial notions of finding a quick fix were soon flummoxed. Section 1 of this collection of chapters, details the impact COVID-19 had and still has on vulnerable populations. Our diverse populations have encountered multifarious challenges. Not surprisingly medical providers were most concerned about their patients who suffered chronic illness. How would they cope with this new threat to their fragile constitutions?

Dr. Dilek Demirtepe-Saygili of Atilim University in Turkey shares her findings concerning the psychological well-being of those who suffer chronic illness and their caregivers. With ten years of work as a researcher and practicing clinical psychologist, she researches their stress and coping mechanisms and adaptation especially in light of the added risks of COVID-19. She goes on to compare similarities and differences between the chronically ill and those without chronic conditions. Look into Chapter 1 to detect some surprising findings.

A less understood vulnerability is ADHD (Attention Deficit Hyperactivity Disorder). Those who have been diagnosed with this disorder may be surprised and pleased to find themselves represented by Justin Vrana who has spent his years at Marymount Manhattan College researching this disorder which he, himself, experiences. He wondered, would those diagnosed with ADHD struggle more in the midst of the COVID pandemic than neurotypical individuals? Could it be that ADHD could be exacerbated by quarantine, Zoom classes, and/or working from home? Would these individuals be somehow more likely to catch the virus? Vrana seeks to learn the best practices for easing the added burden of the virus.

Obsessive Compulsive Disorder (OCD) is another mental condition that, in general, baffles families and friends of the OCD patient. Specifically, though, how would COVID-19 with its directives to wash hands often, to disinfect surfaces constantly and to mask up everywhere affect those individuals who are already driven to repeat these rituals incessantly? Manuella Hounton, raised in Benin, West Africa and long interested in public and mental health issues, examines the assumptions that on one hand, those who indulge in repeated disinfection will probably avoid infection with COVID-19; on the other hand, those directives may trigger more serious obsessions and compulsions or cause an OCD reaction that had not existed before. Tune in to learn more about this debilitating condition and its effects from COVID and possible mitigation.

But how does one mitigate challenges for the deaf and the visually impaired? For the blind, touch, a sense we were asked to particularly avoid during COVID, is one of the most sensitive and helpful sensory tools, especially for those with visual impairment. For those with hearing impairment, that masks cover most of the face but most of all, the lips, obviates the possibility of reading lips. Amanda Hall, who writes about these challenges and more, has grown up among family members with impaired vision. Classes offered at Marymount Manhattan College on Sign Language and Deaf Culture have deepened her interest and desire to help. Ironically, the reader of this study will experience an eye-opening moment: a greater understanding of the hardships that COVID has wrought upon this already challenged population.

The study on Domestic Violence and Child Abuse is equally eye-opening. Under normal living conditions, these topics comprise closely guarded family secrets and can burgeon in lockdown conditions when victims cannot access help by reaching out to friends, family and protective services. Brianna Blackwell, a graduate of Marymount Manhattan College who majored in Psychology, worked at the United Nations, and currently teaches at a Montessori Preschool, has written about this horrific threat and how, unseen and untreated, the exacerbation of ongoing abuse and violence can interfere with overall development.

Isolation during lockdown also wreaks havoc on the vulnerable elderly population, especially upon those whose cognitive abilities have diminished—patients with Alzheimer's and other forms of dementia, even those with MCI (mild cognitive impairment) are a deep concern for me and Ali McClellan. We collaborated on an important review of the literature to describe how COVID has uniquely impacted these communities.

Section 2 of this collection addresses how COVID has affected child development, education and the media—not only in the United States, but globally. Dr. Vincent Agulonye of the University of Lisbon and Dr. Samaila Benedict Bahago of Veritas University—a serving priest of the Catholic Diocese of Minna, Niger State, have joined forces to detail the effects of lockdown on students, gained through copious interviews. Their findings are startling: COVID not only affected children's studies during quarantine, but impoverishment due to significant job loss during COVID, led to reduced access to remote learning educational opportunities, as well.

Nigeria is not alone in experiencing deleterious effects of school closures on children. Ingrid Brussier, an M.A. candidate at the New School for Social Research, examines the effect of school closures in the United States. Her studies highlight pandemic-related stressors that may lead to mood disorders and physical consequences such as obesity. She also touches on predicaments of impoverished families and the teachers of these children. They needed to switch horses in midstream, on a moment's notice, to convert lesson plans to online presentation that would succeed in inspiring their students. What about their mental health?

Though Regina Colie is pursuing an M.A. at Touro College in Clinical Mental Health Counseling, specializing in Eating Disorders and Postpartum Depression, here she writes about the role of children's media during the pandemic. In general, most parents struggle with the issue of controlling their children's exposure to an overdose of screen time. During the pandemic, children needed to sit for many hours a day, months on end—in front of a screen to keep up with schoolwork. Could entertainment companies and schools adapt to offer children a stimulating variety of content and help foster a sense of stability and safety throughout the pandemic?

The final chapter focuses on the way college students have had to adapt to remote learning. Emily Angelillo of Marymount Manhattan College (majoring in psychology and double minoring in Biology and Neuroscience), investigated the correlation between students' mindsets and their adjustment to online classes. Having found a positive correlation between a growth mindset and positive adjustment, Angelillo is passionate about improving adjustment skills, aided by techniques to frame one's thinking in a positive way. The hoped-for result: smoother transitions in the area of work, development, education and life in general.

We cannot be sure that COVID will not raise its ugly, prickly head again in the near future. In fact, most medical experts believe it will never completely leave us. With that indication and the excellent documented studies offered in this text, it would be unthinkable to throw up our hands and offer COVID the victory. So, we soldier on and stockpile creative activities for our school children like weekly outdoor art, science, literacy and music-based adventures, additional and comprehensive supports for our vulnerable populations, those with ADHD, OCD, visual and hearing impairments, chronic illnesses, those being victimized by abuse or neglect and we consider our elderly. Whether in group homes, nursing homes or in their own homes, the elderly need to feel a part of the community despite the medical requirement of keeping them well and sequestered. Most of us could imagine their delight if they received notes or calls from some of the quarantined children, food treats from time to time. There is so much more that needs to be thought of in case of relapse.

We also need to consider our schools. We must conduct a cost-benefit analysis and determine the benefits and limitations of masking, of school closures and of socialization in considering children's current and future development. We must recognize how those who were already impoverished and those who were made even more impoverished due to job loss and illness during COVID reduced even further their own and their children's educational and occupational opportunities We must learn from the past to affect the future. We must arm ourselves with the toolkit of these comprehensive chapters, which have highlighted the significant challenges and at times, creative solutions towards mitigating the impact of this insidious virus, and hopefully offering a much stronger playing field and defense for future viruses, lockdowns, and quarantines. With this knowledge, we can prepare ourselves more thoroughly, especially when considering those disproportionately affected by the pandemic and considering the educational and other institutions which were so substantially impacted.

Nava R. Silton
Marymount Manhattan College, USA

Acknowledgment

This text would not have been possible without a wonderful meeting of brilliant minds. First and foremost, I want to gratefully acknowledge all of the esteemed authors who shared their latest engrossing findings in the important and timely area of the impact of the COVID Pandemic on children, adolescents and adults.

Authors:

Vincent Agulonye, Ph.D. (Lisbon School of Economics & Management (ISEG), University of Lisbon, Portugal)

· **Emily Angelillo** (Marymount Manhattan College, New York, NY)

Samaila Benedict Bahago, Ph.D. (Educational Foundations, Veritas University, Abuja, NG)

Brianna Blackwell (Marymount Manhattan College, New York, NY)

Ingrid Brussier (The New School, New York, NY)

Regina Colie (Touro College, New York, NY)

Dilek Demirtepe-Saygili, Ph.D. (Atilim University, Ankara, TR)

Amanda Hall (Marymount Manhattan College, New York, NY)

Manuella Hounton (Marymount Manhattan College, New York, NY)

Ariana Lopez (Marymount Manhattan College, New York, NY)

Alexandra McCLellan (Marymount Manhattan, New York, NY)

Justin Vrana (Marymount Manhattan College, New York, NY)

I look forward to our future correspondence and collaboration.

Secondly, I'd like to graciously thank the peer reviewers who meticulously evaluated the relevance of content, syntax and empirical rigor of each chapter. Thank you:

Vincent Agulonye, Ph.D. (Vila Franca de Xira, Lisboa, Portugal)

Emily Angelillo (Marymount Manhattan College, New York, NY)

Brianna Blackwell (Marymount Manhattan College, New York, NY)

Ariel Brandwein, M.D. (New York Presbyterian Brooklyn Methodist Hospital, New York)

Ingrid Brussier (The New School, New York, NY)

Karinna Chavez (Marymount Manhattan College, New York, NY)

Regina Colie (Touro College, New York, NY)

Samantha O'Donoghue (Marymount Manhattan College, New York, NY)

Ali McCLellan (Marymount Manhattan, New York, NY)

Mindy Schwartz (Yeshiva University, New York, NY)

Faye Silton (Yeshiva University, New York, NY)

Shira Silton, LCSW, MA (Yeshiva University, New York, NY)

Justin Vrana (Marymount Manhattan College, New York, NY)

Olivia White (Marymount Manhattan College, New York, NY)

Marymount Manhattan College (MMC) students, Emily Angelillo ('22) and Ali McClellan ('22) graciously offered their wonderful assistance with this text. It did not take long before they were inspired and enthused by the innovative research in this area. Marymount Manhattan College (MMC) is one of the most creative and refreshing institutions I have ever had the pleasure of being affiliated with and I thank the whole MMC Community for their constant support and encouragement.

Additionally, I am grateful to Jan Travers, Rowan Rumbaugh, Maria Rohde for their invaluable guidance during the editing process. They were always prompt, comprehensive, patient and gracious in their responses.

Moreover, I would like to thank my incredible husband, Dr. Ariel Brandwein and my charming and hilarious little men, Judah Lior, Jonah Gabriel and Jacob Zeke Brandwein and little ladies, Jordana Leah and Juliet Bella Brandwein, for their good nature, humor, inspiration and patience throughout this endeavor. I want to acknowledge my father, Rabbi Paul Silton and my wonderful siblings, Elana, Michal, Akiva, Tamar, Aviva, and my twin sister Shira for their constant encouragement and support. Finally, I owe the largest debt of gratitude to a consummate renaissance woman and to one of my absolute greatest heroines, my mother, Faye Silton. Her brilliance, creativity, eloquence, wisdom, patience, kindness and love know no bounds. I will cherish this text all the more since her brilliant mind and loving hands painstakingly reviewed its contents.

I want to extend a final note of gratitude to all of the educators, academics, and professionals who

Have researched this important area and to all of the first-responders who have been on the frontlines ever since the pandemic began. We owe all of you such a sincere debt of gratitude and appreciation.

Bravery is not the absence of fear, but action in the face of fear – Mark Messier

Section 1

The Impact of COVID on Vulnerable Populations

Chapter 1
Psychosocial Effects of the COVID-19 Pandemic on Adults With Chronic Illnesses

Dilek Demirtepe-Saygili
Atilim University, Turkey

ABSTRACT

The chapter aims to examine the adaptation to the coronavirus disease-2019 (COVID-19) pandemic process of adults previously diagnosed with a chronic illness. Chronic illnesses negatively affect a person's psychosocial functioning as well as their physical health. When the COVID-19 pandemic entered people's lives, a higher risk was expected for individuals with chronic illnesses. Several studies were conducted to understand their COVID-19 adaptation process and psychosocial consequences. Studies revealed high levels of depressive and anxious symptoms as well as non-compliance, fear of COVID-19, isolation, and loneliness. From another viewpoint, individuals with chronic illnesses were also able to cope with COVID-19-related stressors and some of them experienced better well-being outcomes. Online and telehealth interventions were offered for people in need of psychosocial support. The pandemic experience helped people develop an understanding of the management of health threats and a multidimensional perspective toward health.

INTRODUCTION

Well-being is a multidimensional concept including physical, psychological, and social functioning (World Health Organization (WHO), 2020; American Psychological Association (APA), n.d.). From this holistic perspective, the Coronavirus disease

DOI: 10.4018/978-1-6684-3484-0.ch001

2019 (COVID-19) affected people's lives not just as a physical health risk, but as a psychological and social risk. People with a preexisting chronic health condition might have experienced this risk differently as compared to healthy groups. From a clinical health psychology perspective, psychological functioning interacts with physiological functioning. The aim of clinical health psychology includes developing and providing clinical services for promoting well-being and managing illnesses (APA, 2008). Thus, studies have been conducted to understand the relationship between physical and psychosocial health. It was revealed that being diagnosed with a chronic illness is a risk factor for having psychological symptoms (Brannon & Feist, 2013). Chronic illness is defined as dealing with a health problem for a long period of time. Chronic illnesses, such as cancer, diabetes, or cardiovascular diseases require an adaptation process for individuals to restore their physical and psychological well-being. This adaptation includes changes in the person's self-image, daily life, and relationships as well as dealing with physical symptoms and treatment (Livneh & Antonak, 2005). The adaptation also includes a reorganization of responsibilities, financial arrangements, family roles, and social activities. Although having a chronic illness negatively affects people, it is possible to have a quality of life with a successful adaptation process. For example, an adaptive group of people with chronic illness and disability had lower levels of psychological distress and higher levels of quality of life and life satisfaction as compared to a non-adaptive groups (Livneh et al., 2004). The following section includes psychosocial variables which may play a role as a risk or protective factor in this adaptation process before the COVID-19 pandemic.

PSYCHOSOCIAL ASPECTS OF ADULT CHRONIC ILLNESSES

Researchers examined the predictors of psychological distress for people diagnosed with various chronic illnesses. Various patterns of results were revealed for different illness perceptions depending on the illness characteristics, such as the level of disability, life-threatening nature of the illness, visibility of the symptoms, complexity and side effects of the treatment, needs for assistance in living, and levels of pain (Levendthal et al., 1992). Moreover, it is usually a dynamic process including the interactions between medical, psychological, and coping aspects (Livneh, 2021). Brief information is presented below for psychosocial aspects of chronic diseases, such as asthma, cardiovascular diseases, cancer, and diabetes.

Studies particularly focused on the levels of depressive and anxiety symptoms as the outcome variables. Depression and anxiety disorders are the most common psychological disorders (Kring & Johnson, 2017). Symptoms associated with these disorders are even more common among individuals with chronic illnesses. For example, anxiety symptoms and anxiety disorder diagnoses are more prevalent among people with asthma as compared to non-asthma controls (Ye et al., 2021; Tany & Saha, 2017). Similarly, high levels of depressive and anxiety symptoms were found among people with chronic respiratory disease (Zhou et al., 2017). Sleep problems, limitation of physical activity, and negative life events were revealed as the predictors of these increased levels of psychological symptoms (Zhou et al., 2017). Furthermore, when the patients perceived low control over their illness, they had more panic symptoms (Hallas et al., 2012).

Similar to asthma and chronic respiratory disease, the risk for psychological symptoms also applies to cardiovascular problems and diabetes. As compared to a healthy control group, people with cardiovascular disorders had higher levels of depression, anxiety, and stress (Stankovska & Memedi, 2020). Moreover, for people with cardiovascular disorders, depression, anxiety, and sleep problems were positively related to self-blame, rumination, catastrophization (Mustaţă, 2021), social isolation, and loneliness (Hu et al., 2021). As for diabetes, the complications (e.g. coronary artery disease, neuropathy, and foot problems) predicted future depressive symptoms in a five-year-study (Deschênes et al., 2017).

The psychosocial consequences of having a chronic illness are not always negative. It is possible to grow psychologically after having a chronic illness. For example, although it was revealed that cancer patients had higher levels of depression and anxiety (e.g. Hinz et al., 2010), positive outcomes were revealed, as well. For example, well-being and attribution of meaning to one's life were overlapping factors among cancer survivors (Holtmaat et al., 2019). Similarly, attributing positive meaning to the experience of cancer was related to a decreased level of hopelessness, which in turn was related to improved well-being (Liao et al., 2017). A sense of self-worth, adaptability, and an ability to learn from experiences are the components of resilience (Kralik et al., 2006). It was revealed that resilience serves as a buffer against the negative effects of chronic illness and disability in older adults (Manning et al., 2016). Thus, chronic illness experience is a complex process including positive as well as negative aspects.

As chronic illness adaptation requires special attention by the person, his/her family, and the healthcare system, the protective and risk factors, and possible changes in their well-being should be addressed by researchers (See Stanton et al., 2007; De Ridder et al., 2008 for a review). In general, individuals with chronic illnesses are at risk for psychological symptoms and a high level of stress. When the COVID-19 pandemic is added as a new factor to this ongoing adaptation, it can be expected that people with chronic health conditions would experience a greater impact of the pandemic on their lives. The next section focuses on the studies conducted with people with chronic illnesses during the pandemic between 2020 and 2021.

THE EFFECTS OF THE COVID-19 PANDEMIC ON ADULTS WITH CHRONIC ILLNESSES

When COVID-19 first entered people's lives, it was a novel situation, then it turned into a threat. For some people, it then turned into long-term stress which required change and adaptation regardless of a previous chronic health condition. People's illness representations changed in time according to Shiloh et al.'s (2021) findings in the following way: At the beginning of the pandemic, people perceived COVID-19 as a threat. Four months later, in the second wave of the pandemic, people's perception of COVID-19 worsened and started stabilizing. During the COVID-19 pandemic, people experienced changes in family lives, work lives, daily routines, social lives, and relationships with media regardless of having a chronic health condition. As for people with chronic health conditions, their risk of being affected by COVID-19 was higher, which resulted in more attention and sometimes more limitations in terms of the lockdowns. WHO (2020) at a global level and countries at a national level regarded people with chronic illnesses as one of the vulnerable populations and took more precautions for them. Due to the presence of this threat, people with chronic illnesses had to engage in protective behaviors to a greater degree.

NEGATIVE CONSEQUENCES OF THE COVID-19 PANDEMIC

Pandemic experience included some negative emotions, such as fear of COVID-19, and some behavioral and social limitations, such as lockdowns, and social distancing. Studies conducted with individuals with chronic illnesses revealed important findings. For example, cancer patients reported higher levels of anxiety (Casanova et al., 2020). Cancer screenings, and sometimes treatments were interrupted in the effort to stay away from hospitals. Similarly, people with rheumatoid arthritis reported adherence problems including fewer medical appointments and decreased levels of physical activity (Lévy-Weil et al., 2021). Access to medical care decreased also for people with multiple sclerosis (MS) (Donzé et al., 2021). People with MS reported higher levels of depressive and anxiety symptoms, sleep problems, and fatigue as compared to the general population (Motolese et al., 2020). Similarly, people with MS had higher levels of anxiety and depression when they could not keep their medical appointments, had a diagnosis of COVID-19, and had a perceived progression of their condition (Yunier et al., 2021).

A negative effect of lockdown was reported for physical health as a result of limitations of physical activities. People with diabetes reported self-care difficulties in terms of diet and exercise routines due to lockdowns (Silva-Tinoco et al., 2021). A qualitative study focusing on people with Alzheimer's disease and Parkinson's disease revealed that people's motor symptoms worsened, due to lockdown regulations. Moreover, their access to healthcare services was also disrupted and they experienced social isolation and related psychological symptoms (Macchi et al., 2021). The effects of protective measures on people with asthma were investigated qualitatively by Tyson et al. (2021). The themes included being identified as vulnerable, feeling protected, and becoming more health-conscious, which addresses a change in their illness perceptions. A longitudinal study with people with chronic health conditions, which began before the pandemic, provided a comparison of pre-pandemic conditions with the first two months of the pandemic (Cowden et al., 2021). They revealed that the experience of suffering, i.e. a personal experience of loss of perceived good, before the pandemic was positively related to anxiety and depression levels.

Social support is an important part of well-being, especially for people with chronic illnesses. For example, social support from the family was positively related to coping with diabetes (Karlsen et al., 2004). However, social distancing during the pandemic carried a risk of isolation for everyone (Saltzman et al., 2020). It was revealed before the emergence of the pandemic that as the level of loneliness increases, the levels of pain also increase for people with chronic pain (Oliveira et al., 2015). The social distancing policies during the pandemic may increase the risk of loneliness, which may increase the level of pain in turn (Rhodes et al., 2020). Loneliness among people over the age of 50 with chronic conditions was related to more anxiety (Polenick et al., 2021). Similarly, people with MS reported higher levels of stress and lower levels of social support during the pandemic (Bonavita et al., 2021). Thus, the risk of isolation and decrease in social support were the factors which posed as risks for psychological symptoms.

A global unknown health threat with no empirically supported treatment and vaccination, i.e. COVID-19, resulted in uncertainty and threat. Therefore, it is expected that people would feel fear and anxiety for themselves and their loved ones. A scale specifically designed for COVID-19 fears of people with preexisting medical conditions was developed by Wu et al. (2020). In this study, it was found that fear of COVID-19 positively correlated with stress, depressive, and anxious symptoms. Moreover, financial resources were negatively related to fear of COVID-19 among people with scleroderma (the autoimmune disease systemic sclerosis) (Wu et al. 2021).

POSITIVE CONSEQUENCES OF THE COVID-19 PANDEMIC

Contrary to the findings of studies revealing a negative change for people with chronic illnesses, several studies revealed either no change or positive change. For example, Capuano et al. (2020) revealed no change in depressive and anxiety symptoms before and during the lockdown for COVID-19 and an increase in the quality of life of people with MS. Similarly, Pedrozo-Pupo and Campo-Arias (2020) revealed that depression and post-traumatic stress symptoms of individuals with asthma and chronic obstructive pulmonary disease were similar to those of healthy groups during lockdown for COVID-19. Another qualitative study conducted with people with rheumatoid arthritis found that the participants were able to focus on self-care more while staying at home. They reported having negative emotions and using positive reframing as a part of the management of those negative emotional experiences (Leese et al., 2021). It was found that family resilience and internal locus of control helped during the pandemic process for cancer patients (Brivio et al., 2021).

Zambelli et al. (2021) conducted a comparison study including pre-lockdown and during-lockdown variables for people with chronic pain in the first wave of COVID-19 in the United Kingdom. It was revealed that sleep problems, depressive symptoms, pain severity, and pain interference decreased during the lockdown as compared to before lockdown. The authors attributed this to the possible effects of feelings of security, or changes in the physical activity levels.

People with and without irritable bowel syndrome, a chronic digestive disorder, were compared in terms of COVID-19 related stress, such as fear or financial worries and related psychological variables by Sabate et al. (2020). Both groups showed similar levels of COVID-19 related stress. However, as compared to a control group, people with irritable bowel syndrome reported higher levels of anxiety, depression, and stress (Sabate et al., 2021). Thus, people with chronic illnesses may be affected negatively in relation to their previous characteristics and level of symptoms.

An increasing number of studies have focused on the process of living with the pandemic from different aspects. Considering the importance of people's illness perceptions, the importance of their previous characteristics, and the nature of their chronic conditions, different results can be obtained from well-being studies during the pandemic. Moreover, indirect effects due to possible changes in sleep, level of physical activity, and sociocultural factors, such as financial problems may also contribute to people's pandemic experience (Zvolensky et al., 2020). With an appreciation for individual differences due to the unique characteristics of individuals, an elaboration for the common possible mechanism can be coping with a general health stressor, i.e. COVID-19.

THE STRESS AND COPING PERSPECTIVE ON THE COVID-19 PANDEMIC

Stress and coping theories may enlighten these diverse psychological outcomes. From the perspectives of early physiological theories of stress and coping, stress is regarded as a stimulus that disrupts the body's equilibrium (Cannon, 1932). Moreover, people's resources to cope with stress are limited, which results in depletion of those resources after long-term exposure to the threat. (Selye, 1976). This results in worse health conditions because of stress reactions of the body. Lazarus and Folkman (1984) suggested that stress is an interaction between the person and the environment. Thus, a person's appraisal makes a situation appear stressful. From this viewpoint, COVID-19 is a new stressor added to the previous stressful situation, which makes people more vulnerable. Several studies revealed that people with previous chronic illnesses are affected more negatively in terms of their psychological health as compared to people without a previous diagnosis. The Stress and coping perspective suggesting that limited resources and appraisal of the situation results in worse health consequences, are consistent with these findings.

From another point of view, other stress and coping theories also suggest that when people utilize their previous experience of coping with stress, they can prepare themselves for future stressful situations (Taylor & Aspinwall, 1996; Aspinwall & Taylor, 1997). Proactive coping includes anticipation of potential stressors, accumulation of resources, and initial coping responses (Aspinwall & Taylor, 1997). In terms of COVID-19 experiences, people with chronic illnesses had already encountered a health threat before and they have experience coping with health threats. This perspective is consistent with the findings saying that the well-being of people with chronic illnesses is affected positively. To have a closer look at the stress and coping perspective, it is important to examine research focusing on coping with COVID-19 stress.

COVID-19 is considered a multidimensional stress factor, including worry and isolation (Taylor et al., 2020). It was revealed that people with chronic conditions and disabilities commonly used acceptance and self-distraction to cope with COVID-19 related stress, while denial and substance use were the least commonly used coping mechanisms (Umucu & Lee, 2020), consistent with previous studies (e.g. Burker et al., 2005). The use of active coping, social support, use of humor, and religious coping were positively related to well-being, while less use of self-blame was negatively related (Umucu & Lee, 2020). Likewise, among older adults with cancer, acceptance, self-distraction, and taking action were reported as common coping strategies during the COVID-19 pandemic (Galica et al., 2021). Moreover, these coping strategies were regarded as not new, but "redeployed and repurposed." This means that people with chronic illnesses may have already developed coping strategies for their previous health concerns and adapted them to coping with COVID-19 issues. Thus, the level of their previous functioning, previous levels of stress, depressive and anxiety symptoms interacted with a new multidimensional health threat and resulted in some changes in their well-being.

VACCINATION ATTITUDES AMONG ADULTS WITH CHRONIC ILLNESSES

Research on the COVID-19 pandemic investigated people's pandemic experiences from the beginning. Another important research scope for the pandemic included vaccination studies. Vaccination trials were conducted, resulting in successful results, which are followed by approval by WHO or US Food and Drug Administration (FDA) and applications to the population. The effectiveness and impact of COVID-19 vaccines are also tested for chronic illnesses, such as MS (Apostolidis et al., 2021). The psychosocial aspect of vaccination issues consists of attitudes toward vaccination and behaviors. As the studies mostly include voluntary healthy adult populations, trials were not as commonly applied for people with chronic health conditions. Before the discovery of COVID-19 vaccines, a study was conducted on influenza vaccination attitudes among people with chronic respiratory conditions (Gallant et al., 2021). Side effects, time constraints, and fear of needles were among the perceived barriers to vaccination, while protection, having reminders, and the social influence of others were among enablers for influenza vaccination. Attitudes toward COVID-19 vaccination among people with chronic illnesses was another scope of research that emerged after the use of COVID-19 vaccines. It was reported that half of the participants with chronic illnesses were willing to get vaccines in Saudi Arabia (Al-Hanawi et al., 2021). Similarly, 74% of participants with cancer reported a positive attitude toward vaccination in Poland (Brodziak et al., 2021), while 62% reported willingness to receive the vaccine in Korea (Chun et al., 2021). The effects of vaccination on people's well-being have not been examined yet. It can be expected that vaccination is a new factor to add to the existing dynamic multidimensional system.

INTERVENTIONS FOR ADULTS WITH CHRONIC ILLNESSES DURING THE COVID-19 PANDEMIC

It was suggested that people with chronic illnesses need psychological care as well as physical care during the pandemic (Kang et al., 2020). Positive health outcomes are possible during and after the COVID-19 pandemic for people who need interventions with chronic illness management. In terms of illness management, it was suggested that patients with asthma might have placed more importance on their health, resulting in self-management behaviors (Skene & Pfeffer, 2021). Digital applications for diabetes under the supervision of the clinic of the patients provided a chance for guided management of diabetes, increasing the sense of agency (Gamble et al., 2020). Distance intervention studies including the use of internet and communication devices were employed during the COVID-19 pandemic, such as the telehealth model of acceptance and commitment therapies for chronic pain patients by Rhodes et al. (2020), text messaging system for cancer patients by Agyapong et al. (2020), and online exercise programs for cancer patients (Newton et al., 2020). It was suggested that the experiences of telehealth interventions gained during this compulsory stay-at-home period may help future management of cancer (Paterson et al., 2020) and other chronic conditions. The advantages may include increased access for people living in remote areas (Paterson et al., 2020) or disadvantages include the inability of the physical assessment by the nurses (Paterson et al., 2020), unequal access due to financial issues (Solari-Twadell et al., 2021).

A multidimensional education and support program was developed for people with systemic sclerosis including group videoconferences by Thombs et al. (2021). Although the anxiety symptoms did not change after the intervention, depressive symptoms were lower at six months' follow-up measurements. An epilepsy clinic offered teleconsultation instead of office visits for their 38 registered patients (Olivo et al., 2021). The patients evaluated teleconsultation positively. Moreover, their number of seizures was not different from previous numbers. The authors emphasized the advantage of knowing the patients face-to-face before the pandemic. Thus, first contact via online appointments may have its own problems.

Problems associated with online interventions and self-management include comorbidity of some chronic illnesses with cognitive impairment, increased prevalence of chronic conditions with older age, which may be related to problems with technology use (Archer et al., 2014). Thus, easy-to-use programs and the inclusion of family members may help people use technological devices and online interventions more (Archer et al., 2014). Although telehealth interventions were not new for various physical (e.g. Beatty & Lambert, 2013) and psychological disorders (e.g. Basit et al., 2020) before the COVID-19 pandemic, it can be argued that they became more important than ever.

IMPLICATIONS

The COVID-19 pandemic affected people's lives in many ways. People with a previous chronic illness constitute one of the vulnerable populations in terms of an increased risk for the negative consequences of COVID-19. Considering well-being as a multidimensional construct, their psychological health and social functioning are also affected negatively. The pandemic created a crisis and researchers from various disciplines tried to understand COVID from their own perspectives. Many studies have been conducted and published in this 2-year period. More studies are expected to be published in the near future. Nevertheless, extensive investigation of

COVID-19 related variables is needed. Thus, it is considered as early to reach definite conclusions. Moreover, long-term consequences of the pandemic, psychological outcomes of vaccination, and post-COVID normalization are needed to be addressed by future studies.

The studies revealed that people with chronic illnesses are affected by COVID-19, especially in terms of the limitation of access to medical care and other related treatment responsibilities. They experienced physical limitations because of lockdowns like everyone. However, for some illnesses, the role of physical exercise is more crucial. They had higher levels of depressive and anxiety symptoms. They experienced isolation and fear of getting the virus. On the other hand, they were able to use their existing coping mechanisms. Online interventions were used and tested for effectiveness to help people in need of support. Considering the changes in the well-being of people with chronic illnesses including not only negative but also positive tendencies, the evaluation of the findings from a comprehensive viewpoint is necessary. In this way, the risk and the protective factors affecting the well-being of people with chronic illnesses will contribute to our understanding of clinical health psychology in terms of long-term pandemic experiences. The increase in online resources has the potential to shape intervention programs for people with chronic illnesses via improved access.

Health care professionals, especially mental health professionals working with people with chronic illnesses should focus on the pandemic experience extensively. Adherence issues may need a specific focus because they directly affect people's health. A normalization process may be necessary to deal with the long-term effects. Different ways of seeking social support, such as online gatherings, can be provided as alternatives. While suggesting online systems, professionals should consider access to technology.

CONCLUSION

People from all over the world have been affected by the COVID-19 pandemic in their own ways. One of the most affected groups consists of people with chronic illnesses. The WHO (World Health Organization) (2020) paid special attention to people with chronic illnesses, such as those with lung and heart disease, diabetes, and immune system disorders, during the pandemic. They were also subject to more severe regulations and restrictions as compared to people without chronic illnesses. Some people with chronic illnesses experienced problems with adherence and increased levels of psychological symptoms, while some others coped with this new threat more effectively. The studies offer a better understanding of the pandemic from the perspective of people with chronic illnesses. It is suggested that well-being studies need to consider that it is a multidimensional process and requires long-term monitoring.

REFERENCES

Agyapong, V. I. O., Hrabok, M., Shalaby, R., Mrklas, K., Vuong, W., Gusnowski, A., Surood, S., Greenshaw, A. J., & Nkire, N. (2020). Closing the COVID-19 psychological treatment gap for cancer patients in Alberta: Protocol for the implementation and evaluation of Text4Hope-Cancer Care. *JMIR Research Protocols*, *9*(8), e20240. doi:10.2196/20240 PMID:32750012

Al-Hanawi, M. K., Ahmad, K., Haque, R., & Keramat, S. A. (2021). Willingness to receive COVID-19 vaccination among adults with chronic diseases in the Kingdom of Saudi Arabia. *Journal of Infection and Public Health*, *14*(10), 1489–1496. doi:10.1016/j.jiph.2021.08.002 PMID:34417135

American Psychological Association. (2008). *Clinical health psychology*. https://www.apa.org/ed/graduate/specialize/health

American Psychological Association. (n.d.). Well-being. In *APA dictionary of psychology*. Retrieved October 20, 2021, from https://dictionary.apa.org/well-being

Apostolidis, S. A., Kakara, M., Painter, M. M., Goel, R. R., Mathew, D., Lenzi, K., ... Bar-Or, A. (2021). Cellular and humoral immune responses following SARS-CoV-2 mRNA vaccination in patients with multiple sclerosis on anti-CD20 therapy. *Nature Medicine*, 1–12. doi:10.103841591-021-01507-2 PMID:34522051

Archer, N., Keshavjee, K., Demers, C., & Lee, R. (2014). Online self-management interventions for chronically ill patients: Cognitive impairment and technology issues. *International Journal of Medical Informatics*, *83*(4), 264–272. doi:10.1016/j.ijmedinf.2014.01.005 PMID:24507762

Aspinwall, L. G., & Taylor, S. E. (1997). A stitch in time: Self-regulation and proactive coping. *Psychological Bulletin*, *121*(3), 417–436. doi:10.1037/0033-2909.121.3.417 PMID:9136643

Basit, S. A., Mathews, N., & Kunik, M. E. (2020). Telemedicine interventions for medication adherence in mental illness: A systematic review. *General Hospital Psychiatry*, *62*, 28–36. doi:10.1016/j.genhosppsych.2019.11.004 PMID:31775066

Beatty, L., & Lambert, S. (2013). A systematic review of internet-based self-help therapeutic interventions to improve distress and disease-control among adults with chronic health conditions. *Clinical Psychology Review, 33*(4), 609–622. doi:10.1016/j.cpr.2013.03.004 PMID:23603521

Bonavita, S., Sparaco, M., Russo, A., Borriello, G., & Lavorgna, L. (2021). Perceived stress and social support in a large population of people with multiple sclerosis recruited online through the COVID-19 pandemic. *European Journal of Neurology, 28*(10), 3396–3402. doi:10.1111/ene.14697 PMID:33368849

Brannon, L., & Feist, J. (2013). *Health Psychology: An Introduction to Behavior and Health* (9th ed.). Wadsworth.

Brivio, E., Guiddi, P., Scotto, L., Giudice, A. V., Pettini, G., Busacchio, D., Didier, F., Mazzocco, K., & Pravettoni, G. (2021). Patients living with breast cancer during the coronavirus pandemic: The role of family resilience, coping flexibility, and locus of control on affective responses. *Frontiers in Psychology, 11*, 3711. doi:10.3389/fpsyg.2020.567230 PMID:33519580

Brodziak, A., Sigorski, D., Osmola, M., Wilk, M., Gawlik-Urban, A., Kiszka, J., Machulska-Ciuraj, K., & Sobczuk, P. (2021). Attitudes of patients with cancer towards vaccinations—Results of online survey with special focus on the vaccination against COVID-19. *Vaccines, 9*(5), 411. doi:10.3390/vaccines9050411 PMID:33919048

Burker, E. J., Evon, D. M., Marroquin Loiselle, M., Finkel, J. B., & Mill, M. R. (2005). Coping predicts depression and disability in heart transplant candidates. *Journal of Psychosomatic Research, 59*(4), 215–222. doi:10.1016/j.jpsychores.2005.06.055 PMID:16223624

Cannon, W. B. (1932). *The Wisdom of the Body*. Norton. doi:10.1097/00000441-193212000-00028

Capuano, R., Altieri, M., Bisecco, A., d'Ambrosio, A., Docimo, R., Buonanno, D., Matrone, F., Giuliano, F., Tedeschi, G., Santangelo, G., & Gallo, A. (2021). Psychological consequences of COVID-19 pandemic in Italian MS patients: Signs of resilience? *Journal of Neurology, 268*(3), 743–750. doi:10.100700415-020-10099-9 PMID:32725312

Casanova, M., Bagliacca, E. P., Silva, M., Patriarca, C., Veneroni, L., Clerici, C. A., & .... (2020). How young patients with cancer perceive the Covid–19 (coronavirus) epidemic in Milan, Italy: Is there room for other fears? *Pediatric Blood & Cancer, 67*(7), e28318. doi:10.1002/pbc.28318 PMID:32240567

Chun, J. Y., Kim, S. I., Park, E. Y., Park, S. Y., Koh, S. J., Cha, Y., Yoo, H. J., Joung, J. Y., Yoon, H. M., Eom, B. W., Park, C. M., Han, J.-Y., Kim, M., Lee, D.-W., Kim, J.-W., Keam, B., Lee, M., Kim, T. M., Choi, Y. J., ... Lim, M. C. (2021). Cancer Patients' Willingness to Take COVID-19 Vaccination: A Nationwide Multicenter Survey in Korea. *Cancers (Basel), 13*(15), 3883. doi:10.3390/cancers13153883 PMID:34359783

Cowden, R. G., Davis, E. B., Counted, V., Chen, Y., Rueger, S. Y., VanderWeele, T. J., Lemke, A. W., Glowiak, K. J., & Worthington, E. L. Jr. (2021). Suffering, mental health, and psychological well-being during the COVID-19 Pandemic: A longitudinal study of US adults with chronic health conditions. Wellbeing. *Space and Society*, *2*, 100048. doi:10.1016/j.wss.2021.100048 PMID:34746895

De Ridder, D., Geenen, R., Kuijer, R., & van Middendorp, H. (2008). Psychological adjustment to chronic disease. *Lancet*, *372*(9634), 246–255. doi:10.1016/S0140-6736(08)61078-8 PMID:18640461

Deschênes, S. S., Burns, R. J., Pouwer, F., & Schmitz, N. (2017). Diabetes complications and depressive symptoms: Prospective results from the montreal diabetes health and well-being study. *Psychosomatic Medicine*, *79*(5), 603–612. doi:10.1097/PSY.0000000000000447 PMID:28060138

Donzé, C., Massot, C., Guenot, M., & Hautecoeur, P. (2021). CONFISEP: Impact of the COVID-19 pandemic lockdown on patients with multiple sclerosis in the north of France. *Revue Neurologique*. PMID:34538668

Galica, J., Liu, Z., Kain, D., Merchant, S., Booth, C., Koven, R., Brundage, M., & Haase, K. R. (2021). Coping during COVID-19: A mixed methods study of older cancer survivors. *Supportive Care in Cancer*, *29*(6), 3389–3398. doi:10.100700520-020-05929-5 PMID:33404813

Gallant, A. J., Flowers, P., Deakin, K., Cogan, N., Rasmussen, S., Young, D., & Williams, L. (2021). Barriers and enablers to influenza vaccination uptake in adults with chronic respiratory conditions: Applying the behaviour change wheel to specify multi-levelled tailored intervention content. *Psychology & Health*, 1–20. doi:10.1080/08870446.2021.1957104 PMID:34328044

Gamble, A., Pham, Q., Goyal, S., & Cafazzo, J. A. (2020). The challenges of COVID-19 for people living with diabetes: Considerations for digital health. *JMIR Diabetes*, *5*(2), e19581. doi:10.2196/19581 PMID:32392473

Hallas, C. N., Howard, C., Theadom, A., & Wray, J. (2012). Negative beliefs about breathlessness increases panic for patients with chronic respiratory disease. *Psychology Health and Medicine*, *17*(4), 467–477. doi:10.1080/13548506.2011.626434 PMID:22329594

Hinz, A., Krauss, O., Hauss, J. P., Höckel, M., Kortmann, R. D., Stolzenburg, J. U., & Schwarz, R. (2010). Anxiety and depression in cancer patients compared with the general population. *European Journal of Cancer Care*, *19*(4), 522–529. doi:10.1111/j.1365-2354.2009.01088.x PMID:20030697

Holtmaat, K., Van der Spek, N., Lissenberg-Witte, B. I., Cuijpers, P., & Verdonck-de Leeuw, I. M. (2019). Positive mental health among cancer survivors: Overlap in psychological well-being, personal meaning, and posttraumatic growth. *Supportive Care in Cancer*, *27*(2), 443–450. doi:10.100700520-018-4325-8 PMID:29959577

Hu, J., Fitzgerald, S. M., Owen, A. J., Ryan, J., Joyce, J., Chowdhury, E., Reid, C. M., Britt, C., Woods, R. L., McNeil, J. J., & Freak-Poli, R. (2021). Social isolation, social support, loneliness and cardiovascular disease risk factors: A cross-sectional study among older adults. *International Journal of Geriatric Psychiatry*, *36*(11), 1795–1809. doi:10.1002/gps.5601 PMID:34231940

Kang, C., Yang, S., Yuan, J., Xu, L., Zhao, X., & Yang, J. (2020). Patients with chronic illness urgently need integrated physical and psychological care during the COVID-19 outbreak. *Asian Journal of Psychiatry*, *51*, 102081. doi:10.1016/j.ajp.2020.102081 PMID:32289729

Karlsen, B., Idsoe, T., Hanestad, B. R., Murberg, T., & Bru, E. (2004). Perceptions of support, diabetes-related coping and psychological well-being in adults with type 1 and type 2 diabetes. *Psychology Health and Medicine*, *9*(1), 53–70. doi:10.1080/13548500310001637751

Kralik, D., van Loon, A., & Visentin, K. (2006). Resilience in the chronic illness experience. *Educational Action Research*, *14*(2), 187–201. doi:10.1080/09650790600718035

Kring, A. M., & Johnson, S. L. (2017). *Abnormal Psychology* (14th ed.). Wiley.

Lazarus, R. S., & Folkman, S. (1984). *Stress, Appraisal and Coping*. Springer.

Leese, J., Backman, C. L., Ma, J. K., Koehn, C., Hoens, A. M., English, K., ... Li, L. C. (2021). Experiences of self-care during the COVID-19 pandemic among individuals with rheumatoid arthritis: A qualitative study. *Health Expectations*. Advance online publication. doi:10.1111/hex.13341 PMID:34403189

Leventhal, H., Diefenbach, M., & Leventhal, E. A. (1992). Illness cognition - using common-sense to understand treatment adherence and affect cognition interactions. *Cognitive Therapy and Research, 16*(2), 143–163. doi:10.1007/BF01173486

Lévy-Weil, F. E., Jousse-Joulin, S., Tiffreau, V., Perez, R., Morisseau, V., & Bombezin, A. (2021). Physical activity and quality of life of patients with rheumatoid arthritis at the time of COVID-19 lockdown: Results from Carenity, an online patient community. *Joint, Bone, Spine*. Advance online publication. doi:10.1016/j.jbspin.2021.105212

Liao, K. Y. H., Yeung, N. C., Wong, C. C., Warmoth, K., & Lu, Q. (2017). Fear of cancer recurrence and physical well-being among Chinese cancer survivors: The role of conscientiousness, positive reappraisal and hopelessness. *Supportive Care in Cancer, 25*(4), 1141–1149. doi:10.100700520-016-3504-8 PMID:27924358

Livneh, H. (2021). Psychosocial Adaptation to Chronic Illness and Disability: An Updated and Expanded Conceptual Framework. *Rehabilitation Counseling Bulletin*.

Livneh, H., & Antonak, R. F. (2005). Psychosocial adaptation to chronic illness and disability: A primer for counselors. *Journal of Counseling and Development, 83*(1), 12–20. doi:10.1002/j.1556-6678.2005.tb00575.x

Livneh, H., Lott, S. M., & Antonak, R. F. (2004). Patterns of psychosocial adaptation to chronic illness and disability: A cluster analytic approach. *Psychology Health and Medicine, 9*(4), 411–430. doi:10.1080/1354850042000267030

Macchi, Z. A., Ayele, R., Dini, M., Lamira, J., Katz, M., Pantilat, S. Z., Jones, J., & Kluger, B. M. (2021). Lessons from the COVID-19 pandemic for improving outpatient neuropalliative care: A qualitative study of patient and caregiver perspectives. *Palliative Medicine, 35*(7). doi:10.1177/02692163211017383 PMID:34006157

Manning, L. K., Carr, D. C., & Kail, B. L. (2016). Do higher levels of resilience buffer the deleterious impact of chronic illness on disability in later life? *The Gerontologist, 56*(3), 514–524. doi:10.1093/geront/gnu068 PMID:25063353

Motolese, F., Rossi, M., Albergo, G., Stelitano, D., Villanova, M., Di Lazzaro, V., & Capone, F. (2020). The psychological impact of COVID-19 pandemic on people with multiple sclerosis. *Frontiers in Neurology, 11*, 1255. doi:10.3389/fneur.2020.580507 PMID:33193033

Mustaţă, A. E. (2021). The relationships between coping mechanisms, depression, anxiety and sleep disorders in cardiovascular patients. *Journal of Evidence-Based Psychotherapies, 21*(1), 37–55. doi:10.24193/jebp.2021.1.3

Newton, R. U., Hart, N. H., & Clay, T. (2020). Keeping patients with cancer exercising in the age of COVID-19. *JCO Oncology Practice, 16*(10), 656–664. doi:10.1200/OP.20.00210 PMID:32603253

Oliveira, V. C., Ferreira, M. L., Morso, L., Albert, H. B., Refshauge, K. M., & Ferreira, P. H. (2015). Patients' perceived level of social isolation affects the prognosis of low back pain. *European Journal of Pain (London, England), 19*(4), 538–545. doi:10.1002/ejp.578 PMID:25185789

Olivo, S., Cheli, M., Dinoto, A., Stokelj, D., Tomaselli, M., & Manganotti, P. (2021). Telemedicine during the SARS-Cov-2 pandemic lockdown: Monitoring stress and quality of sleep in patients with epilepsy. *Epilepsy & Behavior, 118*, 107864. doi:10.1016/j.yebeh.2021.107864 PMID:33743345

Paterson, C., Bacon, R., Dwyer, R., Morrison, K. S., Toohey, K., O'Dea, A., & Hayes, S. (2020, October). The role of telehealth during the COVID-19 pandemic across the interdisciplinary cancer team: implications for practice. In *Seminars in oncology nursing* (p. 151090). WB Saunders. doi:10.1016/j.soncn.2020.151090

Pedrozo-Pupo, J. C., & Campo-Arias, A. (2020). Depression, perceived stress related to COVID, post-traumatic stress, and insomnia among asthma and COPD patients during the COVID-19 pandemic. *Chronic Respiratory Disease, 17*, 1479973120962800. doi:10.1177/1479973120962800 PMID:33000648

Polenick, C. A., Perbix, E. A., Salwi, S. M., Maust, D. T., Birditt, K. S., & Brooks, J. M. (2021). Loneliness during the COVID-19 Pandemic among older adults with chronic conditions. *Journal of Applied Gerontology, 40*(8), 0733464821996527. doi:10.1177/0733464821996527 PMID:33641513

Rhodes, A., Martin, S., Guarna, J., Vowles, K., & Allen, T. (2020). A contextual-behavioral perspective on chronic pain during the COVID-19 pandemic and future times of mandated physical distancing. *Journal of Contextual Behavioral Science, 17*, 152–158. doi:10.1016/j.jcbs.2020.07.009

Sabate, J. M., Deutsch, D., Melchior, C., Entremont, A., Mion, F., Bouchoucha, M., Façon, S., Raynaud, J.-J., Zerbib, F., & Jouët, P. (2021). COVID-19 pandemic and lockdown stress consequences in people with and without Irritable Bowel Syndrome. *Ethics, Medicine, and Public Health, 18*, 100660. doi:10.1016/j.jemep.2021.100660 PMID:34150971

Saltzman, L. Y., Hansel, T. C., & Bordnick, P. S. (2020). Loneliness, isolation, and social support factors in post-COVID-19 mental health. *Psychological Trauma: Theory, Research, Practice, and Policy, 12*(S1), S55–S57. doi:10.1037/tra0000703 PMID:32551762

Selye, H. (1976). *Stress in Health and Disease*. Butterworth.

Shiloh, S., Peleg, S., & Nudelman, G. (2021). Making sense of COVID-19: A longitudinal investigation of the initial stages of developing illness representations. *Psychology & Health*, 1–17. doi:10.1080/08870446.2021.1925670 PMID:33998908

Silva-Tinoco, R., González-Cantú, A., De La Torre-Saldaña, V., Guzmán-Olvera, E., Cuatecontzi-Xochitiotzi, T., Castillo-Martínez, L., ... Ochoa-Moreno, J. (2020). Effect in self-care behavior and difficulties in coping with diabetes during the COVID-19 pandemic. *Revista Mexicana de Endocrinología, Metabolismo y Nutrición*, 1-7.

Skene, I. P., & Pfeffer, P. E. (2021). Improved asthma control during the COVID-19 pandemic: Are there lessons to be learnt. *Thorax*, *76*(9), 852–853. doi:10.1136/thoraxjnl-2021-216930 PMID:33837141

Solari-Twadell, P. A., Flinter, M., Rambur, B., Renda, S., Witwer, S., Vanhook, P., & Poghosyan, L. (2021). The Impact of the COVID-19 Pandemic on the future of telehealth in primary care. *Nursing Outlook*. Advance online publication. doi:10.1016/j.outlook.2021.09.004 PMID:34763897

Stankovska, G., & Memedi, I. (2020). Stress, anxiety and depression in patients with cardiovascular diseases. *ACTA MEDICA BALKANICA*, *5*(9-10), 46–52.

Stanton, A. L., Revenson, T. A., & Tennen, H. (2007). Health psychology: Psychological adjustment to chronic disease. *Annual Review of Psychology*, *58*(1), 565–592. doi:10.1146/annurev.psych.58.110405.085615 PMID:16930096

Tany, R. F., & Saha, A. K. (2017). A study on stress and anxiety in relation to asthma. *Journal of Psychosomatic Research*, *12*(1), 117.

Taylor, S., Landry, C. A., Paluszek, M. M., Fergus, T. A., McKay, D., & Asmundson, G. J. (2020). COVID stress syndrome: Concept, structure, and correlates. *Depression and Anxiety*, *37*(8), 706–714. doi:10.1002/da.23071 PMID:32627255

Taylor, S. E., & Aspinwall, L. G. (1996). Psychosocial aspects of chronic illness. In P. T. Costa Jr & G. R. VandenBos (Eds.), *Psychological aspects of serious illness: Chronic conditions, fatal diseases, and clinical care* (pp. 3–60). American Psychological Association., doi:10.1037/10076-007

Thombs, B. D., Kwakkenbos, L., Levis, B., Bourgeault, A., Henry, R. S., Levis, A. W., Harb, S., Tao, L., Carrier, M.-E., Bustamante, L., Duchek, D., Dyas, L., El-Baalbaki, G., Ellis, K., Rice, D. B., Wurz, A., Nordlund, J., Gagarine, M., Turner, K. A., ... Benedetti, A.Scleroderma Patient-centered Intervention Network Investigators. (2021). Effects of a multi-faceted education and support programme on anxiety symptoms among people with systemic sclerosis and anxiety during COVID-19 (SPIN-CHAT): A two-arm parallel, partially nested, randomised, controlled trial. *The Lancet. Rheumatology*, *3*(6), e427–e437. doi:10.1016/S2665-9913(21)00060-6 PMID:33899008

Tyson, L., Hardeman, W., Stratton, G., Wilson, A. M., & Semlyen, J. (2021). The effects of social distancing and self-isolation during the COVID-19 pandemic on adults diagnosed with asthma: A qualitative study. *Journal of Health Psychology*. doi:10.1177/13591053211012766 PMID:33947267

Umucu, E., & Lee, B. (2020). Examining the impact of COVID-19 on stress and coping strategies in individuals with disabilities and chronic conditions. *Rehabilitation Psychology*, *65*(3), 193–198. Advance online publication. doi:10.1037/rep0000328 PMID:32406739

World Health Organization. (2020). https://www.who.int/health-topics/coronavirus#tab=tab_1

World Health Organization. (2020). *Constitution of the World Health Organization*. Available at https://www.who.int/about/governance/constitution

Wu, Y., Kwakkenbos, L., Henry, R. S., Carrier, M. E., Gagarine, M., Harb, S., Bourgeault, A., Tao, L., Carboni-Jiménez, A., Negeri, Z., Patten, S., Bartlett, S. J., Mouthon, L., Varga, J., Benedetti, A., Thombs, B. D., Fortuné, C., Gietzen, A., Guillot, G., ... Ellis, K. (2021). Factors associated with fears due to COVID-19: A Scleroderma Patient-centered Intervention Network (SPIN) COVID-19 cohort study. *Journal of Psychosomatic Research*, *140*, 110314. doi:10.1016/j.jpsychores.2020.110314 PMID:33271402

Wu, Y., Kwakkenbos, L., Henry, R. S., Tao, L., Harb, S., Bourgeault, A., Carrier, M.-E., Levis, B., Sun, Y., Bhandari, P. M., Carboni-Jiménez, A., Gagarine, M., He, C., Krishnan, A., Negeri, Z. F., Neupane, D., Mouthon, L., Bartlett, S. J., Benedetti, A., ... Welling, J. (2020). Validation of the COVID-19 Fears Questionnaires for Chronic Medical Conditions: A scleroderma patient-centered intervention network covid-19 cohort study. *Journal of Psychosomatic Research*, *139*, 110271. doi:10.1016/j.jpsychores.2020.110271 PMID:33096402

Ye, G., Baldwin, D. S., & Hou, R. (2021). Anxiety in asthma: A systematic review and meta-analysis. *Psychological Medicine*, *51*(1), 11–20. doi:10.1017/S0033291720005097 PMID:33431086

Yunier, B. P., Jiménez-Morales, R. M., Monasterio-Ramos, L. O., Vázquez-Gómez, L. A., & Fernández-Fleites, Z. (2021). Fear of COVID-19, problems accessing medical appointments, and subjective experience of disease progression, predict anxiety and depression reactions in patients with Multiple Sclerosis. *Multiple Sclerosis and Related Disorders*. PMID:34119745

Zambelli, Z., Fidalgo, A. R., Halstead, E. J., & Dimitriou, D. (2021). Acute impact of a national lockdown during the COVID-19 pandemic on wellbeing outcomes among individuals with chronic pain. *Journal of Health Psychology*. PMID:33601977

Zvolensky, M. J., Garey, L., Rogers, A. H., Schmidt, N. B., Vujanovic, A. A., Storch, E. A., Buckner, J. D., Paulus, D. J., Alfano, C., Smits, J. A. J., & O'Cleirigh, C. (2020). Psychological, addictive, and health behavior implications of the COVID-19 pandemic. *Behaviour Research and Therapy*, *134*, 103715. doi:10.1016/j.brat.2020.103715 PMID:32891956

ADDITIONAL READING

Beatty, L., & Lambert, S. (2013). A systematic review of internet-based self-help therapeutic interventions to improve distress and disease-control among adults with chronic health conditions. *Clinical Psychology Review*, *33*(4), 609–622. doi:10.1016/j.cpr.2013.03.004 PMID:23603521

De Ridder, D., Geenen, R., Kuijer, R., & van Middendorp, H. (2008). Psychological adjustment to chronic disease. *Lancet*, *372*(9634), 246–255. doi:10.1016/S0140-6736(08)61078-8 PMID:18640461

Livneh, H. (2021). Psychosocial Adaptation to Chronic Illness and Disability: An Updated and Expanded Conceptual Framework. *Rehabilitation Counseling Bulletin*.

Saltzman, L. Y., Hansel, T. C., & Bordnick, P. S. (2020). Loneliness, isolation, and social support factors in post-COVID-19 mental health. *Psychological Trauma: Theory, Research, Practice, and Policy*, *12*(S1), S55–S57. doi:10.1037/tra0000703 PMID:32551762

Stanton, A. L., Revenson, T. A., & Tennen, H. (2007). Health psychology: Psychological adjustment to chronic disease. *Annual Review of Psychology*, *58*(1), 565–592. doi:10.1146/annurev.psych.58.110405.085615 PMID:16930096

Taylor, S. E., & Aspinwall, L. G. (1996). Psychosocial aspects of chronic illness. In P. T. Costa Jr & G. R. VandenBos (Eds.), *Psychological aspects of serious illness: Chronic conditions, fatal diseases, and clinical care* (pp. 3–60). American Psychological Association., doi:10.1037/10076-007

Umucu, E., & Lee, B. (2020). Examining the impact of COVID-19 on stress and coping strategies in individuals with disabilities and chronic conditions. *Rehabilitation Psychology*, *65*(3), 193–198. Advance online publication. doi:10.1037/rep0000328 PMID:32406739

KEY TERMS AND DEFINITIONS

Adaptation to Chronic Illness: Making necessary changes to adjust the chronic illness.

Adherence: Compliance with medical recommendations.

Chronic Illness: A long period of time dealing with a health problem.

Intervention: A structured program to help people with specific problems.

Proactive Coping: Preparation for coping with an anticipated stress.

Chapter 2
ADHD and COVID-19:
Impacts and Best Practices for Mitigation

Justin Vrana
Marymount Manhattan College, USA

ABSTRACT

The COVID-19 outbreak began in December of 2019 and affected many worldwide. Research posited that those with ADHD might struggle more with the conditions of the COVID-19 pandemic than their neuro-typical counterparts. The objective of this chapter was to collect and synthesize much of the present research surrounding those with ADHD and to determine how they have been impacted by COVID-19 in hopes of providing ways to mitigate those impacts. The chapter evaluates the research suggesting that ADHD may be a potential risk factor for contracting COVID-19 and discusses how to reduce the possible increased risk of transmission in both children and adults with ADHD. The chapter also examines the effects of lockdowns and online schooling and working from home on children and adults with ADHD as well as best practices for mitigating these impacts.

INTRODUCTION

The COVID-19 outbreak started in December of 2019 with its origins leading back to Wuhan, China. The disease made its way to the United States in February of 2020 and was officially deemed a global pandemic on March 11, 2020 (Cennimo et al., 2021). With the declaration of COVID-19 as a global pandemic came restrictions such as the stay-at-home orders that began in the United States in mid-March of 2020 (Moreland et al., 2020). Aside from stay-at-home orders, the Centers for Disease Control and Prevention (CDC, 2021) also issued guidelines to prevent the spread

DOI: 10.4018/978-1-6684-3484-0.ch002

of COVID-19. These guidelines included social distancing of six feet from others, washing hands frequently; sanitizing hands when soap and water were unavailable, wearing properly fitted face coverings that covered both the mouth and the nose, and avoiding large gatherings and poorly ventilated areas. While advisories and regulations differed slightly from one place to another, the global scale of the COVID-19 pandemic was unique in that it affected everyone; and as a result the effect it had, especially on individuals with ADHD, can be seen in the literature from all around the world.

Attention-deficit/hyperactivity disorder (ADHD) is one of the most common neurodevelopmental disorders with a lifetime prevalence of around 8.1% in adults and 11.0% in children in the United States (U.S. Department of Health and Human Services, 2017). There are three different presentations of ADHD that include inattentive type, hyperactive type, and combined type. Due to this, individuals struggling with ADHD will often display a variety of different symptoms depending on their presentation. Those with predominantly inattentive type will primarily have symptom profiles that include carelessness, organizational issues, issues with prolonged attention and follow through, forgetfulness, and distractibility. Those with predominantly hyperactive type will primarily have symptom profiles that include impulsivity, fidgeting, restlessness, impatience, and deficits in social as well as pragmatic skills (American Psychiatric Association, 2013). Lastly, those with combined type will have symptom profiles that have characteristics of both the aforementioned presentations.

The many different characteristics that comprise ADHD make it so that those with the disorder may be more greatly impacted by COVID-19 than that of their neurotypical counterparts. The aim of this chapter is to discuss the associations between ADHD and COVID-19 that can be seen in children and adults, as well as to discuss treatment provisions for mitigation of similar situations that may occur in the foreseeable future.

ADHD AS A RISK FACTOR FOR CONTRACTING COVID-19

ADHD, due to its symptomatology, was identified as potential risk factor for contracting COVID-19. This is because the diagnostic criteria for the disorder consists of symptoms that could potentially elevate the risk of disseminating viruses such as COVID-19. This can be seen in certain criteria regarding the aspect of inattention through carelessness, mistake making, forgetfulness, losing things necessary to complete tasks, organizational issues, distractibility, and issues with prolonged attention and follow through. It can also be seen in relation to criteria regarding the component of hyperactivity through impulsivity, restlessness, and impatience. Due to these qualities of ADHD, it is thought that following the guidelines laid out by the Center for Disease Control (CDC), such as social distancing, washing hands, sanitizing, wearing properly fitted face coverings, and avoiding large gatherings and poorly ventilated areas, as well as stay-at-home orders would be harder for individuals with the disorder (Merzon et al., 2021).

Research Surrounding ADHD'S Possible Link To COVID-19

There have been several studies that have put this idea of ADHD's possible link to COVID-19 to the test. Firstly, in a study by Pollak et al. (2020), using a convenience sample of 849 individuals through the use of a survey carried out between March 28 and April 10, 2020, it was found that there was an association between non-adherence to COVID protocols and ADHD profiles with high levels of symptomatology. This is important in that it validates the notion that behaviors associated with ADHD might make it so that individuals with the diagnosis are less likely to comply with the guidelines surrounding COVID-19, and, in turn, may make them more prone to infection. This study also found an association between non-adherence and the male gender, which may prove to be a confounding variable for certain individuals with ADHD. Another variable also found to be associated with non-adherence in this study was risk-taking behaviors at high levels, which are also associated with a diagnosis of ADHD and therefore may also pose a problem for certain individuals in this situation (Shoham et al., 2016).

Secondly, in a study by Merzon et al. (2021), using Leumit Health Services (LHS) of 14,022 individuals in Tel-Aviv, Israel, it was found that there was a statistically significant association between individuals with ADHD ages five to 20 and the COVID-19 infection. The study also found that those who were being treated with anti-ADHD medications were less likely to become infected as opposed to those who were untreated. In a study by Wang et al. (2021), similar findings were noted. The study was carried out by analyzing a US nationwide health records database consisting of sixty-one million adults in the hopes of finding an association between a recent diagnosis of a mental disorder and risk of a COVID-19 infection. Of the 15,100 individuals in the database that were diagnosed with COVID-19, 3,430 (22.7%) had been diagnosed in the year before the COVID-19 pandemic, and 5,450 (36.1%) were individuals with a lifetime diagnosis. Of this COVID-19 population with diagnosed mental health disorders, ADHD was the second most common, at 2.7% after depression, which was the most common disorder noted. These findings are important since they suggest a possible link between ADHD and risk of contraction of COVID-19, and as a result, methods of mitigation should be taken into account when thinking about individuals with the disorder.

Mitigating COVID-19 Transmission in Those with ADHD

In relation to the best methods to protect individuals with ADHD, while there is no formal research on the matter as of yet, it is best to focus on the symptoms of the disorder that are associated with COVID-19, which potentially put them at greater risk. As many know, structure and routines can be extremely beneficial for children with ADHD (Low, 2020). Because of this, it may be helpful to introduce a routine including frequent hand washing, frequent hand sanitization, and practice wearing masks or face coverings for prolonged periods of time as a sort of at-home skills training. Similarly, structure and routines can be extremely beneficial for adults with ADHD, so it might be helpful to introduce a similar routine comprised of the same tasks for them, as well (Tartakovsky, 2013). Individuals should also work to manage their social distancing practices while in public to reinforce the behavior with the help of the parent in the case of children with ADHD. Another possible way to reduce the risk of contracting COVID-19 could be to have the individual do online-schooling or working from home when possible, where the aforementioned risk factors can be managed and largely avoided. That having been said, there might be drawbacks associated with the other symptoms of their ADHD diagnoses that come with online-schooling or working from home that should be taken into account. If going back to school or heading back to work in person, it may be helpful to reach out to teachers, professors, or employers for assistance as a way of managing and avoiding the possible risks facing those with ADHD. Lastly, as was shown in the research above, there is a lower risk of contracting COVID-19 for individuals being treated with medication for ADHD. Therefore, it may be in a child's best interest to stay medicated if he/she is already medicated or to start a medication treatment plan if deemed clinically appropriate.

CHILD ADHD

Child ADHD, in the context of this chapter, is defined as a subgroup of ADHD that includes both children and adolescents, and encompasses those ages 2 to 17. The current research on the COVID-19 pandemic's impact on child ADHD covers several different areas of interest and in this chapter will be broken down into two sections including the impact of lockdowns and the impact of online schooling. Each section is then also broken down into further subsections that contribute to the larger whole.

Impacts of Lockdowns

Lockdowns and their impacts are characteristics of the COVID-19 pandemic that affect everyone worldwide. That said, the characteristics associated with lockdowns such as decreases in physical activity, routine, human interaction, as well as many others, may make the adaptation even more difficult for those with ADHD (Sciberras et al., 2020). Not to mention, many children diagnosed with ADHD also have common comorbidities such as Autism Spectrum Disorder (ASD), Oppositional Defiant Disorder (ODD), and Conduct Disorder (CD) which may, in turn, also contribute to emotional difficulties, behavioral problems, issues in relation to media usage, and impacts on their physical health (Faraone et al., 2015 as cited in Sciberras et al., 2020).

Research Surrounding the Impacts of Lockdowns

There are several studies that have looked at the idea of emotional and behavioral difficulties facing children and adolescents with ADHD in association with the lockdowns due to COVID-19. The first is a study by Sciberras et al., (2020) in which 221 parents in Australia reported on behalf of themselves as well as their 213 children on how they were impacted by the lockdown. This study used questions from the CoRonavIrus Health Impact Survey (CRISIS) to evaluate mental health, physical health, and media use by the child. The six items used asked:

- How stressful the restrictions on leaving home had been for the child
- How stressful changes in family contacts had been for the child
- How stressful changes in friend contacts had been for the child
- Difficulty experienced with cancellation of events
- Child worry about becoming infected
- Child worry about friends or family being infected (Nikolaidis et al., 2020 as cited by Sciberras et al., 2020).

The study also used four items from the COVID-19 Adjustment Survey (CPAS), rated on a 5-point Likert scale. The CPAS asked: how likely parents would be to use an intervention, either online or smartphone-based, for mental health support to their child, parenting support, education support for their child, and sleep support for their child (Westrupp et al., 2020 as cited by Sciberras et al., 2020).

Both positive and negative responses to the different items used to assess the participants in the study were noted. In terms of negative effects, parents reported that 29% of the children in the study were stressed about the possibility of being infected by COVID-19 in the past two weeks, and 27% of the children in the study were stressed about the possibility of a friend or family member being infected by COVID-19 in the past two weeks. It was also noted that 44% of parents responded saying that their child was stressed by the restriction on leaving home. Parents also noted a decline in many areas of their child's functioning. The study found that there were significant associations between COVID-19 stress and social media use, increased negative thoughts, loneliness, irritability, distractibility, fatigue, fidgety behavior, anxiety/nervousness, sadness, general worry, and decreased enjoyment in activities (Sciberras et al., 2020).

In terms of positive effects, it was reported by 64% of parents that some positive adjustments in the life of their child were noted in relation to the restriction on leaving home. The positive changes noted included: being able to spend a greater amount of time with family, the lack of distractions that accompanied at-home learning, parents being able to assist with learning from home, the fact that they were less busy, the fact that they were relaxed, having more time at home, and less stress or pressure in relation to having to attend school.

The demographic criteria of this study should be taken into account in that it may have possibly varied the outcomes of participants in the study. Firstly, the majority of the children in the dataset were males (67%) with a mean age of 11 years (*SD* = 3.09). It is also important to note that many of the children had comorbidities such as an anxiety disorder (59.5%) or a learning disorder (28.3%). The majority of the children in the study were also being medicated, with 84.6% being on an anti-ADHD medication. This last demographic criteria touching on the use of anti-ADHD medications as a means for treatment is also extremely important in that 11% of parents of children who were taking medications reported having problems obtaining their child's medication in the previous month. Similarly, 13% of parents overall noted an issue with their ability to access healthcare services for their child in the previous month (Sciberras et al., 2020).

Secondly, is a study by Nonweiler et al. (2020) in which a parent-report survey was carried out in the United Kingdom from April 2, 2020 until June 2, 2020. The start of the survey was only 10 days after the lockdown began in the UK and included data for 453 children between the ages of 4 and 15. The study used the Strengths and Difficulties Questionnaire by comparing it to the typical responses that had been published previously, as well as by comparing the data to a mental health cohort in the UK that had attributes that were alike. Of the 453 children, 70.6% were males and approximately 40% had ADHD ($n = 183$). Other examined conditions included ASD (23.40%; $n = 106$), which is important to note in that comorbid ADHD and ASD was prevalent in approximately 18% of the sample ($n = 82$). The study found that, compared to their neurotypical peers, those with Neurodevelopmental Disorders (NDD) had a greater frequency of emotional symptoms (42% vs. 15%; $X^2 = 21.0$, $p < 0.001$), a greater frequency of conduct problems (28% vs. 9%; X^2

= 13.2, $p < 0.001$), and lesser pro-social behaviors (54% vs. 22%; $X^2 = 22.5$, $p < 0.001$) (Nonweiler et al., 2020).

Thirdly, is a study by Zhang et al. (2020) in which the symptomatology of school-aged children with ADHD and how it was impacted by the COVID-19 outbreak was investigated. The study consisted of 241 parents whose children's ages ranged from 6 to 15 years old. The mean age of the group was 9.43 with a standard deviation of 2.39 years, and the majority of the group was male (80.5%; $n = 194$) (Zhang et al., 2020). The study used the Swanson, Nolan, and Pelham scale (SNAP-IV)—parent form to gauge the average of the children's behaviors associated with their ADHD (Saxe et al., 2003 as cited by Zhang et al., 2020). The study, through the use of a single sample t-test, noted that the average of ADHD behaviors of the children were significantly worse than they were typically in normal times.

Fourth, is a study by Shah et al. (2021) in which an online survey was carried out over a period of two weeks. There was a baseline survey that 48 parents completed, a treatment intervention that 41 agreed to, and a survey at the completion of the intervention that 29 participants completed. Aside from the intervention, parents were also offered materials to read relating to their child with ADHD as well as optional consultations over the phone. The study noted a higher prevalence (slight/marked) of ADHD symptomatology in the children in the form of level of activity (50.1%), irritability (45.8%), and behavior that was deemed disruptive (47.7%). In relation to findings about parents and family members of the children with ADHD, an increase (slight/marked) of irritability (37.5%), yelling at the child with ADHD (43.8%), verbal abuse (25%), and punishment of the child with ADHD (27.1%) was noted. There was also an increase in praise for the child with ADHD (67.6%), as well as time spent with the child (72.9%).

Lastly, in a study by Bobo et al., (2020), a survey for parents of children with ADHD was carried out in France. The study consisted of responses from 533 parents over a ten-day period with the majority of the respondents being women (95%). The parents responded to questions about how their child was handling the lockdown, how life at home was, if their child had received some sort of telehealth intervention with a mental health provider, as well as their take-away from the experience, and if there was anything else important that they had noticed about their child's ADHD symptomatology in relation to the lockdown. The findings of the study noted a worsening in well-being since the start of the lockdown (34.71%). Parents also stated that 34.33% of the children showed no changes that were significant and that 30.96% were even doing better. Parents also reported problems related to inattention, hyperactivity, and impulsivity as well as anxiety symptoms and sleep issues.

Mitigating the Impacts of Lockdowns

Regarding the best methods to circumvent the impact of lockdowns associated with COVID-19 on children with ADHD, presently there is no formal research on the matter similar to how to mitigate COVID-19 transmission in children with ADHD. Therefore, it is best to focus on the symptoms of the disorder that are associated with the COVID-19 lockdowns that potentially put them at greater risk of worsening symptomatology. Some of the most helpful suggestions on how to navigate ADHD management during COVID-19 come from the European ADHD Guidelines Group (EAGG). In the article by Cortese et al., (2020) many possibly beneficial suggestions are laid out. The first of which touches on the idea that if one is currently seeking treatment for their child's ADHD, it should be continued through the means of either telephone or video calls with the provider as opposed to being discontinued. The EAGG also suggests the utilization of behavioral parenting strategies in that they make parenting easier by minimizing behaviors associated with ADHD such as disruptions and oppositional defiance. They also suggest parents should make use of self-help apparatuses modeled after evidence-based systems, including some online-based tools, while staying vigilant to verify the efficacy of said tools (Cortese et al., 2020). The EAGG also released a list of six tips for parents of children with ADHD to use in lockdown. The tips are as follows:

- "Keep positive and motivated;"
- "Make sure all family members know is expected of them;"
- "Build your child's self-confidence and trust in you;"
- "Help your child to follow instructions;"
- "Promote better behavior;" and
- "Limit conflicts" (Cortese et al., 2020).

In relation to the management of children taking ADHD medication, the EAGG also provides several suggestions to potentially avoid issues associated with the COVID-19 pandemic's impact on ADHD and its treatment. First, children with ADHD should consider starting a medication treatment plan if deemed appropriate by clinical indications and as advised by standard national guidelines. Children on a medication treatment plan should also continue on it as prescribed. Parents should also follow the instructions of their child's prescriber and avoid upping or adding dosages to their child's treatment plan as a method of dealing with the impact of the COVID-19 lockdowns on their child. In relation to following the instructions of their child's prescriber, children with ADHD should also avoid taking drug holidays—stopping one's prescribed medication for a period of time—since continuing treatment through the weekends and other down times may be better to help create structure and routine at a time where the child's ADHD symptoms may be more present.

The EAGG also warns against trying to manage behaviors that are disruptive through the use of sedatives and antipsychotic medications unless indicated clinically. It is also noted that with treatment using anti-ADHD stimulants can come the side effect of headaches, and that due to the guidance surrounding the association of problems with ibuprofen in individuals with COVID-19, paracetamol (acetaminophen) should be used in its place when at all possible. The EAGG also makes it clear that parents should not increase their child's dosage of melatonin past 5-6 mg, and should instead focus on promoting healthy sleep patterns. It is also suggested that children with ADHD who are without any cardiovascular risks should put off in-person clinical cardiovascular monitoring in that the risk of contracting and transmitting COVID-19 exceeds the necessity of these face-to-face examinations at this time. That said, parents should look out for and monitor their child for any concerning cardiovascular symptoms such as difficulties breathing, palpitations that continue for a prolonged period of time, and pain in the chest (Cortese et al., 2020). The EAGG also suggests, if at all possible, for parents to monitor their child's heart rate as well as blood pressure at home by following the guidelines below:

- "Use an age adapted cuff size;"
- "Take the BP at least 2 hours after taking a dose;"
- "Sit down for 10-15 minutes before taking the reading;"
- "Take the reading on the left arm;"
- "Take the lowest of 3 readings, approximately the same time on three separate days and send the readings, alongside the pulse values, to the prescribers;" (Cortese et al., 2020).

All decisions regarding the treatment of one's child with ADHD involving the use of medications as well as the possible change of medications and their dosages should be discussed with their prescriber before being carried out. The best advice for a child with ADHD in these trying times will come from the child's treating physician.

IMPACTS OF ONLINE SCHOOLING

Online schooling due to the COVID-19 pandemic has had an influence on all children globally. However, there are aspects of online schooling that may prove to be especially challenging for children with ADHD, and mental health conditions at large. This is because, for children with ADHD specifically, the adaptation to online schooling may come with more issues. Issues such as, increased hyperactivity, the inability to transfer attention, as well as, the fact that material that is not as engaging (Swick & Jellinek, 2020).

Research Surrounding the Impacts of Online Schooling

While there is currently less research on the impact of online schooling on children with ADHD, there are a couple of studies that are quite comprehensive and that note interesting findings. In a study by Thorell et al., (2021), a group of 6,720 parents were asked questions about their children in the hopes of finding differences between the effect of online schooling on children with mental health conditions and those without. The age range of the children that the parents were responding on behalf of was 5 to 19 years of age, and the data was collected between April 28, 2020 and June 21, 2020. The group of children with mental health conditions (MHC) included neurodevelopmental disorders such as ADHD and ASD. The MHC group consisted of the parents of 2,002 children and the NO-MHC (no mental health conditions) group consisted of the parents of 4,718 children. The study had several series of questions under three different categories. The first category focused on the organization of the online schooling that the child was receiving at home. This category was measured by evaluating the amount of time dedicated to differing tasks such as contact with teachers, contact with classmates/friends, individual study, and contact with parents, as well as questions focused around support received in online learning from home.

The second category looked at both the positive and the negative associations of learning from home. In this category, parents rated the quality of the homeschooling that their child was receiving, the overall positive and negative qualities of the homeschooling, worry and/or stress that they, the parent, were feeling, and the engagement of their child in the homeschooling. Lastly, the study had a category that evaluated the negative changes in the day to day functioning of the child, parent, and family. The responses to this specific category were collected using a 5-point Likert scale in which a rating of one was synonymous with "much less than before" and 5, "much more than before" (Mammarella et al., 2021, p. 4). The questions asked, using this scale, covered areas such as family contact, social isolation, child digital media use, alcohol use, financial problems, and parental work problems. The study noted statistically significant differences in parental experiences of homeschooling between the MHC group and the NO-MHC group, with the MHC group reporting both more negative as well as more positive experiences. The study also found a significant difference between the two groups relating to social isolation, with more parents in the MHC group reporting that their child had struggled with social isolation.

Another study focusing on the impact of online schooling during COVID-19 on children with ADHD is one by Hai et al., (2021). The study consisted of an online survey in Canada that was created using Qualtrics. Responses from the parents of 587 children with ADHD who had a mean age of 10.14 years (*SD* = 3.06) were collected and analyzed. The questions on the survey fit into three main categories. The first category consisted of questions relating to COVID-19's impact on services pertaining to the child's education and learning. The second consisted of questions about the educational challenges facing their children during the pandemic. The third and final category consisted of questions relating to the mental health of the child and used the Swanson, Nolan, and Pelham, Fourth Edition (SNAP-IV), the Generalized Anxiety Disorder-7 (GAD-7), and the Patient Health Questionnaire-9 (PHQ-9). Like many other studies, the majority of the children accounted for in the responses provided by parents were male (70.2%) with the remainder of the study population being 28.3% female, with 1.5% who identify as something other than male/female or preferred not to answer. All schools were closed when the study was carried out and 90% of the parents in the study said that their child was receiving some form of online schooling. That said, of the 69.7% of children in the study who had an individualized education plan (IEP) for their ADHD, parents reported that only 40.5% were getting materials that supported that plan and their child's specific educational needs. Aside from difficulties, children with ADHD were experiencing in relation to their IEP, 60% of parents noted that the adjustment to online schooling was either very or extremely difficult for their child. The main reasons reported for this were the inability to stay focused (80%), distractions (58%), non-engaging material (41%), computer sharing amongst family (18%), no dedicated quiet area (17%), and Internet problems (12%). In addition, 94% of parents said that they tried to implement a routine, but 60.5% of them said that the adjustment to this routine with their child was either very or extremely difficult.

In relation to the mental health of the children that was measured using the SNAP-IV, the GAD-7, and the PHQ-9, many interesting findings were noted. Results from parent responses to the SNAP-IV indicated that 73.6% of the children with ADHD had symptoms of inattention that were clinically significant. The responses also indicated that 66.8% were displaying symptoms of hyperactivity/impulsivity that were clinically significant and that 38.7% were displaying behaviors of Oppositional Defiant Disorder (ODD) that were clinically significant. Results from parent responses to the PHQ-9 indicated that many of the children with ADHD were struggling with depressive symptoms with mild severity (36.5%), moderate severity (27.8%), and severe severity (17.7%). Results from parent responses to the GAD-7 indicated that many of the children with ADHD were also struggling with symptoms of anxiety with mild severity (34.8%), moderate severity (15.0%), and severe severity (13.8%) (Hai et al., 2021).

Mitigating the Impacts of Online Schooling

The best ways of handling the impact of online schooling associated with COVID-19 on children with ADHD is to focus on the symptoms associated with the issues facing these children that potentially put them at greater risk of failing to adapt to the virtual learning environment since there is no formal research on the matter. First off, since it was discovered that the group with mental health conditions had more positive experiences as well as more negative experiences associated with online learning than the NO-MHC group (Non-Mental Health Condition group), it may be beneficial to place greater emphasis on the positive associations as a sort of cognitive restructuring to eliminate some negative thought patterns. In terms of dealing with social isolation for the child with ADHD, one should have their child engage in outdoor physical activity, keep a structured routine, talk to friends and family online or by phone, take part in fun, at-home, family activities, plan for the future, and engage in hobbies or the creation of music, art, or writing (Cuncic, 2020). That said, since difficulty adapting to a structured routine during the pandemic was noted in the literature, it is important to be very vigilant about sticking to the routine created while also making sure to be flexible, in that creating a routine takes time for a child with ADHD to learn. Parents should try to remain positive and patient, remembering that ADHD is a disorder and that the child is likely doing the best that he/she can (Legg, 2018). The EAGG also discussed possible beneficial interventions for students with ADHD in regards to online learning. For example, parents should consider reaching out to their child's teacher and or school and ask if their child with ADHD can be monitored. This is especially true for adolescents with ADHD in that they are at greater risk and are more likely to be disorganized. Characteristics of a child with ADHD that may be helpful for the teacher to monitor are whether the child is engaged in the online learning setting, if the child is turning in his/her work, and if there are any worries related to the child's well-being emotionally and or socially (Cortese et al., 2020).

ADULT ADHD

Adult ADHD, in the context of this chapter, is defined as a subgroup of ADHD that encompasses all those with ADHD aged 18 and older. The current research on the COVID-19 pandemic's impact on adult ADHD is far less vast than that of the research pertaining to ADHD in children. There is not much research specific to how adults have been impacted by lockdowns or online schooling/working from home, but rather possible treatment provisions for adults with ADHD during the COVID-19 pandemic. Because of this, this section on adult ADHD will focus more specifically on an individual study pertaining to lockdowns and treatment provisions for adult ADHD during the COVID-19 pandemic as well as suggested issues that adults with ADHD may encounter and possible solutions.

Impacts of Lockdowns: A Study of Adults with ADHD in Japan

In a study conducted by Ando et al., (2021) using a convenience sample, four participants, all above the age of 20, in Japan, received a treatment intervention for their ADHD during the COVID-19 pandemic. This qualitative study used an interpretive approach and was carried out to look at a coaching intervention that was in progress. The goal was to evaluate how adults with ADHD or suspected ADHD used their time during the lockdown in Japan. Initially the coaching consisted of in-person sessions as well as email support coaching that transferred into online video coaching sessions once the lockdown began. The individuals in this study were clients who had participated in this adaptive coaching intervention since 2014, and the members of the research team were all either researchers or clinicians working in the field of neurodevelopmental disorders with more than 20 years of experience in the clinical setting. The first of four participants was a male in his thirties, deemed A, who worked part-time and lived with a parent. He had combined type ADHD, an average full intellectual quotient (FIQ), and was markedly atypical on the Conners' Adult ADHD Rating Scale (CAARS). The second participant, deemed B, was a female in her forties who worked part-time and lived with her partner. She had combined type ADHD, an average FIQ, and was markedly atypical on the CAARS. The third participant, deemed C, was a male in his twenties who was a student and lived with his parents and siblings. He had inattentive type ADHD, a high average FIQ, and was moderately atypical on the CAARS. The fourth and final participant, deemed D, was a female in her thirties who worked part-time and lived with her partner and children. She had combined type ADHD, a high average FIQ, and was moderately atypical on the CAARS.

Using a codebook developed and adjusted by the researchers of the study, analysis of the coaching sessions led to the synthesis of responses into five themes. They were:

- "Terrible feeling caused by frustration, stress, and anger"
- "Closeness due to the internal difficulties and conflict"
- "Deteriorating ADHD symptoms and executive function-related matters"
- "Condition is the same as usual"
- "Positive aspects associated with the self-lockdown" (Ando et al., 2021, p. 4)

In relation to the terrible feelings that were reported, respondents with hyperactivity noted that they had an excess of energy that they were unable to release, and that they also had problems with their family members who were working from home in that they were unable to remain quiet. Some of the respondents also noted frustration in that they had issues communicating with other individuals. One respondent even mentioned how she got angry more easily than under typical circumstances. In terms of the closeness that was reported, one respondent with hyperactivity noted that it felt as if it were more of a challenge for her to handle the aspect of staying at home that comes with the lockdowns in that she typically is very social and relies on those interactions to get rid of excess energy. When evaluating the deteriorating ADHD symptoms and executive function-related matters, participants found themselves making more absentminded mistakes because they were out of their normal routine. They also found that due to ever-changing circumstances, it was hard for them to keep up with their schedules. On the other hand, those who said that their condition was the same as usual noted no change. For some, this was because they had already been working from home and therefore had already adjusted to the new environment and routine.

The last category is the positive aspects associated with the lockdown in which participants stated that they liked how they were able to maintain an effective rate of productivity since they did not have to contend with aspects of working at the office that would derail or distract them. They also did not have to waste any of their time or energy preparing for school or work, which can sometimes take more out of an individual with ADHD. The last positive aspect that was noted was that many of the participants were working from their own personal spaces in which they were involved in things that may make it so that they are inspired to be more creative in their work (Ando et al., 2021).

Mitigating the Impacts of Lockdowns

The best methods to handle the impact of lockdowns associated with COVID-19 on adults with ADHD is to focus on the symptoms of the disorder that are associated with the COVID-19 lockdowns and that potentially put adults with ADHD at greater risk of worsening symptomatology, since there is no formal research on the matter similar to how to mitigate the impact of lockdowns associated with COVID-19 on children with ADHD. Firstly, a study by Fullen et al. (2020) found clinical significance in a treatment program that used a manual with a form of Acceptance and Commitment Therapy (ACT), "a treatment approach that focuses on radically accepting personal experiences beyond the individual's control and taking committed action towards personal values" (Hayes & Strosahl, 2004 as cited in Fullen et al., 2020, p. 206).

Secondly, in terms of dealing with symptoms of hyperactivity, many individuals with ADHD mention having an excess of energy that they are unable to release due to stay-at-home orders. For individuals such as those mentioned in the Hayes and Strosahl (2004) study, it might be helpful to engage in outdoor activities such as exercise to be able to release their excess energy. Another issue introduced in the Hayes and Strosahl (2004) study was the inability to remain quiet while those around them were working from home. For those individuals, it may be helpful for them to have separate dedicated workspaces away from other family members wherein they can work alone quietly on their own work. If individuals with ADHD are not working themselves, it may still be beneficial for them to be in their own space where they can perhaps work on some sort of creative project or other activity to keep themselves distracted while their family member or members are at work. Another issue that those with ADHD were confronted with was the feeling of being unable to communicate with others.

For those who are having issues communicating, it may be helpful to schedule routine phone or video calls with family members and/or friends as well as planning dedicated times to get together with members of their immediate household to engage in some sort of activity.

With regard to managing their temper, adults with ADHD should: figure out what it is that triggers their outbursts; try to change their way of thinking and eliminate negative thought patterns; take the time to think about the outcome of their outburst; put the situation into perspective; think about ways to solve situations that anger them in a more positive manner; and commend themselves when they respond in a more appropriate and positive way (Maynard, 2021). When it comes to the careless mistake making that has plagued many with ADHD during the COVID-19 pandemic, adults with ADHD should consider creating some sort of routine that makes such careless mistakes less likely. Having some sort of structure and regularity might make it so that one gets comfortable in the tasks that he/she has to achieve and can do them with fewer missteps. In terms of the issue of keeping one's schedule straight, it may be beneficial for adults with ADHD to keep a calendar, either digitally on their phone where it is easily accessible or recorded on paper, in which they can update a change in their daily plans as soon as the change is known to them. This may be especially helpful in that during the COVID-19 pandemic, plans and events are always changing. Lastly, adults struggling with the stress and frustration accompanying the COVID-19 pandemic should try to remember and focus on the positive impacts that the lockdown may have had on them, such as being able to work from home without distraction, not having to waste time and energy getting ready for school or work, and the chance to be more creative.

Working from Home with ADHD During the COVID-19 Pandemic

There are many pitfalls that adults with ADHD can fall into when working from home during the COVID-19 pandemic. Adults with ADHD should know the most common culprits that get in their way of being productive while working from home and the ways to best avoid them. The most common and most obvious issue individuals with ADHD are faced with while working from home is distraction. Adults with ADHD may want to consider setting a timer so that they are able to check in with themselves and get back to what they are supposed to be doing if they find themselves distracted.

Another common issue that some individuals with ADHD working from home have is that they feel unmotivated. There is a good chance that individuals with ADHD are not going to feel as motivated as they do when they are in the office, and for individuals with ADHD, it is often hardest in the initial stage of getting started. Like when trying to avoid getting distracted, it might once again be beneficial to try using a timer to give oneself a deadline for starting to work. Another common barrier that those with ADHD are confronted with while working from home is not having a dedicated workspace. These individuals may want to consider having a space that is clutter-free and that is specific to the workday to avoid crossover between activities/spaces that increase the likelihood of distractions. Then there is the issue of lack of structure, individuals with ADHD may benefit from creating a schedule for their workday start time, scheduled lunch break, and workday end time. This kind of schedule can make it so that one does not work longer or shorter than they should, resulting in this affecting their productivity. Individuals with ADHD should also consider getting fully dressed in work attire to help create some sort of routine that will also help to keep them productive.

Another issue that often arises while working from home is interruptions from other members of the immediate household. To avoid this, those with ADHD should consider setting rules for when they are allowed to talk to other members of their household, and inform those members not to interrupt them unless it is an emergency. The use of noise-cancelling headphones may also prove to be beneficial for some. Many with ADHD also fall into the trap of thinking that they will be able to accomplish more while being at home, having more time, and get distracted doing activities around the house such as chores. For this reason, adults with ADHD who are working from home should perhaps limit themselves to work-related tasks in order to accomplish what it is they need to get done (Rayburn, 2021). It may also be beneficial for those with ADHD who are working from home to continue taking their medication, to remain at their desk, to not spend too much time on one task, and to be active and move during their breaks (ADDitude Editors, 2021). Lastly, those with ADHD may want to avoid using their phone and the Internet (Rayburn, 2021).

CONCLUSION

The impact that the COVID-19 pandemic has had on individuals with ADHD, and the many different characteristics that comprise the disorder, is extremely important. The pandemic has affected many areas of the lives of those with ADHD, from the impact of lockdowns to the impact of online schooling and working from home, to even the possibility of contracting the virus due to their ADHD symptomatology. ADHD is a disorder that affects children as well as adults globally much like the COVID-19 virus, and like the COVID-19 virus, with the right precautions, the effects of the COVID-19 pandemic on those with ADHD can be mitigated. The hope is that this chapter has provided information on ADHD's many different associations with the COVID-19 pandemic and its byproducts that affect those with the disorder, as well as ways to circumvent those possible effects for similar situations that may occur in the foreseeable future.

REFERENCES

ADDitude Editors. (2021, January 19). *ADHD Brains Working at Home: A Beginner's Guide to Telecommuting*. ADDitude. https://www.additudemag.com/working-from-homeadhd/

American Psychiatric Association. (2013). *Diagnostic and statistical manual of mental disorders* (5th ed.). doi:10.1176/appi.books.9780890425596

Ando, M., Takeda, T., & Kumagai, K. (2021). A qualitative study of impacts of the COVID-19 pandemic on lives in adults with attention deficit hyperactive disorder in Japan. *International Journal of Environmental Research and Public Health, 18*(4), 2090. doi:10.3390/ijerph18042090 PMID:33669970

Bobo, E., Lin, L., Acquaviva, E., Caci, H., Franc, N., Gamon, L., Picot, M. C., Pupier, F., Speranza, M., Falissard, B., & Purper-Ouakil, D. (2020). Comment les enfants et adolescents avec le trouble déficit d'attention/hyperactivité (TDAH) vivent-ils le confinement durant la pandémie COVID-19? [How do children and adolescents with Attention Deficit Hyperactivity Disorder (ADHD) experience lockdown during the COVID-19 outbreak?]. *L'Encéphale*, *46*(3, 3S), S85–S92. doi:10.1016/j.encep.2020.05.011 PMID:32522407

Cennimo, D. J. (2021, April 30). *How did the coronavirus outbreak start?* Medscape. https://www.medscape.com/answers/ 2500114-197402/how-did-the-coronavirus-outbreak-start

Centers for Disease Control and Prevention. (2021, March 8). *How to Protect Yourself & Others.* Centers for Disease Control and Prevention. https://www.cdc.gov/coronavirus/2019-ncov /prevent-getting-sick/prevention.html

Cleveland Clinic. (2019, September 25). *ADHD inattentive type in adults: Symptoms, diagnosis & treatment.* Cleveland Clinic. https://my.clevelandclinic .org/health/diseases/15253-attention-deficit-disorder-without-hyperactivity-add-in-adults

Conners, C. K., Erhardt, D., & Sparrow, E. (2002). *Conners' Adult ADHD Rating Scales–Self-Report: Long Version (CAARS–S: L).* Toronto, Ontario, Canada: Multi-Health Systems. https://documents.acer.org/caars-self-l-int1.pdf

Cortese, S., Asherson, P., Sonuga-Barke, E., Banaschewski, T., Brandeis, D., Buitelaar, J., Coghill, D., Daley, D., Danckaerts, M., Dittmann, R. W., Doepfner, M., Ferrin, M., Hollis, C., Holtmann, M., Konofal, E., Lecendreux, M., Santosh, P., Rothenberger, A., Soutullo, C., ... Simonoff, E.European ADHD Guidelines Group. (2020). ADHD management during the COVID-19 pandemic: Guidance from the European ADHD Guidelines Group. *The Lancet. Child & Adolescent Health*, *4*(6), 412–414. doi:10.1016/S2352-4642(20)30110-3 PMID:32311314

Cuncic, A. (2020, March 27). *Ways to Feel Less Lonely During the Coronavirus.* Verywell Mind. https://www.verywellmind.com/how-to-cope-with-loneliness-during-coronavirus4799661

Fullen, T., Galab, N., Abbott, K. A., & Adamou, M. (2020). Acceptance and Commitment therapy for adults with ADHD during COVID-19: An open trial. *Open Journal of Psychiatry*, *10*(04), 205–215. doi:10.4236/ojpsych.2020.104017

Hai, T., Swansburg, R., MacMaster, F. P., & Lemay, J. F. (2021). Impact of COVID-19 on Educational Services in Canadian Children With Attention-Deficit/Hyperactivity Disorder. In *Frontiers in Education* (Vol. 6, p. 32). Frontiers. doi:10.3389/feduc.2021.614181

Jameson, J. (2019, December 5). *Pragmatic social communication: Activities to improve pragmatics*. Jewel Autism Centre Blog. http://jewelautismcentre.com/jewel_blog/pragmatic-social-communication/

Lange, R. T. (2011). Full Scale IQ. In J. S. Kreutzer, J. DeLuca, & B. Caplan (Eds.), *Encyclopedia of Clinical Neuropsychology*. Springer. doi:10.1007/978-0-387-79948-3_1549

Legg, T. J. (2018, September 17). *Parenting Tips for ADHD: Do's and Don'ts.* Healthline. https://www. healthline.com/health/adhd/parenting-tips

Lexico. (n.d.a). *Comorbidity*. https://www.lexico. com/definition/comorbidity

Lexico. (n.d.b). *Neurotypical*. https://www.lexico. com/definition/neurotypical

Low, K. (2020, November 8). *Children With ADHD Need Structure in Their Lives to Stay Focused*. Verywell Mind. https://www.verywellmind.com/why-is-structure-important-for-kids-with-adhd-20747

Maynard, S. (2021, January 20). *Rule #2: Ban Negative Thoughts*. ADDitude. https://www.additudemag. com/anger-management-tips/

McLeod, S. A. (2019, August 3). *Likert scale*. Simply Psychology. https://www.simplypsychology. org/likert-scale.html

Merzon, E., Manor, I., Rotem, A., Schneider, T., Vinker, S., Golan Cohen, A., Lauden, A., Weizman, A., & Green, I. (2021). ADHD as a Risk Factor for Infection With Covid-19. *Journal of Attention Disorders, 25*(13), 1783–1790. doi:10.1177/1087054720943271 PMID:32697120

Moreland, A., Herlihy, C., Tynan, M. A., Sunshine, G., McCord, R. F., Hilton, C. A., Poovey, J., Werner, A., Jones, C. D., Fulmer, E., Gundlapalli, A., Strosnider, H., Potvien, A., García, M. C., Honeycutt, S., Baldwin, G., Clodfelter, C., Howard-Williams, M., Jeong, G., ... Popoola, A. (2020). Timing of state and territorial COVID-19 stay-at-home orders and changes in population movement—United States, March 1–May 31, 2020. *Morbidity and Mortality Weekly Report, 69*(35), 1198–1203. doi:10.15585/mmwr.mm6935a2 PMID:32881851

Nikoladis, A., Paksarian, D., Alexander, L., DeRosa, J., Dunn, J., Nielson, D. M., Droney, I., Kang, M., Douka, I., Bromet, E., Milham, M. P., Stingaris, A., & Merikangas, K. R. (2020). The Coronavirus Health and Impact Survey (CRISIS) reveals reproducible correlates of pandemic-related mood states across the Atlantic. [Preprint]. medRxiv doi:10.1101/2020.08.24.20181123

Nonweiler, J., Rattray, F., Baulcomb, J., Happé, F., & Absoud, M. (2020). Prevalence and associated factors of emotional and behavioural difficulties during COVID-*19 pandemic in children with neurodevelopmental disorders. Children (Basel, Switzerland), 7*(9), 128. doi:10.3390/children7090128 PMID:32899799

Pollak, Y., Dayan, H., Shoham, R., & Berger, I. (2020). Predictors of non-adherence to public health instructions during the COVID-19 pandemic. *Psychiatry and Clinical Neurosciences, 74*(11), 602–604. doi:10.1111/pcn.13122 PMID:32729646

Rayburn, D. (2021, March 11). *6 Perils of Working from Home with ADHD*. Dana Rayburn ADHD Coach. https://danarayburn.com/5-perils-of-working-from-home-with-adhd/

Roth, E. (2018, April 24). *What are the Three Types of ADHD?* Healthline. https://www.healthline.com/health/adhd/three-types-adhd

Saxe, G., Chawla, N., Stoddard, F., Kassam-Adams, N., Courtney, D., Cunningham, K., Lopez, C., Hall, E., Sheridan, R., King, D., & King, L. (2003). Child stress disorders checklist: A measure of ASD and PTSD in children. *Journal of the American Academy of Child and Adolescent Psychiatry*, *42*(8), 972–978. doi:10.1097/01.CHI.0000046887.27264.F3 PMID:12874500

Sciberras, E., Patel, P., Stokes, M. A., Coghill, D., Middeldorp, C. M., Bellgrove, M. A., Becker, S. P., Efron, D., Stringaris, A., Faraone, S. V., Bellows, S. T., Quach, J., Banaschewski, T., McGillivray, J., Hutchinson, D., Silk, T. J., Melvin, G., Wood, A. G., Jackson, A., ... Westrupp, E. (2020). Physical health, media use, and mental health in children and adolescents with ADHD during the COVID-19 pandemic in Australia. *Journal of Attention Disorders*. Advance online publication. doi:10.1177/1087054720978549 PMID:33331195

Shah, R., Raju, V. V., Sharma, A., & Grover, S. (2021). Impact of COVID-19 and lockdown on children with ADHD and Their families-an online survey and a continuity care model. *Journal of Neurosciences in Rural Practice*, *12*(01), 71–79. doi:10.1055-0040-1718645 PMID:33531763

Shoham, R., Sonuga-Barke, E. J., Aloni, H., Yaniv, I., & Pollak, Y. (2016). ADHD-associated risk taking is linked to exaggerated views of the benefits of positive outcomes. *Scientific Reports*, *6*(1), 1–8. doi:10.1038rep34833 PMID:27725684

Sinfield, J. (2020, April 1). *How ADHD Combined Type Has Both Inattention and Hyperactivity*. Verywell Mind. https://www.verywellmind.com/what-is-adhd-combined-type-4135385

Swick, S. D., & Jellinek, M. S. (2020, September 16). *Virtual school is especially difficult for children with ADHD*. MDedge Pediatrics. https://www.mdedge.com/pediatrics/article/228663/mental-health/virtual-school-especially-difficult-children-adhd

Tartakovsky, M. (2013, April 2). *9 Tips for Creating a Routine for Adults with ADHD*. Psych Central. https://psychcentral.com/blog/9-tips-for-creating-a-routine-for-adults-with- adhd#1

Thorell, L. B., Skoglund, C., de la Peña, A. G., Baeyens, D., Fuermaier, A., Groom, M. J., Mammarella, I. C., van der Oord, S., van den Hoofdakker, B. J., Luman, M., de Miranda, D. M., Siu, A., Steinmayr, R., Idrees, I., Soares, L. S., Sörlin, M., Luque, J. L., Moscardino, U. M., Roch, M., ... Christiansen, H. (2021). Parental experiences of homeschooling during the COVID-19 pandemic: Differences between seven European countries and between children with and without mental health conditions. *European Child & Adolescent Psychiatry*, 1–13. Advance online publication. doi:10.100700787-020-01706-1 PMID:33415470

United States Environmental Protection Agency. (2015). America's children and the environment: Neurodevelopmental disorders (Excerpt from the third edition). In C. Croft (Ed.), Environmental hazards and neurodevelopment: Where ecology and well-being connect (pp. 3–39). CRC Press/Routledge/Taylor & Francis Group. doi:10.1201/b18030-3

U.S. Department of Health and Human Services. (2017, November). *Attention-Deficit/Hyperactivity Disorder (ADHD).* National Institute of Mental Health. https://www.nimh.nih.gov/health/ statistics/attention-deficit-hyperactivity-disorder-adhd #:~:text=The%20overall%20prevalence %20of%20current,all%20other%20 race%2Fethni city%20groups

Wang, Q. Q., Xu, R., & Volkow, N. D. (2021). Increased risk of COVID -19 infection and mortality in people with mental disorders: Analysis from electronic health records in the United States. *World Psychiatry; Official Journal of the World Psychiatric Association (WPA)*, *20*(1), 124–130. doi:10.1002/wps.20806 PMID:33026219

Zhang, J., Shuai, L., Yu, H., Wang, Z., Qiu, M., Lu, L., Cao, X., Xia, W., Wang, Y., & Chen, R. (2020). Acute stress, behavioural symptoms and mood states among school-age children with attention-deficit/hyperactive disorder during the COVID-19 outbreak. *Asian Journal of Psychiatry*, *51*, 102077. doi:10.1016/j.ajp.2020.102077 PMID:32315967

KEY TERMS AND DEFINITIONS

Combined Type ADHD: A type of ADHD where both hyperactivity/impulsivity and inattention are present (Sinfield, 2020).

Comorbidities: The presence of one or more disorders alongside the initial diagnosed disorder (Lexico, n.d.b).

Hyperactive and Impulsive Type ADHD: A type of ADHD with a symptom profile consisting predominantly of hyperactivity and impulsivity that can include having trouble sitting still, restlessness, fidgeting, and squirming (Roth, 2018).

Inattentive Type ADHD: A type of ADHD that is characterized by symptoms such as ease of distraction, little attention to detail, and organizational issues, and struggling to complete routine tasks in a timely manner, such as responding to emails or paying bills (Cleveland Clinic, 2019).

Likert Scale: A rating scale consisting of either five or seven points in which an individual can rate how much they agree or disagree with a proposition (McLeod, 2019).

Neurodevelopmental Disorders: Disabilities that center around neurological system functioning and brain functioning (United States Environmental Protection Agency, 2015).

Neurotypical: Someone who does not present with behavior or thought patterns that are neurologically atypical or autistic (Lexico, n.d.a).

Chapter 3
Effects of COVID-19 on OCD Severity and Coping Strategies

Manuella Hounton
Marymount Manhattan College, USA

ABSTRACT

In early 2020, the SARS-CoV-2 Virus made its appearance and has, since then, substantially impacted our lives. Those with mental health issues have been significantly impacted and are still adjusting. Multiple studies since then have been conducted to study its effects. This literature review aims to expand on the research conducted regarding the effects of COVID-19 on patients with obsessive-compulsive disorder (OCD). After briefly reviewing research articles, coping and management techniques were discussed. Lastly, future research suggestions are provided. Five research studies are reviewed, and all of the results reveal that the pandemic has worsened OCD severity. For example, results of the Khosravani et al. study, which included 270 participants, showed that stress reactions related to compulsive checking and contamination exacerbated patient's OCD. A study by Tanir et al., which included 61 participants, discovered that contamination obsessions and cleaning or washing compulsions increased during the pandemic. Additionally, a study by David et al. with 30 participants found that contamination symptoms, particularly along with remitters, showed a worsening of OCD when compared to pre-COVID levels. Regarding coping mechanisms, patients with OCD used instrumental support, religion, denial, and self-blame when dealing with changes to their disorder. Researchers have advised therapists to monitor patients' screen time, since that's one of the ways that OCD levels of those with contamination, hygiene, and cleanliness obsessions tends to worsen. As for future directions, researchers should aim for longitudinal studies, which would fully measure the effects of the pandemic on OCD. The chapter concludes by elaborating on suggestions, since a vaccine is now available.

DOI: 10.4018/978-1-6684-3484-0.ch003

INTRODUCTION

When asked what it's like dealing with Obsessive Compulsive Disorder, Laura McCarthy described it as having an "ever-present nagging feeling that something is just 'not right.' [She] can never really, truly 'make it right.' [She has] to learn to live with the all-consuming feeling of mental discomfort" (Schuster, 2015). Obsessive-Compulsive Disorder is a disorder marked by obsessive thoughts followed by compulsive behaviors. For example, the mental discomfort as mentioned by McCarthy could be preventing obsessive thoughts from becoming a reality; such as the apartment or building complex being set on fire. Through the compulsive ritual of making sure the stove is turned off, one can feel more in control. About 2.3% of the U.S population is affected by OCD and is dealing with these mental discomforts ("Facts about Obsessive Compulsive Disorder," 2018).

HISTORY

Obsessive-Compulsive disorder dates back to the early 1000s when it used to be called "scrupulosity." Many cases were linked to religion. Saint Ignatius of Loyola once said "that devout people need to be sure that they have pleased God and that they have not sinned. If they are unable to convince themselves of this, they may perform acts of penance. If these, too, fail to allay their anxiety, then they will be tormented by doubts and will be preoccupied by rituals" ("The history of OCD," n.d.). Such a case is seen regarding a nun named Kunegond from Johannes Nider's book. Kunegond believed that she remained a sinner despite her confessions, therefore, she turned to excessive fasting which led to her death ("The history of OCD", n.d). Furthermore, clergymen would advise parishioners to stop repressing their obsessive thoughts and encouraged them to distract themselves with other activities (Des Marais, 2020). Des Marais states that the advice given by clergymen is similar to those seen during behavior therapy (2020). However, if that's the case, the type of activities needs to be monitored so that they don't become punishments as in Kunegond's case.

The Enlightenment Period shifted the way many thought. They turned to science, etc. instead of being controlled by the Church. Before people were trying to fix patients with OCD through treatments such as phlebotomy, astrology, etc., but now more insight into possible causes of OCD began to be discussed. Discussions were led by psychologists such as Sigmund Freud, Pierre Janet, etc. For example, Freud believed there is a link between internal conflicts and OCD behaviors. Internal conflicts had to do with the id, ego, and superego. According to Freud, those with OCD have repressed desire which they manifest through uncontrollable maladaptive behaviors (Sigmund Freud, n.d). A case was heard in which he interpreted the possible repressed desire of a young woman with a compulsive bedtime ritual. For example, the young woman either removed or turned off all clocks and watches. Freud then linked the ticking of clocks to arousal, which she confirmed being awakened by during her sleep (Sigmund Freud, n.d).

COVID-19 EFFECTS

As of 2019, we've been dealing with a disease that is worsening OCD symptoms. COVID-19 is an infectious disease caused by a virus, SARS-CoV-2. As of April 28th 2021, there are more than 50 million active cases worldwide and 149 million, if one takes into consideration those who have recovered or died (COVID Live - Coronavirus Statistics - Worldometer, n.d.). Coronavirus is said to be found in both humans and animals. The first COVID case was discovered in December 2019. The virus is said to be transmitted through contact, cross-contamination and can be air-borne, as well. Most symptoms are similar to the flu because they include fever, cough, loss of taste and smell, headache, shortness of breath, etc. But COVID affects all aspects of life whether mental, physical, social, political, or economic.

While looking into participants' dysfunctional and functional beliefs associated with COVID-19, a study found that 36% of participants endorsed the saying that "other people are now realizing how dangerous viruses and germs are (Jelinek, et al. 2021)." Behaviors such as disinfecting surfaces or washing hands frequently were considered excessive; however, it has become normalized since the rise of COVID-19 and the implementation of prevention techniques (Silva et al., 2020). The cleaning aspect of preventing COVID aligns with the compulsive behaviors of one with OCD. Several researchers have been studying changes in OCD symptoms during the pandemic (Khosravani et al., 2020, Tanir et al., 2020, Benatti et al., 2020, Davide et al., 2020, Jelinek et al. 2020). All studies were conducted abroad and they were able to support the theory that COVID-19 has exacerbated OCD symptoms.

The Study of Khosravani and Colleagues (2020)

Khosravani et al. (2020) studied the effect of the COVID-19 pandemic across symptom dimensions of patients with obsessive-compulsive disorder. They hypothesized that there would be an increase in OCD symptoms when comparing its severity before and after COVID-19 (Khosravani et al., 2020). It was also hypothesized that OCD symptoms would increase and causes wouldn't be limited to fears of contamination (Khosravani et al., 2020).

As a method, they reached out to OCD patients whom they examined pre-Covid, but few people responded, due to the fear of being infected by face-to-face interviews or for not having the equipment required to participate online or on the phone (Khosravani et al., 2020). Previously 764 participated, but now only 270 participants responded (Khosravani et al., 2020). Of the 270 participants, 120 had a comorbid disorder, all of them were on medication and less than half (30%) received psychological treatment (Khosravani et al., 2020).

For self-report measures, they used a COVID-19 stress scale (CSS) which measures COVID-19 stress reactions across sub-dimensions broken down into five sections: Danger and contamination, socio-economic consequences, xenophobia, traumatic stress, and compulsive checking). The Yale-Brown Obsessive-Compulsive scale (Y-BOCS) was used to determine OCD severity and the dimensional obsessive-compulsive scale (DOCS) was used to examine OCD symptom dimensions (contamination, responsibility of harm, unacceptable obsessional thoughts, and symmetry) (Khosravani et al., 2020).

Khosravani and his colleagues (2020) measured differences of severity pre vs post Covid using Paired T-tests. Hierarchical regression analysis was then used to examine how much of an effect CSS subscales had in changes or severity of symptoms from COVID-19 (Khosravani et al., 2020). All T-tests were significant ($p < .001$), results showed that there is a significant difference between symptoms' dimensions measured by DOCS and OCD severity measured by Y-BOCS before and after COVID-19 (Khosravani et al., 2020). The study was able to show that stress reactions relating to danger and contamination, compulsive checking, xenophobia, traumatic stress, and socio-economic struggles were causing the worsening of OCD severity, as well.

Khosravani et al. (2020) believed that self-reports may be subject to response bias since distress may cause them to exaggerate their symptoms. Factors affecting results may also be that the severity is higher now due to limited access or accountability to therapy (Khosravani et al., 2020). They offered multiple suggestions for future research, like conducting another study post-Covid to see if there would be a change in severity compared to during Covid (Khosravani et al., 2020).

The Study of Tanir and Colleagues (2020)

Tanir et al. (2020) studied the effects of COVID-19 on children and adolescents with obsessive-compulsive disorder. They hypothesized that there would be an increase in the severity of symptoms during the pandemic lockdown compared to the pre-Covid period (Tanir et al., 2020).

Participants were between the ages of 6 to 18 years old and had to meet certain criteria such as OCD diagnosis according to the DSM-5 criteria (Tanir et al., 2020).

They interviewed participants via telephone and online programs for a week to collect data for the increase in possible exacerbation of symptoms during the pandemic period (Tanir et al., 2020). A total of 61 participants participated, but 29 were excluded since they didn't meet the criteria (Tanir et al., 2020).

Tanir and his colleagues (2020) used three forms of measurement. The two most important measures were: The Clinical Global Impression-Severity Scale (CGI-S) and The Children's Yale-Brown Obsessive-Compulsive Scale (CY-BOCS) (Tanir et al., 2020). The CGI scale measured symptoms based on severity, improvement, and efficacy, while the CY-BOC scale measured obsession and compulsion, which were scaled using a 5-point Likert (Tanir et al., 2020). As for statistical analyses, they used different sorts of tests such as the Wilcoxon test, Cohen's Kappa Coefficient, etc.

As a result, they found out through the CYBOCS and CGI-S scales that more than half of participants stated that they noticed an increase in symptom severity (Tanir et al., 2020). The frequency of contamination obsessions and cleaning or washing compulsions increased during the pandemic and were the top two that increased in obsessions versus compulsions categories (Tanir et al., 2020). Before and after findings of contamination obsessions CGI-S scores ($z: -4.339$, $p<0.001$), and pre and post findings of cleaning compulsions ($z: -4.196$, $p<0.001$) were both significantly high (Tanir et al., 2020). Since the study was cross-sectional, they recommended that future studies include larger samples and should be conducted for a longer time frame to best discern whether severity was linked to COVID-19 (Tanir et al., 2020).

The Study of Benatti and Colleagues

The Benatti et al. (2020) study investigated the impact of COVID-19 on outpatients with OCD. They hypothesized that patients would experience worsening clinical and behavioral OCD symptoms. They also hypothesized that there would be an increase in pre-existing symptoms, the development of new symptoms, or a switch to different phenotypes (Benatti et al., 2020). The study was cross-sectional and was conducted via three different tertiary clinics. Nearly four percent of the participants participated in the study by being interviewed through the phone while the remainder did in-person interviews (Benatti et al., 2020). In total, 123 outpatients with OCD participated in the study (Benatti et al., 2020). They started with demographic questions and then went in-depth with questions pertaining to the development of new symptoms like, a tic (Benatti et al., 2020). An exploratory analysis was used to compare patients with OCD who had symptoms that did or did not worsen (Benatti et al., 2020). Statistical analysis such as Pearson Chi-square and ANOVA tests were used (Benatti et al., 2020).

As a result, the researchers in the Benatti et al. (2020) study discovered that more than one-third of patients experienced an exacerbation of clinical OCD. There was a significant difference between the development of new obsessions and the recurrence of old ones in the OCD worsening group versus those who were not in the worsening group (Benatti et al., 2020). Those whose OCD worsened reported having an increase in avoidance behaviors [OW vs without OW: 65.9% vs 20.3%; $p<.05$] (Benatti et al., 2020). Similar to other studies, the researchers were aware that severity may be subject to change post-Covid. They advised future studies to employ specific psychometric measures and to perhaps avoid only conducting cross-sectional studies (Benatti et al., 2020).

The Study of Davide and Colleagues (2020)

The study of Davide et al. (2020) aimed to find changes in OCD symptoms during quarantine for patients who had undergone psychiatric care for OCD pre-COVID. They also looked at the effects of contamination symptoms and remission state pre-COVID on OCD symptoms that had changed during quarantine (Davide et al., 2020). They hypothesized that patients with contamination symptoms and those who had not achieved a remission state pre-quarantine would have worsening OCD symptoms, as a whole, compared to other symptoms (Davide et al., 2020).

Participants were outpatients who had a diagnosis of OCD according to the DSM-5 (Davide et al., 2020). They were under psychiatric care during the last six months before the outbreak (Davide et al., 2020). Participants were excluded if they had other medical conditions (Davide et al., 2020). Y-BOCS-SC severity scores were used to measure the severity of obsession and compulsion before and six weeks after the lockdown period (Davide et al., 2020).

In terms of statistical analyses, they used paired samples t-tests and independent samples t-tests with significance set at $p<.01$ (Davide et al., 2020). Twelve out of the 30 participants were remitters on OCD symptoms before the quarantine period (David et al., 2020). Final results showed that overall OCD symptoms worsened when they compared pre and post-quarantine, but contamination symptoms and those who were remitters showed an exacerbation of OCD. Other factors which will be discussed later were also linked to OCD worsening.

Since the study only included thirty participants, they advised future studies to examine larger sample sizes. They advised comparing patients with OCD with a non-clinical control group without OCD to see whether OCD symptom worsening was only specific to those with OCD (Davide et al., 2020).

The Study of Jelinek and Colleagues (2020)

The study of Jelinek et al. (2020) explored the effect of COVID-19 on those with OCD, especially those with washing compulsions and they analyzed the reason behind the changes in severity, if any. This study was conducted in Germany. Unlike past studies, they wanted a larger sample size. Participants were recruited between March 23rd and May 18th, 2020 (Jelinek et al., 2020). An online survey was sent out to participants who receive services from an OCD nonprofit organization (Jelinek et al., 2020). A total of 394 people completed the survey though 1905 had access to it (Jelinek et al., 2020).

The German version of Obsessive-Compulsive Inventory-Revised (OCI-R) was used to measure the severity of participants' OCD while the German version of the Patient Health Questionnaire was used to measure the severity of Depression (Jelinek et al., 2020). Five OCD experts then personalized a questionnaire to determine the effect of COVID-19 on individuals with OCD (Jelinek et al., 2020). For example, participants had to state their predominant OCD symptoms [obsessions, washing/cleaning, checking, symmetry/ordering, hoarding, and others), why there was a change in severity [reduced mobility, availability of cleaning/hygiene products, economic factors, lack of availability of doctors/therapist, interpersonal conflicts], etc. (Jelinek et al., 2020).

Participants reported having moderate to severe OCD severity while Depression severity was moderate (Jelinek et al., 2020). The majority of participants reported the typical core OCD symptoms (obsession, washing/cleaning, and checking) being at the core of theirs too (Jelinek et al., 2020). However, since the goal was to focus on those with washing compulsions; they divided the group into two (Jelinek et al., 2020). Those with, versus those without, washing or cleaning compulsions (Jelinek et al., 2020). Washers reported having a greater increase in the severity of OCD symptoms (Jelinek et al., 2020). Washers more than non-washers associated the availability of cleaning products and interpersonal conflicts with a change in the severity of their OCD symptoms (Jelinek et al., 2020). Washers more than non-washers also reported having severe compulsions and avoidance behavior but not obsessions (Jelinek et al., 2020).

They advised that future studies be longitudinal and have comparisons of OCD severity before the outbreak (Jelinek et al., 2020). Future studies should also take into consideration other reasons which would account for symptom change (Jelinek et al., 2020).

Why the Study Results are Important

Results conducted using statistical measures demonstrated that COVID-19 was affecting the lives of patients with OCD. For example, the study by Tanir et al. (2020) discovered that before and after findings of contamination obsessions and cleaning compulsions were significantly high. As expected, everyone was worried about contracting the virus, but that only heightened the cleaning compulsions of patients with OCD. Those who were remitters showed OCD worsening, as well (Davide et al., 2020). That finding is important because therapists are now facing a new challenge. They will have to look into creating a new treatment plan, to reduce severity levels to what they were before COVID.

Khosravani et al. (2020) study emphasized stress reactions being at the root of OCD severity. Not only stress reactions attributed to OCD, but stress reactions associated with social and economic struggles. Knowing that socio-economic aspects of their lives also affected OCD severity is a telltale sign that treatment options have to consider and address overall wellbeing, as well. When COVID cases were rising, individuals were advised to stay inside. Benatti et al. study (2020) discovered that those whose OCD worsened had an increase in avoidance behaviors, but since things have been opening back up, they will have to decrease those avoidance behaviors. Lighter activities such as socializing and going on walks can improve wellbeing and avoidance of these activities due to a fear of contamination can be limiting.

WAYS PATIENTS WITH OCD HAVE BEEN COPING

During moments of distress, coping strategies can provide temporary relief. Coping strategies such as cognitive-behavioral techniques can be used to manage or ease stressful situations. The study of Rosa-Alcázar et al. (2021) explored the various ways patients with OCD and control groups of healthy individuals are coping during this COVID-19 pandemic. Some of the coping dimensions were measured and provided by the Spanish Version of the Brief COPE. The Brief COPE includes techniques such as positive reframing, denial, humor, emotional support, active coping, substance use, etc.

The T-test conducted yielded a significant effect on emotional strategies such as positive reframing, humor, and acceptance (Rosa-Alcázar et al., 2021). When looking at the coping techniques used most when anxiety and depression were significantly different between the groups, Rosa-Alcázar et al. (2021) study discovered that the control group made more use of planning as a coping strategy for anxiety compared to patients with OCD. Thirty-six percent of patients with OCD had comorbidities and differences were found in coping strategies such as denial, self-blame, avoidance coping, and substance use compared to those with no comorbidities (Rosa-Alcázar et al., 2021). Patients with OCD found themselves using instrumental support, religion, denial, and self-blame during the pandemic while individuals in the healthy group made use of more positive strategies such as humor, reframing, and acceptance (Rosa-Alcázar et al., 2021).

MANAGEMENT OF OCD DURING COVID-19 AND CHANGES NEEDED

Due to the pandemic, most therapy sessions have been virtual. Since therapy has been online, those contending with mental health issues can seek out therapists who don't necessarily live in their hometown. Therefore, it's advised that therapists become more cognizant of world-wide events that might be impacting their patients and particularly sensitive regarding what they choose to discuss (Fineberg et al., 2020).

The Media: Positive or Negative?

Studies reviewed pinpoint potential reasons that OCD symptoms could have worsened during the pandemic. One of the reasons related to what was discussed in the early stages of the outbreak, whether on TV or between friends and family. Though TV news can be informational, studies have shown how it can be detrimental, as well. A study found that "watching a predominately negatively valence news program raised self-reported measures of anxious and sad moods, and subsequently led to the enhanced catastrophizing of personal worries (Johnston & Davey, 1997).

Khosravani et al. (2020) discovered that for someone with OCD, excessively checking the news can increase the viewer's concerns about responsibility for harm and checking behaviors. The media has been a great source to promote and remind citizens of the benefit of washing one's hands, however, it has been negatively affecting those with OCD; especially those who have concerns about contamination, hygiene, and cleanliness (Tanir et al., 2020). Therefore, researchers have been advocating for less screen time or monitoring screen time, to either limit or avoid exposure to COVID-19 related news (Fineberg et al., 2020).

Cognitive Behavioral Therapy

Khosravani et al. (2020) study advised that therapists provide cognitive behavioral therapy aimed at reducing COVID-19- related stress. The plan can include things such as distress tolerance, relaxation techniques, participating in positive activities, etc. (Khosravani et al., 2020). An important component of cognitive-behavioral therapy (CBT) is exposure and ritual prevention therapy (ERP). Silva et al. (2020) suggested that the cleaning aspect of protecting against the virus could reinforce irrational beliefs of patients with OCD and poor insight.

As it's named, ERP includes a mix of exposure and ritual prevention therapy. Whether the exposure is in-vivo (real-life) or imagined, patients are exposed repeatedly and over time to the stimuli evoking their obsessive thoughts one less minute each time so they reach the average time spent. Ritual prevention would be prescribed for patients to see how long they can last before reaching for disinfectant or washing their hands after touching surfaces with germs. With time, one then realizes that anxiety is the culprit and one can control it. Exposure and ritual prevention therapy has been helpful pre-COVID. It's said that therapist-aided exposure is more effective than self-exposure (Foa, 2010). Also, both exposure and ritual prevention should take place concurrently since each done at different times can yield different results (Foa, 2020).

Due to COVID restricting measures, exposure and ritual prevention therapy may not in effect be possible and that could impact the long-term prognosis for OCD (Silva et al., 2020). Instead, some researchers are advising therapists to use hours toward supporting patients and preventing them from deteriorating through techniques (e.g. behavioral activation and activity scheduling), especially those whose exposure is contamination-related (Fineberg, et al. 2020). It's said that activity schedules can be fulfilling, it gives patients feelings of mastery and pleasure (Fineberg et al., 2020). Davide et al. (2020) found that participants who weren't working, were in school remotely during the quarantine, or were living with parents or those with COVID-19 symptoms experienced worsening OCD symptoms. Therefore, perhaps not having anything to do leads to feeding into the negative aspects of the pandemic (deaths, rise of cases, etc.) which worsens disorders.

Distraction is useful to cope with anxiety, depression, etc. However, distraction is used to shift focus, it doesn't mean we should use it to suppress thoughts. For example, engaging in physical activities will help decrease the level of anxiety. While being occupied in school, work will be a confidence-booster, since patients are not letting disorders get in the way of living and fulfilling purposes. Another healthy distraction that aids in overcoming loneliness is maintaining contact with loved ones through text, face-time, etc. It's said that circadian rhythm disruptions could increase anxiety and worsen OCD symptoms, therefore, it's been recommended that individuals maintain a regular wake time and bedtime every day (Fineberg et al., 2020). Doing it the wrong way will only make matters worse. To prevent backsliding, avoidance and accommodation should be assessed (Fineberg et al., 2020).

Pharmacological Treatment

Pharmacological treatment paired with cognitive behavioral therapy remains effective. It's said that pharmacotherapy should be the first option for patients with OCD, especially those with contamination, washing, or cleaning symptoms (Fineberg et al., 2020). SSRI antidepressant drugs such as paroxetine, fluoxetine, etc. have been helpful. More studies need to be done to see how it helps with the management of OCD. However, we do know that it affects a chemical named serotonin in the brain. Serotonin aids in stabilizing our emotions as well as enables communication within brain cells.

In Benatti et al. (2020), participants with worsening OCD reported having higher rates of suicide ideation and sleep disorders such as insomnia. During the lockdown, it may have been difficult to achieve therapeutic adjustment [such as a change in dosage] due to limited access to non-priority medical services (Benatti et al., 2020). Considering that SSRI antidepressant drugs aren't limited to treating OCD, they could be more in need due to people developing anxiety, etc.

Relapsing

Relapse occurs when one falls back into old routines; for someone who struggles with alcoholism, it could be accidentally walking past a favorite bar. As for OCD, it can be as simple as engaging in a compulsion they were able to manage due to the appearance of obsessive thoughts. Feeling reassured or accepted from dysfunctional beliefs regarding COVID can also be a way to slip into relapse. For example, a study conducted by Jelinek and colleagues (2021) found that washers more than non-washers agreed to dysfunctional hygiene related beliefs such as "My fears about the dangers in the world are confirmed," "The threat associated with coronavirus makes me realize how exaggerated my compulsions are," and "The general panic about the coronavirus calms me down" (Jelinek et al., 2021).

Though the percentage of OCD relapse is low, it appears that the longer one goes without therapy, the more he or she is likely to relapse. Braga et al. (2005) looked at the effectiveness of Cognitive Behavioral Therapy over a one-year follow-up. Out of the original forty-two participants they selected, they subsampled thirty-one who improved with therapy to study how long it would take for relapse to take place. They discovered that only three of the thirty-one participants relapsed after three months; four of them relapsed after six months, and twelve relapsed after 12 months (Braga et al., 2005). Another study conducted by Fisen and her colleagues (2013) took the longitudinal approach in which they looked at OCD patients' progress overtime. Regarding remission and relapse, they found out that those who weren't fully remitted, were more likely to relapse (Fisen et al., 2013). They also found out that participants with comorbid OCD had a higher chance of relapsing.

With little to no access to effective therapy during the pandemic, it wouldn't be a surprise if relapse percentages were to increase. Davide et al. (2020) highlighted an important point regarding relapse: since OCD symptoms are worsening among patients during the pandemic, therapists should include relapse prevention techniques and not just focus on treating patients who report OCD symptoms.

BUT PLOT TWIST, THERE'S VACCINE!

As of early 2021, the United States, as well as Europe, have authorized vaccines given by Pfizer and Moderna. The two companies were able to develop a vaccine using mRNA technology. The vaccine works by making proteins that trigger the immune response in our bodies. Since the authorization, they have distributed it in multiple phases. During phase 1, vaccines were given to frontline healthcare workers as well as to those who were 75 years and older. According to Our World in Data, about 4.6% of the population worldwide has been vaccinated.

What Does This Mean for Future Research?

Due to the virus and quarantine, patients with OCD have been experiencing worsening symptoms. However, with the vaccine out; it will be interesting to see how that will change the mindsets of not only those with OCD, but those with mental health disorders, more generally. There have been discussions about new variants of COVID-19, but getting the vaccine has been comforting for people's mental health. However, having a vaccine doesn't mean that things will automatically go back to how they were. Therapy sessions could still be conducted online and patients may choose to continue virtually just for precautions. Researchers weren't considering a vaccine when conducting their studies; they just advised that future studies do a comparison of effects pre-Covid and post-Covid to see if the symptoms' severity are back to pre-Covid levels.

Though researchers have good suggestions, it's hard to know when 'post-Covid' will be. Things won't go back to normal for at least another year. Therefore, longitudinal studies need to be conducted. As time-consuming as it may seem, that sort of study will be best to keep progress over time. Not only a longitudinal study but one with a large group of participants, who have different OCD levels and types. Another one can piggyback off of the study of Fineberg, et al. (2020) to see just how detrimental the effects have been in those with OCD when compared to healthy individuals. Also, the vaccine may change the mindset of those with OCD regarding contamination. Therefore, a study needs to be done to see if vaccination decreases severity levels in any way.

REFERENCES

Benatti, B., Albert, U., Maina, G., Fiorillo, A., Celebre, L., Girone, N., Fineberg, N., Bramante, S., Rigardetto, S., & Dell'Osso, B. (2020). What Happened to Patients with Obsessive Compulsive Disorder During the COVID-19 Pandemic? A Multicentre Report from Tertiary Clinics in Northern Italy. *Frontiers in Psychiatry*, *11*, 720. Advance online publication. doi:10.3389/fpsyt.2020.00720 PMID:32793008

Braga, D. T., Cordioli, A. V., Niederauer, K., & Manfro, G. G. (2005). Cognitive-behavioral group therapy for obsessive–compulsive disorder: A 1-year follow-up. *Acta Psychiatrica Scandinavica*, *112*(3), 180–186. doi:10.1111/j.1600-0447.2005.00559.x PMID:16095472

Darvishi, E., Golestan, S., Demehri, F., & Jamalnia, S. (2020). A Cross-Sectional Study on Cognitive Errors and Obsessive-Compulsive Disorders among Young People During the Outbreak of Coronavirus Disease 2019. *Activitas Nervosa Superior*, *62*(4), 137–142. doi:10.100741470-020-00077-x PMID:33163111

Davide, P., Andrea, P., Martina, O., Andrea, E., Davide, D., & Mario, A. (2020). The impact of the COVID-19 pandemic on patients with OCD: Effects of contamination symptoms and remission state before the quarantine in a preliminary naturalistic study. *Psychiatry Research*, *291*, 113213. Advance online publication. doi:10.1016/j.psychres.2020.113213 PMID:32535508

Damirchi, E. S., Mojarrad, A., Pireinaladin, S., & Grjibovski, A. M. (2020). The Role of Self-Talk in Predicting Death Anxiety, Obsessive-Compulsive Disorder, and Coping Strategies in the Face of Coronavirus Disease (COVID-19). *Iranian Journal of Psychiatry*, *15*(3), 182. doi:10.18502/ijps.v15i3.3810 PMID:33193766

Fineberg, N. A., Van Ameringen, M., Drummond, L., Hollander, E., Stein, D. J., Geller, D., Walitza, S., Pallanti, S., Pellegrini, L., Zohar, J., Rodriguez, C. I., Menchon, J. M., Morgado, P., Mpavaenda, D., Fontenelle, L. F., Feusner, J. D., Grassi, G., Lochner, C., Veltman, D. J., ... Dell'Osso, B. (2020). How to manage obsessive-compulsive disorder (OCD) under COVID-19: A clinician's guide from the International College of Obsessive Compulsive Spectrum Disorders (ICOCS) and the Obsessive-Compulsive Research Network (OCRN) of the European College of Neuropsychopharmacology. *Comprehensive Psychiatry*, *100*. Advance online publication. doi:10.1016/j.comppsych.2020.152174 PMID:32388123

Fisen, J. L., Sibrava, N. J., Boisseau, C. L., Mancebo, M. C., Stout, R. L., Pinto, A., & Rasmussen, S. A. (2013). Five-year course of obsessive-compulsive disorder: Predictors of remission and relapse. *The Journal of Clinical Psychiatry*, *74*(3), 233–239. doi:10.4088/JCP.12m07657 PMID:23561228

Foa, E. B. (2010). Cognitive behavioral therapy of obsessive-compulsive disorder. *Dialogues in Clinical Neuroscience*, *12*(2), 199–207. doi:10.31887/DCNS.2010.12.2/efoa PMID:20623924

Jelinek, L., Moritz, S., Miegel, F., & Voderholzer, U. (2021). Obsessive-compulsive disorder during COVID-19: Turning a problem into an opportunity? *Journal of Anxiety Disorders*, *77*, 102329. Advance online publication. doi:10.1016/j.janxdis.2020.102329 PMID:33190017

Johnston, W. M., & Davey, G. C. L. (1997). The psychological impact of negative tv news bulletins: The catastrophizing of personal worries. *British Journal of Psychology*, *88*(1), 85–91. doi:10.1111/j.2044-8295.1997.tb02622.x PMID:9061893

Khosravani, V., Aardema, F., Samimi Ardestani, S. M., & Sharifi Bastan, F. (2021). The impact of the coronavirus pandemic on specific symptom dimensions and severity in OCD: A comparison before and during COVID-19 in the context of stress responses. *Journal of Obsessive-Compulsive and Related Disorders*, *29*, 100626. Advance online publication. doi:10.1016/j.jocrd.2021.100626 PMID:33520614

Matsunaga, H., Mukai, K., & Yamanishi, K. (2020). The acute impact of the pandemic of COVID -19 on the phenomenological features in the full or partial remitted patients with obsessive–compulsive disorder (OCD*). Psychiatry and Clinical Neurosciences*, *74*(10). Advance online publication. doi:10.1111/pcn.13119 PMID:32697002

Rosa-Alcázar, Á., García-Hernández, M. D., Parada-Navas, J. L., Olivares-Olivares, P. J., Martínez-Murillo, S., & Rosa-Alcázar, A. I. (2021). Coping strategies in obsessive-compulsive patients during Covid-19 lockdown. *International Journal of Clinical and Health Psychology*, *21*(2), 100223. Advance online publication. doi:10.1016/j.ijchp.2021.100223 PMID:33519939

Saya Des Marais. (2020, December 4). *A Comprehensive History of OCD: From Religious Scruples to Modern Treatment*. Impulse Therapy. https://impulsetherapy.com/a-comprehensive-history-of-ocd-from-religious-scruples-to-modern-treatment/

Schuster, S. (2015, October 12). *17 Quotes That Prove OCD Is So Much More Than Being Neat*. The Mighty. https://themighty.com/2015/10/what-ocd-feels-like/

Silva, R. M., Shavitt, R. G., & Costa, D. L. (2020) Obsessive-compulsive disorder during the COVID-19 pandemic. *Brazilian Journal of Psychiatry*. doi:10.1590/1516-4446-2020-1189

Sigmund Freud. (n.d.). *OCD History*. https://www.ocdhistory.net/20thcentury/freud.html

Tanir, Y., Karayagmurlu, A., Kaya, İ., Kaynar, T. B., Türkmen, G., Dambasan, B. N., Meral, Y., & Coşkun, M. (2020). Exacerbation of obsessive compulsive disorder symptoms in children and adolescents during COVID-19 pandemic. *Psychiatry Research*, *293*, 113363. Advance online publication. doi:10.1016/j.psychres.2020.113363 PMID:32798931

KEY TERMS AND DEFINITIONS

Brief COPE: A 28-item self-report questionnaire that measures effective and ineffective ways of coping with stressful life events.

Circadian Rhythm: An internal process that regulates sleep-wake cycles. It repeats every 24 hours.

Cross-Sectional Study: The study of data from a population taken at a specific point in time.

Ego: Aids in keeping the Id in check. It's based on the reality principle which seeks to satisfy the Id's desires in realistic and appropriate societal ways.

Hierarchical Regression Analysis: A statistical procedure used to control variables and measure effects when other variables are added.

Id: One's animalistic instinct. It's driven by the pleasure principle that sought to gratify desires, needs, and wants.

Longitudinal Study: A study that takes place over an extended period of time.

Phlebotomy: The process of using a needle to draw blood from a vein.

Superego: Based on idealistic standards. It provides guidelines for making judgments such as moral standards or ideals acquired from parents and society.

Xenophobia: Dislike or prejudice against those from other countries.

Chapter 4
The Hardships of COVID-19:
The Deaf and Visually Impaired Experience

Amanda Hall
Marymount Manhattan College, USA

ABSTRACT

The past two years have been a learning curve for everyone around the world. The waves of COVID-19 took the world by storm and threw our way of life upside down. As humans, we adapt rather quickly to changing environments due to our evolutionary genetic makeup, but for some, the adaptations were harder to process and execute. Communities with disabilities had to take additional steps to accommodate to these new norms for our society. Specifically, the deaf and visually impaired communities were some of the groups of individuals who struggled the most. With the overuse of video broadcasting and online meetings, as well as the now taboo-like sense around touch, COVID-19 has worsened the living experience for many individuals in these vulnerable groups.

INTRODUCTION

Covid-19

Coronavirus 2019 (Covid-19) is a contagious disease caused by severe acute respiratory syndrome coronavirus 2 (SARS-CoV-2). It is a new strain of RNA viruses that first emerged in Wuhan, China from the Pangolin Armadillos and Bats which were sold at China's "wet-markets." The two animal versions of Covid-19 were apparently spread

DOI: 10.4018/978-1-6684-3484-0.ch004

and passed through these market trades, while simultaneously being transferred to the Civets (small, nocturnal mammals found in Africa and Asia) that lived in the area. The worldwide virus-strand ended up cultivating in humans starting at the end of 2019, hence the Covid-19 number origin. The people of Wuhan had referred to the virus as the "Wuhan pneumonia" and passed it around to foreign travelers unknowingly. Once these foreign travelers returned to their countries of origin after their visit to this region, they passed it onto their family members, co-workers and friends. The coronavirus is highly contagious due to the genetic makeup of our RNA system, and by March of 2020, the world was overcome with a wave of hospitalizations and deaths, shutting down cities and countries across the globe.

Within the first four months of global spreading, the virus had led to about 700,000 deaths in countries like Italy, China, the United States, and more. At this time, Covid-19 has been the primary cause of over 5,000,000 deaths around the world in just a little more than two years. When these statistics started to increase rapidly, we witnessed the shutdown of international travel, international shipping, and then even local traveling. The world was at a standstill for months, waiting for the virus to die down. The only countries who had a handle on Covid-19 by 2021 were provinces in China, New Zealand, Australia, North Korea, and a number of island territories in the ocean. To this day, the rest of the world still battles the virus despite the distribution of vaccinations. Multiple countries are still under strict lockdown, mask wearing and social distancing rules that do not seem to be letting up until herd immunity (meaning around 80% of the population is vaccinated) is achieved.

This global pandemic has brought about a whole new set of norms set by the World Health Organization (W.H.O.) and the Centers for Disease Control and Prevention (C.D.C.). New regulations such as the "social distancing" (six feet or two meters apart at all times), regulated indoor dining, the requirement of masks, and the televised rollout of new information became the basic standard of living in this new Covid-19 world. Every store had a mask requirement, and some took it a step further by only allowing a certain number of customers in the store at any given time. People could not meet in large gatherings or events, and if they planned on doing so, they were encouraged to quarantine for 10 to 14 days prior to and afterwards to ensure there would be no spread of the disease. The same directives applied to traveling. If traveling, you were required to take a Covid-19 test before leaving and quarantine for 10 to 14 days upon arrival at your destination before interacting with the new environment. You were also encouraged to quarantine again upon your return. These were all new lifestyles that were encouraged to protect ourselves and others from the deadly virus.

As lockdowns lifted and vaccinations from Moderna, Pfizer, Johnson & Johnson, and others were rolled out in different neighborhoods, Covid-19 restrictions began to loosen to the point of allowing 50% capacity in indoor dining, traveling opened up for some, and even schools started to meet in person again (at least a few times per week, as long as they were practicing Covid-19 guidelines). The loosening of these strict restrictions reflected progress in the fight against the virus, but did not mean the world was out of the danger zone just yet. Covid-19 rates are still fluctuating in many parts of the world, preventing them from opening the local economies back up completely in most countries, and there is no clear end date in sight. It has been projected that the world could face at least another year or more before even returning to a semblance of what "normal" used to be.

THE DEAF COMMUNITY

To be "deaf" is to not be able to hear or to have impaired hearing abilities. Hearing loss can be caused by many things such as diseases, hereditary and or genetic disposition, trauma, exposure to specific chemicals, age, and more. Rising above all of these causes are the two categories in which hearing loss falls: conductive hearing loss and sensorineural hearing loss (American Speech-Language-Hearing Association. n.d.). Conductive hearing loss has to do with the transmission between the inner and outer portion of the ear. In such a case that one has impacted ear wax or fluid blocking sound waves, one could go to a doctor and receive treatment to improve hearing quality. Sensorineural hearing loss is not as easily treatable. "Sensorineural" means that there is damage to the cochlea (inner ear). This form of hearing loss is what one would see in movies. The electrical impulses that would normally send the soundwaves to the brain to process are not functioning properly. Due to the highly sensitive area, many cases do not respond well to treatment.

Children in the Deaf Community

Children born into the Deaf Community are a part of a group of individuals with "congenital hearing loss." These children had a genetic disposition to being deaf and were born with no ability to hear. They grow up learning about deaf culture and are typically taught sign language to communicate at an early age. To the child, nothing seems wrong, these children have developed in a way to accept the unfairness of the world around them. There aren't many fully deaf-specialized schools and for this reason, many deaf children end up in a mixed-class or a classroom filled with children who don't showcase any disabilities. This tends to bring out the disparities and differences between the deaf child and their classmates, many times resulting in the child falling victim to bullying or negligence at school. The rate of bullying for children in the Deaf Community is two to three times higher than in their typical-hearing classmates (Bauman, S. & Pero, 2011). It is also more common for the school to not intervene in these cases; failing to confront these behaviors.

For these children, the biggest obstacle in academics is not the social-interactive part, it is the perception and understanding of the English language in print format. Children in the Deaf Community have never heard the language before, so it is marginally harder for them to understand the concept of, what is seemingly, a bunch of letters thrown together to make a "word." There is no connection to sound for them, so there is also no connection to writing, phonetics, etc. To teach a deaf child how to read and write is to first make a connection between print and hand-sign. Many hand signs when relating to a specific action, all happen in the same area (the arm, the head, the mouth, etc.). This can make certain sentences confusing when they are translated verbatim. So, children will continue to memorize these words and make associations to get by. Or, they learn how to read lips and get information from another person, rather than through a printed source. Despite this amazing skill, many deaf students don't read past the sixth-grade reading level (Goldin-Meadow et. al., 2001). This makes life for these students exceedingly challenging in school, causing many of them to rely on aides and other tools to succeed.

Fortunately for children, there is a way to be able to hear by the time they reach their first major school years. Parents can have their children get a "cochlear implant." A cochlear implant is a surgically implanted device that helps those with severe hearing loss. The device has been a game-changer for parts of the Deaf Community. The cochlear implant was designed to be implanted in a child, about one-year of age, to help with the development of language and speech that is a struggle for others in the deaf community. When implanted at this age, there is only a 0.02% chance of it being rejected by the body. It allows the body time to adjust to sound, making it a normal part of the child's life by the time phonetic connections are generally made. The cochlear implant can be implanted later in a child's development, but there tends to be a significantly higher chance of the implant being rejected by the body.

The controversy surrounding the cochlear implant and its usefulness lies solely in "deaf culture." Many members of the Deaf Community believe that children who are born deaf should grow up deaf. They are born into this community and there is nothing wrong with that, so there is no reason to change them or push them into the hearing world. Aligned with this notion, if the parents decide to give their child the surgical hearing aid, it would seem as if they were ashamed of the community their child was born into or that they dislike the idea of their child knowing sign language. This is not the case for many of the parents who pursue the implant. Many of the parents are a part of the community themselves and just want their child to have a better life in a world designed for those in the hearing world. The implant helps with the development of speech, language, vocabulary, and much more. To the willing parents, their child would just become a hearing child in the Deaf Community.

They would still learn sign language, be a part of gatherings, and would be able to combine these two "worlds."

General Hardships of the Deaf Community

In a pre-Covid-19 world, the Deaf Community had, what now seem like, a few obstacles. Being deaf in and of itself is difficult, but also having to adapt to a more-or-less non-conforming society adds a new level of stress and obstacles for one to traverse. Individuals in the Deaf Community rely on facial expressions, lip reading, and interpreters to get information from the hearing world. Without being able to pick up on these minute clues or having access to someone who understands sign language, the Deaf Community is closed off in their own sanctuary.

Other than information gathering, many in the Deaf Community are looked down upon in society and have a hard time facing the public eye. The rate of bullying for those in the Deaf Community is much higher, specifically on online forums. The fact that those in the community are encouraged to use technology to communicate opens up more vulnerabilities online (Bauman, S. & Pero, 2011). As also stated in Bauman and Pero's article, the rates of cyberbullying are high within the Deaf Community too. The adults of the community tend to experience discrimination in the workplace and have a hard time landing jobs or bookings, putting some in the community in a financial bind. There is a huge gap in unemployment rates between the Deaf Community and the hearing due to the discrimination, misconceptions, and hiring practices. Even those who acquired a higher degree of education are turned down as often as the rest of the community.

Covid-19 Related Hardships

Covid-19 has taken away many of the Deaf Community's forms of communication. With the mask mandate in place, those who are hard of hearing can no longer rely on facial cues or lip reading to get by in a social encounter. Many in the Deaf Community have now exhibited higher levels of stress and anxiety when pursuing mundane tasks like going to the grocery store because they have no mode of responding (Taylor, 2020.). If one were to look at them the wrong way or even ask if they needed help, a person in the community would never know and this could lead to image-anxiety. Children in the community have also experienced a spike in stress and anxiety around school (Office for Civil Rights, 2021.). Tools and guides aren't available and many children who relied on these tools are at a loss. Along with that, as mentioned prior, some deaf children at a young age will have a cochlear implant. These cochlear implants help a child hear and acclimate to the world with a new range of sounds. Children with this implant are typically taught to speak, and with this new online-learning system. The Zoom teaching style can be less effective than teaching in person, which causes the child's skills to regress.

Another issue that has come up during the Covid-19 era is rates of poverty and those in the community losing their jobs and sources of income. In 2018, it was found that up to 8% of those in the Deaf Community who were eligible to work, did not have jobs and only one in ten people had health insurance (Correll, 2021.). Since then, those numbers have dropped even lower due to the economic climate of this era. A large part of the community has to depend on programs like Medicaid, Social Security Disability, and Supplemental Security Income to get them through the month. These programs are difficult to apply for and go through changes all the time, making a steady income hard to achieve. Furthermore, those in the Deaf Community have reported being more isolated and noted that they receive more volatile looks when outside.

Isolation

The Deaf Community is a very "hands-on" group and almost all interactions happen in person, face-to-face. Like previously stated, sign language relies on facial expressions, body movement, and subtle gestures. To be stripped of their facial expressions is a huge detriment to their ways of communicating with one another. Taking it a step further, the two-meters-apart mandate rules out a number of the subtle gestures that would typically come into play (Podsada, 2020.). During the beginning of the Covid-19 pandemic, and in some places presently, the 'stay-at-home' mandate has completely shut off a person in the Deaf Community's normal way of communicating. They were already cut off from society in a way, and now they were being ripped away from their circle. So, like everyone else throughout 2020 and 2021, they turned to online forms of contact.

Online chatting is an isolating experience for anyone who undertakes it. For those in the everyday world, while unsettling, it can still bring a sense of togetherness and unity; to be able to speak with friends, family, peers, etc. It's not like that for those in the Deaf Community. Even if they are able to get online and start a meeting call with others, there are obstacles they have to overcome. For example, if one's internet connection is not perfectly stable, the video feed will freeze and cut out, causing one to miss signs and whole chunks of a story a friend is trying to convey. In conjunction with that, sometimes signing just won't get picked up by the computer camera because of how fast the motions are. The signs will just blur together making them hard to decipher.

Another obstacle when using virtual methods of communication is information gathering. Everyone was restricted at home now for news reports, important live feeds with the heads of state or C.D.C. representatives. While this typically wouldn't be an issue, because of the two meters mandate, it has become one. There were no sign language interpreters inside the White House or at government recordings until October of 2020, seven months after the start of lockdowns here in the United States. This further isolated those in the Deaf Community since people did not have access to new information at the same time everyone else did. They had to wait hours for someone to transcribe the full report and post it online just so they could sit down and read through it. Plus, for those whose first language was not English, there was an even greater delay until they could read the latest updates on Covid-19.

New Technology/Services for Covid-19 Accessibility

For the duration of the pandemic, associations like the National Association for the Deaf and the Hearing Loss Association of America have made step-by-step guidelines for those in the community to help them prepare for a doctor or hospital visit, how to communicate with said doctors, and how to ensure they keep themselves safe (National Association of the Deaf, 2020). The C.D.C. has put out a playlist of videos (all in A.S.L.) of everything they would need to know about Covid-19, how to manage the pandemic at home, and risk factors. There has also been a Covid-19 Hotline for the Deaf Community to call into, run by the Communication Service for the Deaf and C.S.D. Neighborhood for the group to call into if they need assistance or just have inquiries that need to be answered.

Another big turning point for the Deaf Community on conference calls is the use of audio-captions. On meeting platforms like Zoom, there is a new feature that allows the host to turn on audio captions. These audio captions work just like captions on televisions or on YouTube. There is a bit of a delay, but they translated the spoken sentences into words, sentence by sentence towards the bottom of one's screen. While not always the most accurate, they have been a huge help to the community during the pandemic and when turned on have given them some sense of inclusion. This feature gives those in the community the opportunity to be a part of the conversation and to get caught up on whatever is being discussed.

In just over two years, there's been a bountiful number of new ideas and start-ups planned to help the Deaf Community. Companies like Nuear and SoundSense Learn have come up with ways to have hearing-aids act like tracking devices for one's vitals and make apps that allow the user to change their hearing-aid settings to adapt to their current environment (Humanitas University, 2021). There's also been advancements in how a hearing-aid can look, going from the stereotypical design to more fashionable, colorful pieces that make people feel like they are wearing an accessory rather than a piece of technology.

THE VISUALLY-IMPAIRED COMMUNITY

The idea of being "visually-impaired" covers a broad range of eyesight and conditions that affect the orbital area. This could include astigmatisms, bacterial infections, albinism, being completely blind, lesions to the retina, and more. It encompasses all types of vision loss. For the sake of specificity, we will be referring to those who are legally blind, completely blind or on the border of either type. To be legally blind is to have 20/200 vision. This means one's field of vision is less than 20 degrees and to see an object 200 feet away, you would have to be in a 20-foot radius. To be completely blind is to have no form of vision at all.

Typically, many people consider being "visually impaired" a nuance of life. After all, "everyone gets there eventually." People will brush it off saying that one just needs to put glasses on or undergo surgery to correct the problems and challenges those in the community encounter. In recent years, the number of eye-related surgeries has gone up as technology advances. For example, depending on how one is visually-impaired, they can get laser in-situ keratomileusis (LASIK), cataract removals, and or artificial lens implants. With the progressing technology, being a part of this community does not seem dire.

Kids in the Visually-Impaired Community

For children, like all humans, there is a separation between being blind, legally blind, or just visually-impaired. Approximately 6.8% of children under the age of 18 tend to have a visual impairment that tends to permanently set in by 9 or 10 (amblyopia, a weaker eye, etc.) (Centers for Disease Control and Prevention. (n.d.). This statistic is a drawn conclusion of genetics, a child's screen time (on a technological device or in front of a television), and or just weak orbital nerves. This makes the group the hardest, yet easiest to treat because while they haven't started running into huge problems, they have a lot of sensitive nerve-endings that are challenging to get around as they develop.

Children, in a way, have it the easiest compared to their community when it comes to environmental interactions. When they're just on the visually impaired side, they can get fitted for glasses easily and can-do eye-training or get eye drops to help strengthen their focus. For the children who are blind at a young age, there's time to teach them Braille and in our modern world, getting voice-to-text devices isn't the hardest thing to do. Children are also typically in classroom environments where there is a teacher or supervisor to help guide them if needed. Parents can also arrange for their children to have a service dog or walking stick early on to lessen the environmental stress and to build social skills. If all goes well, they will continuously acclimate to the surrounding environments and will be able to successfully live a fully-independent life.

General Hardships of the Visually-Impaired Community

Like any other disabled community, the Visually-Impaired Community faces a fair share of hardships in life. In many aspects of media, you'll see the community with walking sticks, service animals, and note-takers to help them traverse their environments. You have also seen in the media how damaging these objects can sometimes be to a visually-impaired person's safety. For instance, people will fight to pet a service animal and that, in of itself, can disturb the animal and the owner. There have been cases where you see the service animal alerting their owner of a psychological attack when faced in these situations. There's also the prospect of a walking stick being taken or pushed away from someone because they're "faking it" or because "it's funny." These experiences can stir up old or new challenges for the Visually-Impaired Community that they can't completely manage.

This leads right into the rates of other mental illnesses that are often found in those who are a part of the community. Those in the Visually-Impaired Community have a higher chance of being diagnosed with an anxiety disorder in comparison to individuals who do not have a visual-impairment. The rates of displaying anxiety symptoms and being diagnosed can reach anywhere up to 30% higher than average (Demmin, et al. 2020). Their rates of depression are also higher in comparison to their typically-sighted peers. There have been studies that reveal visually-impaired elders exhibiting high rates of suicidal ideation; the risk being correlated with how severe the impairment is. Those with poor eyesight are two to three times more likely to report suicidal thoughts and actions (Demmin, & Silverstein, 2020.).

Another hardship that people of the community encounter is relevant to their need to touch and use their hands as their eyes. In the Visually- Impaired Community, there is a language called 'Braille" which consists of six dots arranged in differing patterns to represent letters. Braille was introduced in 1824 by Louis Braille while studying at the Nationale des Jeunes Aveugles in France. Louis Braille was blind by the age of three and when studying to help kids like him, he created a touch-sensitive language to replicate the alphabet. The language was popular among blind communities all over the world for over 100 years, but with the invention of text-to-voice items, the language hasn't been taught as much. This makes it difficult for those who don't have a guide with them to walk around banks or medical centers that use Braille to help people get around. And while there are braille-readers to help translate, not many are widely used. This makes the younger generation very dependent on others and that can be anxiety-provoking, lonely, and can stress them out (emotionally and monetarily).

Aligned with the notion that text-to-voice items have taken over the community, the internet and services they provide should be discussed, as well. While these ideas are built into most of the latest computer models, they don't work with every website or every search option. The website designers would need to encrypt a feature that allows for such tools. As the world progresses, website designers need to take disabilities into account when formatting their code. For example, instead of color-coding sections or areas to create a relationship between the two, just use text boxes or symbols to eliminate the inaccessibility and confusion for people who have a form of colorblindness. Sadly, these ideas and seemingly simple fixes are still being worked towards, making those with disabilities, like those with visual-impairments, try and push that much harder to be able to access what others can easily access (Ingram, 2021).

Covid-19 Related Hardships

In comparison to the Deaf Community, the Visually-Impaired Community is actually more dependent on help during these times. Members of the Visually-Impaired Community are being subjected to a world where their main sense, touch, can't be used. Touch is so important to a visually-impaired person because it offers an idea of what the world looks like, helps one navigate, and is basically their new set of eyes. Going back to the idea of Braille, many places that utilize the dotted language have covered it up in plastic wrapping or cloth to keep the space clean and sanitary. This makes it harder for those who do know Braille or use a Braille-reader to explore. Now the language that they can see is being taken away from them. This can introduce new anxieties in the sense that they are being thrust into a world where they have little direction or visibility.

Along with the loss of touch, the community is now very co-dependent on others to maintain a normal state. They lose all sense of autonomy because they need to interact with others for any form of direction and, during Covid-19, to see where the social distance markers are. Many in the community have opted to wear pins or badges to indicate that they are blind and would appreciate assistance. They have also opted to call stores and transportation lines ahead of time to see what hours they are running, if any changes are occurring, if there is someone willing to help, etc. These new routines are limiting and a waste of time for those in the community. To take more steps in an already difficult situation, frustrates these individuals, brings a sense of loneliness and exacerbates their lifestyle.

As mentioned in the prior section on Visually-Impaired hardships, the topic of the internet is once again brought up, and specifically web designs in this case. Even with new inventions and web design ideas coming about to help those who need them, there's still a severe lack of accessibility in programs like Zoom or Google

Meetings, which have become heavily-used during Covid-19. There's no built-in help or artificial Intelligence (A.I.), making navigating the App hard. People in the community have to get into the meeting the same way as everyone else, with a link or code and password. While a link may be easier to navigate, having to manually enter a code or password can be more difficult when not knowing where to input it or being unable to identify the correct spot. When in a meeting, there are multiple buttons and options to press that are needed when in a class or meeting setting. With the lack of direction, for some people in the Visually-Impaired Community, the use of these programs becomes slightly uncomfortable and can cause a certain amount of frustration for the user and others.

There have been general challenges for children during the pandemic. Covid-19 has seriously impacted children's schooling; creating a number of setbacks in academic progress and inequalities in academic achievement. But children who live with a visually-impaired guardian are more deeply affected and have less time outside with other children since their guardian can't keep full watch over them. In conjunction with that, these children are being put in a position of being their guardians' eyes. These children are isolated from their peers and the outside world because there is no guarantee that someone will help their guardian or that the child will be okay. And then there are children who live with a visual-impairment of their own that can run into the same problems of not being able to traverse an online learning environment without the appropriate tools. Many of the inventions to help the Visually-Impaired Community are expensive and a number of the sites that teachers use to help their students learn don't offer text-to-voice features, inconveniencing and isolating the child even further.

Isolation

As previously stated, this particular community is practically being forced to interact and put themselves out there just so they can go grocery shopping. Yet in a sense that can also be very isolating to a human. A huge part of human nature is a desire for independence and a sense of pride when we can accomplish things ourselves. The fact that there is a period in one's life where that independence becomes dependence, and that pride turns to shame is frustrating. Not to be able to fend for oneself or one's family goes completely against the natural human instinct. So, these feelings of frustration quickly affect one's mood and behaviors in day-to-day life. A person can become irritated quickly, suffer higher levels of depression and alcohol intake, possibly develop a multitude of destructive behaviors, or completely isolate themselves from everyone in their lives. All of this threatens their mental health, physical health, and family life.

Children, as well, also show more negative behaviors from the isolation. They cannot interact as well with peers and are not free to explore the world. Children in developmental phases such as Erikson's Industry vs. Inferiority Stage are struggling to find those solid successes in academia and social relationships due to their disabilities and the presence of Covid-19. In Erikson's psychosocial theory, failure of this stage leaves a child with a deep sense of inferiority and doubt in themselves. The isolating life a child with a visual-impairment lives in this time period can be detrimental to his/her developmental growth. With these feelings of doubt and isolation, one may further isolate him/herself when getting back into the real world due to overthinking and social anxiety.

New Technology for Covid-19 Accessibility

Fortunately, a number of resources have become available during Covid-19 to help the community improve their life experience at this time. Many eye doctors have taken up the online meeting method and opened access to those who needed to get prescribed glasses or other eye-related prescriptions, virtually. This allows parents and their children to stay Covid-19 safe and to ease some of the anxiety that would come with going to a doctor's office. Along with doctors, many organizations, like the American Optometric Association, have opened up service hotlines, meetings, and created guidelines for the community to help answer any and all questions. One group, the National Federation of the Blind, has even started distributing free white canes and visually-impaired friendly instruction guides to all those who can't afford walking sticks on their own.

In a time where the internet is such a valued place, the community has acquired some advancements to make it easier to navigate. Screen readers have become vastly popular, allowing the user to adjust the screen to fit their needs, whether that be enlarging text or spacing text out. The issue that follows is when icons or symbols are used (in interactive and non-interactive ways) and cannot easily be deciphered by people. To help with that issue, a program labeled WAI-ARIA or just simply, 'ARIA' exists. ARIA is a "web standards suite that makes web content and apps more accessible" (Ingram, L. 2021.). ARIA fills the user in on what screen readers cannot, those interactive points. These updated and remodeled interface structures help make the digital world easier to navigate through.

There's also an upcoming invention from OrCam Technologies called the OrCam MyEye Pro, which is a small device that sits on one's glasses. This device helps those who are blind or who have low vision read print and digital text, recognize faces, and more, all while audibly relaying the info in real time (OrCam Technologies. 2022). It can also connect to the user's laptop with command keys, giving them a "Smart Reading" option. The "Smart Reading" option allows users to optimize their reading by formatting whatever is in front of them to the user's preferences, enlarging words or respacing paragraphs. An invention like this could really change how the world is perceived by the visually-impaired and better improve their lifestyles.

Unfortunately, many of the recommended items that are necessary to help the visually impaired community manage Covid-19 are costly. Portable magnifiers and motion-sensor bands, which can help identify small print and nearby heat-signatures, start at around $300 and could go up to around $2,000. These prices are wildly out of reach since many individuals during the pandemic were unemployed and living off the $600 to $1,400 stimulus checks provided by the government. These checks had to last a person through the month, and for those with children, had to provide for multiple individuals on this bare bones funding source. Even thinking about getting a motion-sensor band would put one down almost a fourth of their income. So, while new inventions, or things already on the market coming to the limelight, are being brought up, they are inaccessible for many at this time and leave those in the Visually-Impaired Community with no recourse.

DISCUSSION

Covid-19 has adversely impacted multiple communities. This pandemic is something no one has ever experienced before, throwing everyone into uncharted territory. The weight it has put on everyone's shoulders is excessive and it has affected people in every aspect of their lives. Compared to their peers on the outside, the disabilities communities have been substantially more adversely impacted. Those with a disability have had to face new adversities and obstacles. The adversities and obstacles faced include, but are not limited to anxiety, depression, isolation, technology, loss of a major sense, need for information-gathering, and threatened interactions with the outside world. The obstacles for the disability community are formidable, forcing them to manage new and difficult living conditions.

Those specifically in the Deaf and Visually-Impaired Communities have overcome these hurdles in their own unique ways, resulting in noticeable differences in their behaviors and routines. Many individuals in the Deaf Community have become overwhelmed by outdoor interactions, to the point of avoiding going into stores when possible. The fear of being judged and confronted is too great a risk to chance. While for the Visually-Impaired Community, their anxiety lies within the fact that they're shut out from the world and can't tell if they're complying with Covid-19 regulations. In comparison to the Deaf Community's increase in social anxiety, there was a spike in frustration and loneliness in the Visually-Impaired Community as described in interviews and online forums. Those in the Visually-Impaired Community are more willing to encounter people on the outside, because they need a helping hand to maneuver in a socially-distanced world.

Another comparison can be drawn in how children are in each community during this time. In general, both communities' children are struggling with not being able to interact with their peers in a face-to-face setting. Children all over are showing increases in screen time and rowdy behaviors because of the loss of structure and routine typically set for school-age kids (Imran, N. et. al. 2020.). But, for the children in the Deaf and Visually-Impaired Communities, their behaviors differ because they're even more isolated and pressured to assist around their home. For children in the Deaf Community, hearing children can still participate in online interactions and, while they help their hard-of-hearing parents, they tend to follow more closely with their friends and classmates' behavioral changes. Children in the community who are also hard-of-hearing have a deeper sense of isolation since they are still learning hand signs, Braille, and the use of deaf-friendly devices to get around. In comparison, the youth of the Visually-Impaired Community, who are able to see well, are their parent or guardian's guide around the home, taking on more roles. When children in the community have a visual-impairment, they struggle with the feeling of isolation, because it is harder for them to go outside to play and to use items around the house to entertain themselves, without needing a text-to-voice translator.

Still, there have been commonalities among various communities during Covid-19. One big similarity they seem to share is their unhappiness in using online forms of contact and technology, in general. As we know, the whole year of 2020 and 2021 learning was transferred online. School, work meetings, birthday parties, and even weddings were all conducted virtually. The Internet has always been hailed as one of the greatest inventions in our technological evolution as a species, but it still does not give a full range of opportunity to everyone who needs it. The Deaf and Visually-Impaired Communities need specific modifications made to keyboards, websites, and computer applications to be able to freely use the internet. The Deaf Community needs closed captions on video-sharing sites and up-to-date transcripts of any form of news. The Visually-Impaired Community needs Braille indentations on their keys and an option to have a website, or at the very least, important features on websites, spoken aloud to them. Both communities have shown frustration over the necessary usage of technology as it has just become another obstacle that they have to learn to traverse.

Future Directions

For further accessibility and research, if a pandemic like Covid-19 is to ever occur again, it is necessary to produce and invent disability-oriented items. These items need to be accessible, affordable, and widely distributed. Along with the physical objects needed, more technological advances should be made to further ensure that individuals in the Deaf or Visually-Impaired Community, do not have to rely on others to glean information. Websites and app owners, like Amazon, are looking into getting closed-captions on all important video feeds, recording info drops in advance, have transcribers at the ready, and give the option to have highlighted sections be read out loud or have someone read out the page and save it in a media link at the top of a page, resembling a number of podcast sites. Just recently, Google has started creating devices that can single out one person's voice or one specific sound while there's a myriad of sounds around the user (Humanitas University. 2021.). The idea of connecting hearing-aids to the world wide web has also been thrown around in recent months, making the future look that much brighter.

Other innovations that help these communities and can be updated, include 'Siri' and 'Cortana.' 'Siri' and 'Cortana' are computer and phone A.I.s that can be used to look things up, generally programmed to read texts and google searches out loud to the user. Their voice-recognition feature also allows people to open apps and use specific commands within the app by just saying a key phrase. With updates to their text-to-voice/voice-to-text feature, applying it to most Safari site-openings could be an incredibly useful feature to the disabilities community and could reduce a number of their initial hardships. An example of this progression is Microsoft's Seeing Artificial Intelligence and Humanware's Advanced Technology devices which are in the process of being made to give more accessibility online to individuals who need it.

With companies creating devices and looking to support the Deaf and Visually-Impaired Communities, and others with special online-needs, if another virus were to come around in our society that forced us to go remote, there would not be as many hurdles to overcome. In conjunction with the improvement of online interfaces, due to the research and experience the world now has around Covid-19, if another pandemic were to occur, we would be better equipped to handle it, decreasing mass hysteria and anxiety.

REFERENCES

American Speech-Language-Hearing Association. (n.d.) *Types of Hearing Loss.* American Speech-Language-Hearing Association. https://www.asha.org/public/hearing/types-of-hearing-loss/

Basner, M., Dinges, D. F., Mollicone, D. J., Savelev, I., Ecker, A. J., Di Antonio, A., . . . Sutton, J. P. (2014, March 27). *Psychological and behavioral changes during confinement in a 520-day simulated interplanetary mission to mars*. Retrieved from https://www.ncbi.nlm.nih.gov/pmc/articles/PMC3968121/

Battistin, T., Mercuriali, E., Zanardo, V., Gregori, D., Lorenzoni, G., Nasato, L., & Reffo, M. E. (2021). Distance support and online intervention to blind and visually impaired children during the pandemic COVID-19. *Research in Developmental Disabilities*, *108*, 103816. doi:10.1016/j.ridd.2020.103816 PMID:33271446

Bauman, S., & Pero, H. (2011). Bullying and Cyberbullying Among Deaf Students and Their Hearing Peers: An Exploratory Study. *Journal of Deaf Studies and Deaf Education*, *16*(2), 236–253. doi:10.1093/deafed/enq043 PMID:20855432

Cacioppo, J. T., Hawkley, L. C., Norman, G. J., & Berntson, G. G. (2011, August). *Social isolation*. Retrieved from https://www.ncbi.nlm.nih.gov/pmc/articles/PMC3166409/

Cacioppo, J. T., Hawkley, L. C., & Thisted, R. A. (2010, June). *Perceived social isolation makes me sad: 5-year cross-lagged analyses of loneliness and depressive symptomatology in the Chicago Health, Aging, and Social Relations Study*. Retrieved from https://www.ncbi.nlm.nih.gov/pmc/articles/PMC2922929/

Centers for Disease Control and Prevention. (n.d.). Retrieved from https://www.cdc.gov/

Correll, R. (2021). *Challenges that still exist for the Deaf Community*. Verywell Health. https://www.verywellhealth.com/what-challenges-still-exist-for-the-deaf-community-4153447

COVID-19 (Coronavirus) Eye Health Care Guide for Patients. (n.d.). https://www.aoa.org/healthy-eyes/caring-for-your-eyes/covid-19-eye-health-care-guide-for-patients?sso=y

COVID-19: Medical Communication Access for Deaf and Hard of Hearing. (2020). *National Association of the Deaf.* https://www.nad.org/covid19-communication-medical-access-for-deaf-hard-of-hearing/

Demmin, D., & Silverstein, S. (2020). *Visual Impairment and Mental Health: Unmet Needs and Treatment Options*. PubMed Central. https://www.ncbi.nlm.nih.gov/pmc/articles/PMC7721280/

Goldin-Meadow, S., & Mayberry, R. I. (2001). How do profoundly deaf children learn to read? *Learning Disabilities Research & Practice*, *16*(4), 222–229. https://doi.org/10.1111/0938-8982.00022

Guo, M., Wu, C. F., Liu, W., Yang, J. Y., & Chen, D. (2004). Sex difference in psychological behavior changes induced by long-term social isolation in mice. *Progress in Neuro-Psychopharmacology & Biological Psychiatry*, *28*(1), 115–121. doi:10.1016/j.pnpbp.2003.09.027

Humanitas University. (2021). *How technology could turn US into superheroes: The Future of Hearing*. Hunimed. https://www.hunimed.eu/news/how-technology-could-turn-us-into-superheroes-the-future-of-hearing/

Imran, N., Aamer, I., Sharif, M., Bodla, Z., & Naveed, S. (2020). Psychological Burden of quarantine in children and adolescents: A rapid systematic review and proposed solutions. *Pakistan Journal of Medical Sciences*, *36*(5). https://doi.org/10.12669/pjms.36.5.3088

Ingram, L. (2021). Integrating the visually impaired into the virtual future. In *Visually Impaired in the Digital Age*. IEEE Computer Society. https://www.computer.org/publications/tech-news/trends/integrating-the-visually-impaired-into-digital

Lourens, H. (2021). The politics of touch-based help for visually impaired persons during the COVID-19 pandemic. *The COVID-19 Crisis: Social Perspectives*, 17.

Office For Civil Rights. (2021). *Education in a pandemic*. https://www2.ed.gov/about/offices/list/ocr/docs/20210608-impacts-of-covid19.pdf?tpcc=nlcapsule

OrCam Technologies Personal AI Solutions. (n.d.). https://www.orcam.com/en/article/orcam-technologies-personal-ai-solutions-ces-2022-innovation-award-and-2021-time-best-invention/

Owen, N., Healy, G. N., Matthews, C. E., & Dunstan, D. W. (2010, July). *Too much sitting: the population health science of sedentary behavior*. Retrieved from https://www.ncbi.nlm.nih.gov/pmc/articles/PMC3404815/

Pagel, J. I., & Choukèr, A. (2016). Effects of isolation and confinement on humans-implications for manned space explorations. *Journal of Applied Physiology*, *120*(12), 1449–1457. doi:10.1152/japplphysiol.00928.2015

Patton, R. M. (1963). *Behavioral Testing During a 7-day Confinement*. Academic Press.

Podsada, J. (2020). *Masks, Social Distancing Challenge Interpreters for the Deaf.* www.heraldnet.com/business/masks-social-distancing-challenge-interpreters-for-the-deaf/

Rizzo, J. R., Beheshti, M., Fang, Y., Flanagan, S., & Giudice, N. A. (2020). COVID-19 and Visual Disability: Can't Look and Now Don't Touch. *PM & R.*

Senjam, S. S. (2020). Impact of COVID-19 pandemic on people living with visual disability. *Indian Journal of Ophthalmology, 68*(7), 1367.

Sorenson, M. (2020). *The Impact of the Coronavirus on the Deaf Community.* doorinternational.org/the-impact-of-the-coronavirus-on-the-deaf-community

Taylor, D. B. (2020). For the Deaf, Social Distancing Can Mean Social Isolation. *The New York Times.* www.nytimes.com/2020/06/04/us/coronavirus-deaf-culture-challenges.html

KEY TERMS AND DEFINITIONS

Braille: A tactile writing system made up of small circular bumps, in sections of up to six, traditionally on embossed paper. Was made for and mostly used by the Visually-Impaired Community.

Cochlear Implant: A device that electrically stimulates the cochlear nerve. Has a microphone that picks up sounds, processes it, and then transmits it to the main device. Is typically implanted as a toddler.

Conductive Hearing Loss: When sounds cannot get through the outer and middle ear. Can be reversed with medical/surgical intervention and/or corrected with hearing aids.

Congenital Hearing Loss: When hearing loss is present at birth.

Industry vs. Inferiority: The 4th stage in Erik Erikson's eight psychosocial stages. This stage is known to occur from ages six to eleven, where a child is learning to be productive and to accept criticism. Some kids don't take well to the criticism and end up feeling inferior and incompetent in areas of their life.

Norms: A standard or pattern, especially of social behavior, that is typical or expected of a group.

Sensorineural Hearing Loss: When there is damage to the inner ear or the nerve from the ear to the brain, causing sound to not travel. Can be helped with hearing aids or Cochlear Implants.

Visually Impaired vs. Legally Blind: A visual impairment is any decreased ability to see to a degree that causes issues. Legally blind is the state of being unable to see due to injury, genetics, etc.

Chapter 5
Domestic Violence and Child Abuse:
The Unforeseen and Ongoing Consequences of the COVID-19 Pandemic

Brianna Victoria Blackwell
Marymount Manhattan College, USA

ABSTRACT

The COVID-19 pandemic revealed unforeseen consequences for those already experiencing domestic abuse, violence, or child abuse with intensified, new, and recurring stressors, which made individuals more susceptible to abuse. The stressors covered in this literature review include isolation, mental health issues, economic or job instability, parental stress or burnout, global social and economic crisis, school and protective services closures, limited access to childcare, the threat of contagion, grief, and increased alcohol and drug consumption or abuse. Due to the nature of government-mandated stay-at-home orders and mass closures intended to stop the spread of COVID-19, victims have had few options for outreach to friends, family, or to protective services. This literature review identifies the current stressors throughout the COVID-19 pandemic that can increase risk factors for domestic abuse, violence, and child abuse.

DOI: 10.4018/978-1-6684-3484-0.ch005

INTRODUCTION

The COVID-19 pandemic has introduced many new, inadvertent consequences, manifesting the perfect concoction of stressors, intensifying previous abusive circumstances, and evoking some individuals to react with abusive behaviors. Due to this public health crisis, adults and children are more vulnerable to abuse, leading to drastic increases in domestic abuse or intimate partner violence during the lockdown mandates in many countries (Bradbury-Jones & Isham, 2020). New public safety orders in the United States include physical distancing, self-quarantine, masking, and "stay-at-home" orders (Kofman & Garfin, 2020), which created novel circumstances for many families, disrupting normal life. Homes are typically places where violence escalates, and due to the unusual nature of the "stay-at-home" orders, these endangered individuals or families facing violence or threatening situations (Bradbury-Jones & Isham, 2020; Kofman & Garfin, 2020). Accordingly, victims in abusive circumstances prior to the pandemic were trapped with their abuser through mandated at-home isolation (World Health Organization, 2020). With one in four women and one in ten men experiencing domestic violence (Megan et al., 2020), the pervasive nature of this issue needs to be addressed. Typically, domestic violence and child abuse coexist, significantly increasing the risk for child maltreatment under COVID-19 quarantine or self-isolation at home (Herrenkohl et al., 2008, as cited in Humphreys et al., 2020).

As the initial escalation of COVID-19 cases arose and government-mandated isolation began, domestic violence hotlines prepared for the influx of calls and demands for services (Megan et al., 2020). However, many organizations identified a more than 50% decrease in hotline calls in some regions, not due to the decrease of cases; rather the option for safe reporting (Megan et al., 2020). This trend is predicted to continue throughout the COVID-19 pandemic as waves of infection continue to increase and governments extend public health policies intended to stop the spread (Megan et al., 2020). Unfortunately, these restrictions jeopardize victims' ability to safely report violence, potentially subjecting them to repeated abuse (Megan et al., 2020). As our society has witnessed the uncovering of some harsh realities throughout the COVID-19 pandemic, significant inequalities continue to be heightened by the social determinants of health, as stay-at-home orders have not affected everyone equally (Megan et al., 2020). This literature review examines the new and existing stressors that amplify the prevalence of domestic abuse, violence, and child abuse through a unique set of circumstances outlined by the consequences of the COVID-19 pandemic.

OVERVIEW OF DOMESTIC VIOLENCE AND ABUSE

Domestic abuse is between intimate partners where one person in the relationship attempts to control the other through using fear and intimidation tactics and potentially threatening physical violence (De Benedictus & Jaffe, 2004). Patterns of domestic abuse tend to be seen in cycles; the building tension phase, the incident of abuse, and the honeymoon phase (De Benedictus & Jaffe, 2004). In De Benedictus and Jaffe (2004), researchers note domestic violence escalates from threats to verbal abuse and lastly to physical violence, sometimes even ending up in serious bodily harm or murder. Victims of domestic violence are men, women, non-binary, and transgender people, and it is prevalent in heterosexual and same-sex partnerships (De Benedictus & Jaffe, 2004; Rogers, 2020). Domestic abuse has many facets, with a wide range from only violent encounters, to those including emotional, physical, sexual, economic, psychological, or spiritual abuse (De Benedictus & Jaffe, 2004).

Domestic violence is separated into non-sexual and sexual forms; sexual forms including sexual assault, rape, and stalking; non-sexual forms including abuse, threats, and physical contact (Walby, 2004). According to De Benedictus and Jaffe (2004), researchers suggest a powerful predictor of domestic violence in adulthood is a child's exposure to violence within the household. As seen in the current research, this can spark the continuation of the cycle of violence between generations since the parents or caretakers have modeled violence as normative behavior, especially in romantic partnerships. The COVID-19 pandemic has prompted unusual circumstances that have greatly endangered victims already in abusive scenarios and has likely elicited new cases through the unforeseen stressors of government-mandated public health regulation.

STRESSORS

As seen around the world, domestic and child violence have strikingly increased due to the COVID-19 pandemic. Many of the restrictions, essential to uphold public health policies, are a dangerous combination for those families experiencing violence or individuals on the brink of a violent episode (Usher et al., 2020). Psychological stressors challenge an organism's adaptability in unknown social or physical environmental circumstances (Monroe & Slavich, 2016). Stressors are the actual or perceived threat to an individual, and the response to that stressor is known as the stress response (Schneiderman et al., 2005). Some unique or intensified stressors in the COVID-19 pandemic include isolation, mental health issues, economic or job instability, parental stress or burnout, global social and economic crisis, school and protective service closures, limited access to childcare, the threat of contagion, grief, and alcohol and drug consumption or abuse (Usher et al., 2020; Griffith, 2020; Sharma & Borah, 2020; Brown et al., 2020; Baron et al., 2020; Cullen et al., 2020). This literature review will assess the current stressors in the COVID-19 pandemic, exacerbating domestic abuse, violence, and child abuse situations.

CHILD VIOLENCE AND ABUSE

Child violence and abuse continue to be a discreet, yet pervasive part of society, and during the COVID-19 pandemic, new circumstances have increased the risk of incidence. The COVID-19 pandemic has suddenly disrupted children's daily lives, significantly changing their routines and increasing family violence risk (Lawson et al., 2020). Pre-pandemic research has shown that one in eight children reported maltreatment to Child Protective Services (CPS) in the United States, further accompanied by high recurrence rates (Wildeman et al., 2014, as cited in Humphreys et al., 2020; Kim & Drake, 2019, as cited in Humphreys et al., 2020).

During the pandemic, rates of child abuse reports have decreased as families have had to self-isolate or abide by "stay-at-home" orders, reducing contact with mandated reporters and reducing the chances of school or teacher intervention (Lawson et al., 2020). School closures naturally forgo the largest source of child protective services (CPS) reports, meaning there is less detection of maltreatment (Humphreys et al., 2020). Child maltreatment is associated with psychological, behavioral, and physiological deficits throughout their lives, raising public health concerns (Cicchetti & Toth, 2005, as cited in Lawson et al., 2020; Cicchetti, 2016, as cited in Lawson et al., 2020). Childhood sexual abuse victims have a higher risk of developing extreme psychological disturbances and higher levels of general distress (Polusny & Follett, 1995, as cited in Schneiderman et al., 2005). Children exposed to chronic stress during crucial developmental periods can have adverse effects like "increased risk for anxiety and mood disorders, aggressive dyscontrol problems, hypo-immune dysfunction, medical morbidity, structural changes in the CNS, and early death" (Shaw 2003, as cited in Schneiderman et al., 2005).

According to the ecological-transactional model of child maltreatment (Cicchetti & Lynch, 1993, as cited in Brown et al., 2020; Cicchetti & Rizley, 1981, as cited in Brown et al., 2020), there are different risk and protective factors that influence vulnerability at each level of ecology. The macrosystem (cultural factors), exosystem (community factors), microsystem (family factors), and ontogeny (individual factors) are the primary ecology levels affecting maltreatment outcomes. When children and families experience multiple risk factors across the different levels of ecology, it can increase their risk for maltreatment (Brown et al., 2020). Subsequently, some protective factors included in the ecology may effectively decrease the risk of child maltreatment by shielding families from additional stress (Brown et al., 2020).

With parents' pressure to continue working full-time throughout the pandemic, limited access to childcare, school closures, and attempting to meet online school demands, children face multitudes of vulnerabilities previously supported by our normal systems (Humphreys et al., 2020). If parents are essential workers or need to work outside of the home, children may face supervisory neglect, though if parents work from home, balancing childcare on top of a full-time job is not feasible (Humphreys et al., 2020). Children may also experience an increased risk of online abuse due to extended time online for remote learning and sustaining a need for entertainment (World Health Organization, 2020). Humphreys et al. (2020) suggest that parental anxiety and stress compounded with increased child oppositional behavior and other stressors like financial instability and isolation may provoke abuse or violence. Typically, multiple stressors combine to instigate child abuse and violence that are all substantially heightened due to the repercussions of the COVID-19 pandemic.

ECONOMIC CRISIS

Job instability, layoffs, and income loss have abruptly increased due to government-mandated public health restrictions and self-isolation policies implemented to slow the spread of the COVID-19 virus (Sharma & Borah, 2020). "Stay-at-home" orders mandating that individuals only leave their homes for essential items has resulted in an economic crisis as businesses are shut down or forced to run at reduced capacity (Department of Labor, 2020, as cited in Lawson et al., 2020; Dunn et al., 2020, as cited in Lawson et al., 2020). Unemployment rates have soared from 3.5% (5.7 million people) pre-pandemic to 14.7% (23.1 million people) in April of 2020 (Department of Labor, 2020, as cited in Lawson et al., 2020). Uncommon events like the COVID-19 pandemic imposing stay-at-home or lockdown circumstances can increase rates of domestic violence and the severity of abuse (Sharma & Borah, 2020). Through statistical tracking of domestic violence cases in economically struggling regions, researchers confirm that economic issues caused by the COVID-19 pandemic have contributed most significantly to the rise of domestic violence rates (Sharma & Borah, 2020).

Economic strain and other factors during a stressful world event can provoke violent outbreaks, with research suggesting that low income is related to increases in domestic violence (Peprah and Koomson, 2017, as cited in Sharma & Borah, 2020). Poor neighborhoods have the highest prevalence rates of domestic violence, with socioeconomic status factoring into this. (Bonomi et al., 2014, as cited in Sharma

& Borah, 2020; Kiss et al., 2012, as cited in Sharma & Borah, 2020). Therefore, domestic violence rates are expected to significantly increase due to income loss in the COVID-19 pandemic, as our society has already witnessed. (Purvin, 2003, as cited in Sharma & Borah, 2020; Williams & Mickelson, 2004, as cited in Sharma & Borah, 2020). In the family stress model, outlined in Conger and Elder (1994), as cited in Lawson et al. (2020), researchers identify economic stress as putting substantial stress on the family relationships; stress significantly increases the risk for child abuse (Lawson et al., 2020). Facing economic strain is observed as a component of harsh parenting (Conger & Elder, 1994, as cited in Lawson et al., 2020; Evans, 2004, as cited in Lawson et al., 2020) and may add to the development or dynamic of child abuse.

Economic abuse can also be prevalent in domestic abuse situations; withholding economic or physical resources, stealing money or assets from a partner, and preventing a partner from working or having an occupation are examples of economic abuse (De Benedictus & Jaffe, 2004). The growing economic crisis of the COVID-19 pandemic intensifies these potential forms of economic abuse within partnerships. These global economic losses may further justify an abuser's tendencies to withhold individual financial freedom. Governments need to prevent and alleviate domestic violence occurrences; implementing safeguarding would help provide security for those in abusive circumstances (Sharma & Borah, 2020). Providing safeguarding will thereby demand governmental investment, leading to further economic strain (Heath, 2012, as cited in Sharma & Borah, 2020; Houghton, 2009, as cited in Sharma & Borah, 2020). There are various "costs" of domestic violence, including the use of public services (criminal justice system, health care system, social services, and other legal services), loss of financial yield to employment disruption, and the physical, psychological, and social suffering at the victim's expense (Walby, 2004). Economic issues throughout the COVID-19 pandemic are both the "causes and consequences" of domestic violence, since there are many other stressors to include in this dynamic that ultimately spark abusive incidences (Sharma & Borah, 2020).

SOCIAL CRISIS

Since lockdown mandates have been enforced, victims have little to no option to escape potential violence, since individuals experiencing abuse pre-pandemic likely had more access to social support (Sharma & Borah, 2020). Family, friends, relatives, sheltered homes, and legal administrations for protective services are now less accessible due to restrictions and stay-at-home orders (Sharma & Borah, 2020). There are few possibilities for creating or strengthening social support networks with lockdown or "safer-at-home" mandates (Marques et al., 2020). Therefore, reaching out for help through familiar relationships is risky; abusers may keep watch of texts, phone calls, or other online activity to ensure victims' compliance (World Health Organization, 2020). The lack of childcare and school closures creates additional stress and responsibility for victims and abusers, and children encounter further challenges in their home environment. These challenges can include access to food and education, affecting overall aspects of development, and heightened negative interactions between parents affecting the mental health of children (Sharma & Borah, 2020).

Travel restraints, social services, school, and work closures have all prompted detrimental effects to individuals and children experiencing abuse and violence at home. Almost all schools in the United States paused in-class instruction, transitioning to remote learning, to slow the spread of COVID-19 (Baron et al., 2020). While academic effects are destined to be measured (Kuhfeld et al., 2020, as cited in Baron et al., 2020), school closures removed the link between mandated reporters and child maltreatment victims (Baron et al., 2020). Mandated reporters include teachers, school psychologists, guidance counselors, and other school staff, providing the most significant pool of child maltreatment reports (Administration for Children and Families, 2020, as cited in Baron et al., 2020). In Baron et al. (2020), researchers gather data to determine the impact of COVID-19 school closures on child maltreatment reports in Florida. Current researchers obtained data for child maltreatment allegations through the Florida Child Abuse Hotline, pulling the available statistics from January 2004 to April 2020 (Baron et al., 2020). With the absence of a natural control group due to country-wide school closures, researchers predicted the number of allegations in March and April of 2020 solely based on previous data trends, finding that actual reported allegations were 27% lower than they predicted (Baron et al., 2020). Researchers validate that their results, a 27% decrease from their predicted statistic, may be a conservative estimate since unprecedented stressors of the COVID-19 pandemic have likely increased cases of child maltreatment overall (Baron et al., 2020). The observed decrease in reporting numbers in March and April 2020 closely parallels the decline in allegations during school breaks (Baron et al., 2020). Similarly, domestic violence cases are usually spotted in the workplace (De Benedictus & Jaffe, 2004). In many cases, an abuser may make threatening phone calls, show up at the workplace, or victims may show physical signs of abuse (De Benedictus & Jaffe, 2004). With workplace closures and mass shifts to online workplaces, support for victims and spotting potential abuse have significantly decreased (Sharma & Borah, 2020).

Black or African American and Latinx individuals are disproportionately more likely to acquire COVID-19, be hospitalized, and die from the illness, significantly increasing the disease burden on minority populations (Center for Disease Control and Prevention, 2020, as cited in Brown et al., 2020). Ethnic minority women are disproportionately affected by domestic violence (Black et al., 2011, as cited in Kofman & Garfin, 2020; Renninson & Welchans, 2000, as cited in Kofman & Garfin, 2020), further increasing their vulnerability to enduring abuse or violence during the COVID-19 pandemic. Similarly, Indigenous populations, LGBTQ+ persons, migrant or refugee populations, and those living in poverty generally experience high rates of violence, potentially encountering disadvantages in access to protective services (World Health Organization, 2020). Social determinants of health like income, access to resources, and education are all affected by privilege and influence the impact of domestic violence on victims (Megan et al., 2020).

ISOLATION

The unique circumstances of the COVID-19 pandemic have created the ideal conditions for abusers to maximize harm. Abusers use the strategy of social isolation to distance victims from their friends, family, and other support networks; isolation throughout the lockdown mandates has generated these ideal incidents (Coohey, 2007, as cited in Sharma & Borah, 2020; Menjívar & Salcido, 2002, as cited in Sharma & Borah, 2020). Changes in responsibilities put families in close quarters for extended periods, ultimately increasing the chances of violence occurring because of reduced safe time available (Sharma & Borah, 2020). Increased time with partners or families may expose non-compatible qualities or habits that exacerbate tensions and domestic violence occurrences (Sharma & Borah, 2020). Since there is limited chance for victim outreach and identification of abuse through mandated reporters, friends, family, or co-workers, confinement also helps keep the abuse hidden (Stark, 2009, as cited in Usher et al., 2020).

Families and partnerships are likely to experience social isolation due to restrictions of the COVID-19 pandemic, which has been shown to exacerbate stress in households (Brown et al., 2020). Families remaining in close contact and faced with social isolation, high stress, and high demands are more vulnerable to at-home aggressive behaviors and violence (Brooks et al., 2020, as cited in Brown et al., 2020; Greenaway et al., 2014, as cited in Brown et al., 2020; Reynolds et al., 2008, as cited in Brown et al., 2020). Sexual coercion and unwanted sex are heightened risks for victims during stay-at-home orders that may increase an abuser's frequency of sex demands (World Health Organization, 2020). Abusers have also capitalized on the fear of COVID-19 or "threat of contagion," further excusing and inciting control over the whereabouts of family members and partners (Usher et al., 2020). Disease-related concerns allow abusers to induce further control, restricting access to resources, forms of communication, economic needs, and any social interactions (World Health Organization, 2020). Isolation and self-quarantine have become standard components of the COVID-19 pandemic; therefore, the prolonged seclusion of an individual may look precautionary rather than potentially cohered from an outside perspective.

PHYSICAL AND MENTAL HEALTH

There are multitudes of adverse physical and mental health effects due to domestic violence and child abuse that have been outlined throughout the literature. The result of domestic violence can be devastating to the victim, with long-lasting effects like depression, anxiety, low self-esteem, abandonment issues, anger, lack of trust in others, and diminished mental and physical health (De Benedictus & Jaffe, 2004). Physical symptoms of domestic violence may be seen through bruises, cuts, or other injuries on the individual (De Benedictus & Jaffe, 2004). However, violence or physical injury is not necessary for domestic abuse to remain present in a partnership and may also be discreetly inflicted to remain inconspicuous (De Benedictus & Jaffe, 2004). Even in just witnessing domestic violence, children may develop serious emotional, behavioral, developmental, or academic problems, manifesting symptoms in inconsistent ways (De Benedictus & Jaffe, 2004). Children and teens growing up in households with domestic violence are more likely to commit suicide, use drugs, commit crimes, use violence as a social response, and even become abusers in their own relationships (De Benedictus & Jaffe, 2004).

Mental illness can be considered a factor in the propensity for an individual's violence or abusive tendencies. Recent literature has suggested that serious mental illness is associated with violence, predominately if there is a comorbidity of substance use disorder (Volavka & Swanson, 2010). Researchers Volavka and Swanson (2010) stated that attempting to create a broad relationship between mental illness and violence is inaccurate because many other elements come into play when an individual is violent. Instead, mental illness may factor into the abuse dynamic, especially in the unique circumstances of the COVID-19 pandemic. Many individuals have experienced the development and heightened mental illness symptoms through lockdown mandates and a disturbance to normal life (Cullen et al., 2020). Recent research suggests substance use has increased in those undergoing quarantine or "stay-at-home" orders; additional evidence of increased anger and posttraumatic stress symptoms have been revealed (Brooks et al., 2020, as cited in Humphreys et al., 2020). Alcohol and drug use are associated with escalated violence, and extended isolation can increase alcohol consumption or other substances (World Health Organization, 2020).

The restrictions of the COVID-19 pandemic intensifies new and existing stressors associated with depressive behavior, and research has proposed that stressful life events can be a factor in the development of depression (Hammen, 2005, as cited in Schneiderman et al., 2005; Kendler et al., 1999, as cited in Schneiderman et al., 2005). As cited in Schneiderman et al. (2005) article, Kessing et al. (2003) tracked first-time admission patients in Denmark with a diagnosis of depression and found more unemployment, recent divorces, and suicides by relatives compared to control groups. With the potential for tensions rising in home lives and global distress from the pandemic, these stressful life events can compound one another in an individual's life. Since the COVID-19 pandemic has exposed some mental health challenges, families with higher risk factors for mental health issues may be more vulnerable to child maltreatment (Brown et al., 2020). Children who endure abuse during childhood are found to have higher rates of depressive symptoms and suicidal ideation during adolescence (Wolfe et al., 2001, as cited in Liu et al., 2021) and adulthood (Dube et al., 2001, as cited in Liu et al., 2021; Widom, 1998, as cited in Liu et al., 2021). There are substantial physical and mental health effects victims can sustain through violence and abuse, in addition to overall heightened rates of mental illness observed by restrictions of the COVID-19 pandemic (De Benedictus & Jaffe, 2004; Cullen et al., 2020).

BATTERED WOMAN SYNDROME

In some responses to violence, women can develop "battered women's syndrome," a psychological condition that can develop due to violent abuse (Dutton, 1993). Battered woman syndrome is most importantly utilized in criminal or civil legal contexts in which a woman may be charged with a crime where domestic violence is present in the dynamic (Dutton, 1993). Battered women are acutely aware of their abusers' behavior and may perceive imminent danger from the behavioral or verbal cues of their abusers' previously shown patterns (Dutton, 1993). Victims of abuse may lash back at abusers or intend to harm an abuser to escape the cyclical violence (Walker, 1992). In Walker (1992), the researcher outlines how attorneys have used battered woman self-defense to demonstrate the extreme psychological torment a victim endures, convincing the court to justify some criminal acts. As cited in the Liu et al., (2021) article, Golding (1999) researched mental disorder susceptibility in battered women and found that 47.6% suffer from depression; additionally, more than 17.9% of them have attempted suicide. There are extreme mental and physical consequences to domestic violence and battered woman syndrome that can alter every aspect of the victims' lives. Battered woman syndrome has been compared to the symptomology of posttraumatic stress disorder (PTSD), a disorder where individuals experienced or witnessed a traumatic event and have difficulty recovering from it (Dutton, 1993). Although victims can develop PTSD and have each of the principal symptoms, the PTSD diagnosis might not thoroughly clarify the woman's psychological reaction to violence in the legal context since it defines the issue as merely a clinical dilemma (Dutton, 1993). In addition, if a woman does not meet the clinical criteria for a PTSD diagnosis, battered woman syndrome can act in legal contexts (Dutton, 1993). As outlined in battered woman syndrome, the cycle of violence on individual experiences can bring up unique circumstances in which the individual must act based on the fear that she might lose her life or the life of her child.

PARENTAL AND CHILD STRESS

Throughout the COVID-19 pandemic, our modified life circumstances to protect our individual and public health have proven stressful, particularly for parents. In Brown et al. (2020), researchers studied the impact of stress and parenting during the pandemic, finding that 21%-47% of parents indicated that their children had changes to their health and learning due to the consequences of the COVID-19 pandemic. Stress is a factor in the potential for child maltreatment (Rodriguez-Jenkins & Marcenko, 2014, as cited in Brown et al., 2020; Whipple & Webster-Stratton, 1991, as cited in Brown et al., 2020), and exposure to stressors can put a strain on the child-parent relationship (Deater-Deckard, 2004, as cited in Brown et al., 2020). There is no single stress determinant that prompts child maltreatment, rather compounding risk factors including economic hardship, low education, and single parenthood (Center for Disease Control and Prevention, 2020, as cited in Brown et al., 2020; Sedlak et al., 2010). Brown et al. (2020) suggest that poor parenting behaviors may result from the individuals' perception of these co-occurring stressful events. Throughout the pandemic, research has shown increased parenting stress and, therefore, the risk of harsh parenting correlating with parents' perceived impact of COVID-19 (Chung et al., 2020, as cited in Brown et al., 2020). Previous research has demonstrated that parental stress is a significant risk factor in domestic violence and child abuse, suggesting a positive correlation between abusive behavior and parental stress (Abidin, 1997, as cited in Griffith, 2020; Curtis et al., 2000, as cited in Griffith, 2020). Another strong predictor for the potential of child abuse is elevated parental stress with co-occurring anxious and depressive symptoms, typically exhibiting less responsiveness to their child's needs (McPherson et al., 2008, as cited in Brown et al., 2020).

Social distancing requirements, which resulted in school, workplace, childcare agencies, and business closures, have aggravated stress in households due to increased social isolation (Brown et al., 2020). Social isolation increases an individual's vulnerability to experiencing stress (Hawkley & Cacioppo, 2010, as cited in Brown et al., 2020). With parents challenged by various demands, susceptibility to stress may be exceptionally high (Brown et al., 2020). Correlations between stress and poverty have also commonly been associated with child maltreatment. However, research has indicated specific economic factors that may be more indicative than others, like unemployment and foreclosure rates (Frioux et al., 2014, as cited in Brown et al., 2020). The COVID-19 pandemic is a unique global experience that has altered most features of our societies lives; even if families do not face a direct impact from COVID-19, indirect consequences are still likely to affect them (Van Bavel et al., 2020, as cited in Brown et al., 2020).

PARENTAL BURNOUT

Many parents experience stress related to parenting and their adequacy of care, even without the looming fears surrounding the COVID-19 pandemic (Abidin, 1997, as cited in Griffith, 2020; Raphael et al., 2010, as cited in Griffith, 2020). During the COVID-19 pandemic, daily life changes have been implicated to ensure the relative safety of each individual. Due to these drastic life changes, parents may experience parental burnout, which is "a prolonged response to chronic and overwhelming parental stress" (Mikolajczak et al., 2019 pg. 1319, as cited in Griffith, 2020). Stressors have been maximized during the COVID-19 pandemic, including financial insecurity or job loss, access to childcare, and lack of leisure time, increasing the risk of parental burnout (Griffith, 2020). Also, grandparents have commonly helped parents with childcare; however, due to the "high risk" for COVID-19 in the older population (Aronson, 2020, as cited in Griffith, 2020) and other disease-related restrictions, this care is no longer safe. Routine grandparent visits and other forms of social support are important variables to preventing parental burnout (Parkes et al., 2015, as cited in Griffith, 2020).

Lack of leisure time has also become a problem since at-home parental duties have extended to all day hours, every day of the week (Griffith, 2020). Additionally, balancing work from home, virtual school activities, and managing childcare poses significant stress on parents (Griffith, 2020). Both self-oriented perfectionism and socially prescribed perfectionism have been associated with increased parental burnout risk (Sorkkila & Aunola, 2020, as cited in Griffith, 2020). Self-oriented perfectionism is the parent's self-expectations as caretakers, and socially prescribed perfectionism is the parent's perception of societal expectations (Hewitt & Flett, 1991, as cited in Griffith, 2020). Attempting to balance all parental responsibilities during the global uproar the pandemic provoked has proven exceedingly demanding; therefore, striving for these forms of parental perfectionism may imply a higher risk for parental burnout (Griffith, 2020).

Researchers found that parents experiencing higher levels of parental burnout report higher rates of suicidal ideation, partner estrangement ideation, and increased levels of child abuse and maltreatment (Griffith, 2020). Researchers note that the relationship between parental burnout and propensity for child abuse and neglect have similar effects across demographic variables like education and income level (Mikolajczak et al., 2019, as cited in Griffith, 2020). These findings suggest that parental burnout's adverse effects do not discriminate, significantly impacting parent-child interactions (Griffith, 2020). Interventions implemented to reduce parental burnout have been shown to successfully decrease child abuse and neglect (Brianda et al., 2020, as cited in Griffith, 2020). Some studies have also shown links between child abuse and parenting style, suggesting that parents subscribing to authoritarian parenting styles may be more likely to carry out abusive behaviors (Rodriguez, 2010, as cited in Griffith, 2020). Child abuse and neglect can have long-term physical and psychological effects on the child, leading to a series of disorders and interrupting their quality of life (Griffith, 2020). Children may also experience detrimental psychological effects because of the unpredictability the COVID-19 disease presents for their older family members, even though the virus poses a lower risk for children developing serious illness complications (Sinha et al., 2020, as cited in Griffith, 2020).

GRIEF

Throughout the COVID-19 pandemic, our society has experienced both individual and collective grief through unified hardships worldwide. COVID-19 has not only become a leading cause of death worldwide (Zhai & Du, 2020) but grief is elevated because people may not be able to say a proper goodbye to loved ones. Frontline healthcare workers are also encountering exorbitant rates of patient loss, resulting in the psychological and physical symptoms of grief (Li et al., 2020, as cited in Zhai & Du, 2020). Anticipatory grief may be felt by individuals or families experiencing a loved one suffering from COVID-19 complications, and disenfranchised grief can result in the absence of death rituals like a funeral (Zhai & Du, 2020).

Loss and grief are more encompassing than just death itself (Zhai & Du, 2020), since our society has also lost a sense of our "old lives" or normalcy. Individuals suffering from loss and grief must manage their needs to prevent deterioration of mental and physical health (Kang et al., 2020, as cited in Zhai & Du, 2020). As outlined in Elisabeth Kubler-Ross's "On Death and Dying," she proposes a five-stage theory of grief: "denial, anger, bargaining, depression, and acceptance" (Elisabeth Kubler-Ross, 1969, as cited in Stroebe et al., 2017). These stages are distinct and linear though an individual's experience can warrant differences like coexisting stages and fluctuations between stages (Stroebe et al., 2017). Anger is a common and seemingly necessary aspect of the grieving process for most people (Kubler-Ross & Kessler, 2005, as cited in Stroebe et al., 2017). Though it manifests differently in each individual, it may prompt a verbal or violent outburst. Rather than grief being the sole cause of domestic abuse, grief can act as a compounded stressor looming over both abusers and victims, potentially aggravating heightened tensions.

CONCLUSION

Throughout this literature review, new and existing stressors prompted by the COVID-19 pandemic are evaluated as risk factors in the potential for domestic abuse, violence, and child abuse. Economic and social crises, school and work closures, parental stress and burnout, and isolation are some of the main risk factors for inciting abuse or sparking abusive behavior. The restrictions of the COVID-19 pandemic have caused numerous complications for many individuals and families across the world. The psychological, physical, and social consequences that result from sustaining abuse pervade the victim long-term. As our society begins to heal from the uncertainty and hardship the pandemic has posed, we will continue to remedy the ramifications.

DISCUSSION

As outlined in this literature review, many new and recurring stressors exacerbated by the COVID-19 pandemic have generated perfect circumstances to cultivate perilous outcomes for domestic abuse, violence, and child abuse. Domestic violence has commonly been a camouflaged aspect of societal concern, and as prevalence rates increase, we must address the circumstances at hand. The restrictions of the COVID-19 pandemic have endangered millions of adults and children in abusive conditions, facing at-home violence with little chance of escape (Kofman & Garfin, 2020). The main stressors outlined in the literature review are isolation, mental health issues, economic or job instability, parental stress or burnout, global social and economic crisis, school and protective services closures, no access to childcare, the threat of contagion, grief, and increased alcohol and drug consumption or abuse (Usher et al., 2020; Griffith 2020; Sharma & Borah, 2020; Brown et al., 2020; Baron et al., 2020; Cullen et al., 2020). These stressors are interconnected, typically compounding risk factors that make individuals, children, or families more susceptible to abuse. This abuse could result in the victims' bodily, psychological, sexual, economic, and social harm, potentially perpetuating a cycle of violence throughout generations to come (De Benedictus & Jaffe, 2004). Each stressor outlined also has the capacity to help identify families at-risk for violence or abuse (Lawson et al., 2020).

These consequences require government safeguarding and preemptive prevention measures to ensure the protection of victims (Sharma & Borah, 2020). Much of public health policy enacted within the first surge of the COVID-19 pandemic was intended to slow the spread; with that objective remaining transparent, the United States continued to lack preparation and foresight for the unforeseen consequences that may have long-term, pervasive effects. In light of these unprecedented times, there has been no comprehensive direction to mitigate the malignant effects of this public health disaster without severe tactics to adjust our realities and sense of normalcy. Nevertheless, as the victims endure the uproar of unforeseen effects of domestic abuse, violence, and child abuse resulting from the COVID-19 pandemic, one would argue that relief programs, as well as justice reform, must assist in the rebuilding process for those most gravely impacted (Sharma & Borah, 2020).

FUTURE DIRECTIONS

As our society begins to remedy the change, loss, and unparalleled times of the COVID-19 pandemic, we will likely continue to see an influx of unforeseen consequences emerge as a result of this massive global disruption. Unfortunately, domestic abuse, violence, and child abuse will likely be among those consequences encountered. Our society must remain aware of the risk factors posed by the public health mandates of the COVID-19 pandemic and address the immense ramifications placed on individuals and families worldwide.

Further research will need to be conducted to understand the full effects of children facing at-home abusive circumstances combined with the global public health disaster of the COVID-19 pandemic (Griffith, 2020). These compounded negative events may pose significant physical, psychological, and social effects in developing children that may not be fully known until adulthood (Griffith, 2020). Similarly, the research could look into child educational neglect or gaps in education retention due to the transition to remote learning. Additional statistical research must be done to realistically grasp the true number of domestic violence cases at the peak of the pandemic. Understanding how the compounding of these unique stressors associated with increased risk for domestic violence will play out after the pandemic is deemed over will also be an important line of research. Current research should observe the promotion of our "new normal," since it may continue to foster domestic violence risk factors even after governmental mandates are lifted. The COVID-19 pandemic has generated uncharted territory for our global community, setting forth massive turmoil and collective dismay about our impending future. Further research in domestic violence, abuse, and child abuse is vital to address the fluctuations and detrimental consequences introduced by the pandemic and this new adjusted reality.

REFERENCES

Baron, E. J., Goldstein, E. G., & Wallace, C. T. (2020). Suffering in silence: How COVID-19 school closures inhibit the reporting of child maltreatment. *Journal of Public Economics*, *190*, 104258. doi:10.1016/j.jpubeco.2020.104258 PMID:32863462

Bradbury, C., & Isham, L. (2020). *The pandemic paradox: The consequences of COVID-19 on domestic violence*. Academic Press.

Brown, S. M., Doom, J. R., Lechuga-Peña, S., Watamura, S. E., & Koppels, T. (2020). Stress and parenting during the global COVID-19 pandemic. *Child Abuse & Neglect*, *110*(Pt 2), 104699. doi:10.1016/j.chiabu.2020.104699 PMID:32859394

Cullen, W., Gulati, G., & Kelly, B. D. (2020). Mental health in the COVID-19 pandemic. *QJM: Monthly Journal of the Association of Physicians*, *113*(5), 311–312. doi:10.1093/qjmed/hcaa110 PMID:32227218

De Benedictus, T., & Jaffe, J. (2004). Domestic violence and abuse: Types, signs, symptoms, causes, and effects. *Helpguide: Mental Health Issues*.

Dutton, M. A. (1993). Understanding women's responses to domestic violence: A redefinition of battered woman syndrome. *Hofstra Law Review*, *21*(4), 2.

Griffith, A. K. (2020). Parental burnout and child maltreatment during the COVID-19 pandemic. *Journal of Family Violence*, 1–7. doi:10.100710896-020-00172-2 PMID:32836736

Humphreys, K. L., Myint, M. T., & Zeanah, C. H. (2020). Increased risk for family violence during the COVID-19 pandemic. *Pediatrics*, *146*(1). doi:10.1542/peds.2020-0982 PMID:32317306

Kofman, Y. B., & Garfin, D. R. (2020). Home is not always a haven: The domestic violence crisis amid the COVID-19 pandemic. *Psychological Trauma: Theory, Research Practice and Policy*.

Lawson, M., Piel, M. H., & Simon, M. (2020). Child maltreatment during the COVID-19 pandemic: Consequences of parental job loss on psychological and physical abuse towards children. *Child Abuse & Neglect*, *110*, 104709. doi:10.1016/j.chiabu.2020.104709 PMID:32893003

Liu, M., Xue, J., Zhao, N., Wang, X., Jiao, D., & Zhu, T. (2021). Using social media to explore the consequences of domestic violence on mental health. *Journal of Interpersonal Violence*, *36*(3-4). doi:10.1177/0886260518757756 PMID:29441804

Marques, E. S., Moraes, C. L. D., Hasselmann, M. H., Deslandes, S. F., & Reichenheim, M. E. (2020). Violence against women, children, and adolescents during the COVID-19 pandemic: Overview, contributing factors, and mitigating measures. *Cadernos de Saude Publica*, *36*, e00074420. doi:10.1590/0102-311x00074420 PMID:32374808

Megan, L., Evans, M. D., Margo, M. P. H., Lindauer, J. D., Maureen, E., & Farrell, M. D. (2020). A pandemic within a pandemic— Intimate partner violence during COVID-19. *The New England Journal of Medicine*, *383*(24), 2302–2304. doi:10.1056/NEJMp2024046 PMID:32937063

Monroe, S. M., & Slavich, G. M. (2016). Psychological stressors: overview. Academic Press.

Rogers, M. M. (2020). Exploring the Domestic Abuse Narratives of Trans and Nonbinary People and the Role of Cisgenderism in Identity Abuse, Misgendering, and Pathologizing. *Violence Against Women*. PMID:34448660

Schneiderman, N., Ironson, G., & Siegel, S. D. (2005). Stress and health: Psychological, behavioral, and biological determinants. *Annual Review of Clinical Psychology*, *1*(1), 607–628. doi:10.1146/annurev.clinpsy.1.102803.144141 PMID:17716101

Sedlak, A. J., Mettenburg, J., Basena, M., Peta, I., McPherson, K., & Greene, A. (2010). Fourth national incidence study of child abuse and neglect (NIS-4). Washington, DC: US Department of Health and Human Services.

Sharma, A., & Borah, S. B. (2020). Covid-19 and domestic violence: An indirect path to social and economic crisis. *Journal of Family Violence*, 1–7. doi:10.100710896-020-00188-8 PMID:32836737

Stroebe, M., Schut, H., & Boerner, K. (2017). Cautioning Health-Care Professionals. *Omega*, *74*(4), 455–473. doi:10.1177/0030222817691870 PMID:28355991

Usher, K., Bhullar, N., Durkin, J., Gyamfi, N., & Jackson, D. (2020). *Family violence and COVID-19: Increased vulnerability and reduced options for support*. Academic Press.

Volavka, J., & Swanson, J. (2010). Violent behavior in mental illness: The role of substance abuse. *Journal of the American Medical Association*, *304*(5), 563–564. doi:10.1001/jama.2010.1097 PMID:20682936

Walby, S. (2004). *The cost of domestic violence*. Academic Press.

Walker, L. E. A. (1992). Battered women syndrome and self-defense. *Notre Dame Journal of Law and Ethics*, *6*(2), 321–334.

World Health Organization. (2020). Addressing violence against children, women and older people during the COVID-19 Pandemic: Key actions (No. WHO/2019-nCoV/ Violence_actions/2020.1). World Health Organization.

Zhai, Y., & Du, X. (2020). Loss and grief amidst COVID-19: A path to adaptation and resilience. *Brain, Behavior, and Immunity*, *87*, 80–81. doi:10.1016/j.bbi.2020.04.053

KEY TERMS AND DEFINITIONS

Battered Woman Syndrome: Battered woman syndrome develops in women who are victims of domestic abuse (physical, sexual, and psychological abuse), in which they develop psychological symptoms making it hard for them to regain control. Battered woman syndrome is labeled as a subcategory of posttraumatic stress disorder, with many women also meeting the clinical criteria for diagnosis.

Child Abuse: Child abuse is when an adult, parent, or caretaker causes injury, death, emotional or sexual harm, or risk of serious harm through action or failing to act.

Domestic Abuse: Domestic abuse closely resembles domestic violence yet broadens the definition of domestic violence to encompass other family members like children, older adults, and non-related parties. Domestic abuse includes the same manipulation patterns to ensure victims' compliance so an abuser can maintain control.

Domestic Violence: Domestic violence is used by abusers to control a spouse or intimate partner through maintaining power and abuse behavior patterns. This violence can include physical, emotional, sexual, psychological, economic, or spiritual abuse in the form of action, threats, or other behaviors intended to manipulate, injure, intimidate, or humiliate someone.

Economic Abuse: Economic abuse is when an abuser controls their partner's economic resources, forcing the victim to depend on their abuser financially. Examples of economic abuse can be withholding financial resources like money, preventing someone from having a job or obtaining the necessary education, or stealing money or assets from their partner.

Sexual Abuse: Sexual abuse is any unwanted or non-consensual sexual activity that may use force or threats. Sexual abuse also includes perpetrators taking advantage of victims not able to give consent like minors and highly intoxicated people.

Spiritual Abuse: Spiritual abuse can occur in intimate partner relationships as ridiculing, insulting, or manipulating their partner's religious beliefs and preventing their partners from practicing beliefs. Forcing the children to be raised in a faith the other partner has not agreed to and using religious texts or beliefs to minimize abusive behavior can also be examples of spiritual abuse.

Stay-at-Home Orders: Varying on a state-by-state basis, the stay-at-home orders or safer-at-home orders were enacted to slow the spread of COVID-19. Many states shut down non-essential businesses to encourage self-quarantine and slow the spread of the virus. Many states and cities also enforced mask mandates and social distancing regulations.

Chapter 6
The Impact of COVID on Elderly Adults With Dementia and Other Cognitive Disabilities

Nava R. Silton
Marymount Manhattan College, USA

Alexandra McClellan
https://orcid.org/0000-0002-9347-0911
Marymount Manhattan College, USA

ABSTRACT

The COVID-19 pandemic was particularly problematic for vulnerable populations. Elderly individuals with cognitive disabilities were a particularly high-risk group. The present review utilized the findings of previous studies to examine the implications of COVID-19 on the lives of elderly populations living with cognitive disabilities, such as mild cognitive impairment (MCI), dementia, Alzheimer's disease, and Parkinson's disease. The findings of this literature review revealed significant changes in psychological and cognitive health, as well as the mortality rate of patients with cognitive disabilities. Analysis of the study results suggested that the effects of COVID-19-induced isolation led to notable adverse changes in the psychological and cognitive health of those presenting with mild cognitive impairment, dementia, Alzheimer's disease, and Parkinson's disease. Additionally, findings revealed the substantial impact of the COVID-19 virus infection on the mortality of these populations. In many cases, COVID-19 led to a worsening of emotional, behavioral, and cognitive symptoms and to an increase in mortality.

DOI: 10.4018/978-1-6684-3484-0.ch006

INTRODUCTION

The COVID-19 pandemic undoubtedly left lasting effects on populations across the globe. The months of isolation and restrictions forced individuals, communities, and societies, to alter their everyday functioning. Though humanity is adaptable and resilient, even the smallest changes brought upon by Covid-19 were significantly felt. At-risk populations, such as immunocompromised individuals, children, elderly individuals, and those presenting with mental illness, were of high concern regarding both the effects of the virus itself, and the results of the COVID-19 lockdown and isolation measures. The present review focused on a particularly high-risk group: elderly individuals with cognitive disabilities. Four primary cognitive impairment diagnoses were discussed, including Mild Cognitive Impairment, Dementia, Alzheimer's Disease, and Parkinson's Disease.

In January 2020, the World Health Organization (WHO) addressed the various implications of lockdown for these specific populations, stating that elderly individuals with cognitive decline/dementia may encounter an increase in psychological symptoms such as anxiety and stress, as well as other behavioral changes. This review features over a dozen publications that discuss the substantial effects of COVID-19 on elderly individuals with cognitive disabilities and specifically highlights three key themes: changes in psychological and psychiatric health, shifts in cognition/ cognitive symptoms, and the effect of Covid-19 infection on mortality rates. The publications featured in this review generally contain hypotheses that predict COVID-19 will negatively impact populations with cognitive disabilities, whether emotionally, cognitively, or regarding mortality rate.

COVID-19 LOCKDOWN'S EFFECT ON MENTAL HEALTH: PSYCHOLOGICAL AND PSYCHIATRIC CHANGES

A common theme in the present literature included the impact of the COVID-19 lockdown on one's psychological health. One of the first studies to emerge on COVID-19 and elderly populations with cognitive decline included a 2020 study of patients with Alzheimer's Disease who were facing lockdown in retirement homes in France (El Haj, et al. 2020). The study recorded the patients' levels of anxiety and depression before and during the COVID-19 lockdown. Previous records of cognitive states, measured by a "Mini Mental State Exam" prior to COVID-19, were used for a Pre-Covid analysis of cognitive state. A self-assessment using the Hospital Anxiety and Depression Scale (Zigmond and Snaith 1983), which was completed with the assistance of caregivers, was used to determine the patients' cognitive state during Covid. Even without the presence of COVID-19 related effects, individuals with cognitive impairment or with a disability were more predisposed to an increase in anxiety and depression due to their diagnosis. Studies revealed that throughout the course of Alzheimer's disease, anxiety was experienced by 25 to 71 percent of individuals (El Haj, et al. 2020, as cited in Mintzer et al. 2005) and depression occurred within 50 percent of patients (El Haj, et al. 2020, as cited in Starkstein et al., 2005). Therefore, the disruption of these individuals' everyday routines and the isolation due to COVID-19, certainly exacerbated these previously prevalent emotional experiences, while often inducing others, as well. The results of the study indicated a substantial difference in pre and post self-assessment scores of patient anxiety and depression levels before and during COVID-19; anxiety and depression levels of patients with Alzheimer's Disease were higher during the lockdown than they had been before (El Haj, et al. 2020). Similarly, Tsapanou, et al. (2020) discussed the psychological decline of 204 patients with Mild Cognitive Impairment (MCI)/ dementia in Greece. Through caregiver self-report questionnaire responses on their patients, studies' results revealed a significant decline in the patients' communication, mood, movement, and compliance with COVID-19 measures. Patients' psychological health and wellness were disrupted by the lockdown.

Throughout the months of lockdown, which somewhat varied across countries, social interaction and typical day-to-day activities were halted. Subsequently, the physical isolation of these populations led to feelings of emotional isolation and a sense of loneliness. A third publication, a review by Manca, De Marco, and Venneri (2020), compiled 15 articles that examined COVID-19's infection and social isolation effects on psychiatric and neuropsychiatric symptoms of individuals with cognitive disabilities. Results of these studies indicated that delirium, a disturbance in mental abilities that can result in confused thinking and a decreased cognizance of the environment, was the most recognized behavioral change seen among patients with dementia, who contracted the COVID-19 virus (Bianchetti et al. 2020, as cited in Manca, et al., 2020). Further, Varatharaj et al. (2020; as cited in Manca et al. 2020) discovered that those with dementia experienced severe worsening of mental health symptoms while having the virus; there were enough symptoms to meet the criteria for a psychiatric diagnosis. Their study suggested the results of the compiled research indicated that social isolation was a leading factor in the "exacerbation or manifestation of a variety of neuropsychiatric symptoms in cognitively healthy older adults (especially stress, mood, and anxiety) and those with dementia (mainly agitation and apathy)." A study by Suarez-Gonzalez et al. (2021) revealed similar findings. Fourteen out of the fifteen collected studies of patients with dementia, showed a worsening of psychological symptoms, such as an increase in anxiety, depression, apathy, and agitation. Additionally, six of the reviewed studies revealed an increase in pharmaceutical drug use for psychiatric symptoms, most commonly antipsychotics and benzodiazepines (Suarez-Gonzalez et al., 2021). Further evidence of social isolation as a key influence was apparent in a qualitative study by Farhang et al. (2021), that used thematic analysis to investigate the struggles of MCI patients in Chile, while in quarantine. Results indicated a strong association between isolation and the occurrence of negative emotional states, most notably anger, fear of contracting the virus or transmitting it to family, anxiety, sadness, and emotional loneliness (Farhang et al., 2021). Congruently, Shankar et al. (2013) as cited in Manca et al., 2020, explained the pre-established link between loneliness and cognitive decline even among populations without cognitive decline. Their study provided results that indicated a positive association between older adults experiencing isolation, and the occurrence of depressive symptoms and a number of comorbidities. In other words, as isolation among older adults increased, their symptoms of depression did as well, along with other comorbid disorders. Therefore, the discussion of Farhang et al. (2020) and Manca et al. (2020) regarding isolation as a prime force in mental, emotional, and cognitive decline of both elderly people with cognitive disabilities and those without, helps emphasize the impact of the COVID-19 lockdown and quarantine on further mental health decline.

Goodman-Casanova et al. (2020) present another example of the adverse impact of isolation on mental health. Through a telephone-based survey in Spain, 93 patients diagnosed with Mild Cognitive Impairment (MCI) and mild dementia, were interviewed during lockdown quarantine to determine how they were most affected. Results from this study found a difference between participants living with others, and those living alone. The physical aspect of being alone appeared to adversely impact individuals more in certain measurement categories than those living with others. For instance, findings included reports of greater negative feelings including anxiety, sadness, boredom, lack of well-being, and more issues with sleep (Goodman-Casanova et al., 2020). Based on these findings, the authors of this study suggested that living alone was a risk factor for mental health.

In further examining the psychological and behavioral effects of COVID-19 on populations with cognitive disabilities, Simonetti et al. (2020) reviewed the findings of previous studies. Their analysis of the compiled studies indicated notable shifts in emotions and behavior due to COVID-19 and the lockdown. The researchers highlighted a number of reasons why elderly individuals with cognitive challenges might be particularly at risk for these changes. The lockdown interrupted their routine activities, which is particularly perilous for elderly individuals with cognitive impairment. They are highly sensitive to environmental changes and a disruption of routine can initiate an exacerbation of neuropsychiatric symptoms which can then increase their risk of self-injury, personal distress, COVID-19 contagion and death.

A more specific example of this relates to the Canavelli (2020) study, which was cited by Simonetti et al., 2020, and reported that within the first month of lockdown, patients with dementia showed an increase in depressed mood, feelings of apathy, and agitation. Canavelli et al. (2020) reported that apathy was present in more than one-quarter of quarantined individuals with dementia within the first month of lockdown. Patients with apathy were less likely to pursue behaviors that would prevent the transmission of COVID-19, like participating in self-care, personal hygiene, washing hands, or covering their mouths while coughing. Moreover, continued apathy could lead patients to spend more of their time bed-ridden and could therefore lead to the risk of hospitalization, pressure ulcers, and other physical ailments. Therefore, the neuropsychiatric symptoms of depression and apathy, which were already present within the first month of lockdown, had the potential to exacerbate the physical health and functioning of individuals with cognitive decline and dementia.

As highlighted in each of these studies, the COVID-19 lockdown had a significant adverse impact on the psychological well-being of elderly populations with the cognitive disabilities of Dementia, Alzheimer's, and Mild Cognitive Impairment and many of these neuropsychiatric challenges, also impacted their physical health, as well.

COVID-19 LOCKDOWN'S EFFECT ON COGNITION

In addition to changes in psychological wellbeing, elderly individuals with dementia and cognitive decline showed notable changes in cognition due to the COVID-19 lockdown, as well.

The disruption in one's everyday routine and a lack of social interaction introduced by the lockdown were challenging aspects for everyone, however, even more so for those who were already experiencing cognitive decline. Researchers Ismail, Kamel, and Al-Hashel (2021) examined the role of the COVID-19 lockdown on the cognitive decline of patients with Mild Cognitive Impairment, Alzheimer's, Parkinson's, and Dementia at an outpatient hospital in Kuwait. Through a cross-sectional observational study, their findings revealed statistically significant data that showcased the cognitive decline among those with MCI and Dementia throughout the course of the lockdown (Ismail, Kamel, Al-hashel, 2021). Eleven of the 36 patients in the study faced a progression of cognitive impairment and were moved to the "severe decline" category. The results suggested a notable decline in cognition categories of "memory" and "attention."

Similarly, Tondo et al. (2021) utilized a retrospective study design and compared the cognitive decline of patients with dementia in previous years (2018 and 2019) to that of 2020, to determine a possible change in the rate of decline. Results of the 132 participants indicated a significant decline in cognition when comparing their 2018 to 2019 decline to their decline from 2019 to 2020 (Tondo et al., 2021). The five-year cognitive decline trajectory showed a significant worsening of cognitive decline between 2019 and 2020 ($p < 0.001$), while the decrease in the Mini Mental State Exam (MMSE) scores were not statistically significant between previous time points. This study demonstrated how pandemic measures due to COVID-19, have initiated a significant exacerbation of cognitive decline in people with dementia, which suggested the need for more careful assistance to reduce the negative effects of social isolation in the event of future lockdowns

When on-site studies were not possible, the use of phone interviews with patient caregivers were a common methodology for assessing cognitive decline in patients, as seen through the studies of Borges-Machado (et al., 2020) and Rainero (et al., 2021). Borges-Machado (2020) analyzed the effects of home confinement on patients with Dementia through phone interviews with their respective caregivers. They utilized various indexes to assess their patients' functionality levels, their activities of daily living (ADL), and neuropsychiatric states. A comparison of pre and post confinement data suggested a decline in ADL scores and an increase in neuropsychiatric symptoms (Borges-Machado, 2020). Specifically, 80% of caregivers reported observing cognitive declines within their respective patients.

Similarly, Rainero (2021) conducted a similar study in which caregivers engaged in a telephone interview and reported significant cognitive changes in their patients with Alzheimer's Disease and various types of Dementia. Eighty-seven Italian Dementia centers (4913 total patients) participated in the study and findings revealed that approximately 60 percent of all patients encountered a worsening of cognitive symptoms throughout the quarantine. Statistical analysis reported three rapidly increasing symptoms among patients, including forgetfulness, confusion, and temporal disorientation. Upon further analysis, the results were not found to be associated with age, gender, duration of quarantine, disease severity, or changes in caregivers' psychological features. Interestingly, the data results did, however, reveal that patient's levels of awareness had an impact on levels of cognitive decline; the more awareness that a patient possessed regarding quarantine, the less likely he/she was to face a worsening of cognitive symptoms.

COVID-19 INFECTION IMPACT ON MORTALITY OF POPULATIONS WITH COGNITIVE DISABILITIES

A third noteworthy theme was revealed within the literature: the influence of COVID-19 on mortality rates of populations with cognitive disabilities. COVID-19 and its various strains have proved highly transmissible and deadly, affecting all populations. As discussed in multiple studies, including the aforementioned Simonetti (2020) study which noted that those with apathy, which is defined as a lack of interest, enthusiasm or concern, may be less likely to participate in self-care and in behaviors that would prevent them from contracting the virus. Those with cognitive disabilities were found to be much more vulnerable to infection, hospitalization, and death by the virus.

Drawing upon previous studies, Bianchetti (et al., 2022) discussed why populations with cognitive disabilities, specifically dementia, faced an increased risk of the virus' negative consequences. Data from Azarazhooh, (et al., 2020, as cited in Bianchetti, et al., 2022) suggested that patients with dementia are inherently more susceptible than others to facing poor outcomes from any form of infection and are more often faced with comorbidities. Due to this, these populations would face a two to five times greater risk of contracting and facing death due to the COVID-19 virus than a person without dementia (Bianchetti, 2022). A potential reason for this greater risk could relate to the pre-established declining health of those with dementia coupled with the aggressive nature of the virus, which may require intense medical intervention (Zuin et al., 2020, as cited in Bianchetti, 2022). Concurrently, Kuo et al.'s (2020) study as cited in Hariyanto et al., 2020, discusses a notable factor contributing to the increased risk of infection. An ApoE e4 genotype, which "modulates the pro/anti-inflammatory phenotypes" is abundant within several cells found in the lungs and is also largely associated with dementia (Kuo et al., 2020 as cited in Hariyanto et al., 2020). Since COVID-19 is a respiratory infection that infiltrates the lungs, this pre-existing presence of ApoE e4 genotype may be increasingly affected by the COVID-19 infection and can lead to greater mortality. Additionally, a retrospective study conducted by Wan (et al., 2020, as cited in Bianchetti et al., 2022) revealed that in comparison to other neurological conditions, individuals with dementia had a higher COVID-19 related mortality rate.

Further supporting the notion that COVID-19 more strongly affects those with dementia than other populations, in another study, Hariyanto et al. (2021) performed a meta-analysis of 24 studies, that upon a pooled analysis, suggested associations between dementia and a high-risk of COVID-19 infection, severe COVID-19 infection, and increased mortality rate from COVID-19 infection (Hariyanto, 2021). Proposed explanations for these findings included age in combination with comorbid conditions, and non-presenting COVID-19 symptoms that may result in illness being detected too late or not at all, thus increasing the possibility of mortality.

Similarly, an observational study of 848 home-dwelling patients with dementia in Italy examined the impact of COVID-19 on overall health (Caratozzolo et al., 2020). The results of this study indicated a substantial difference in hospitalization and death rates of patients with dementia with COVID-19 (44.2 percent hospitalized and 33.7 percent died) and patients with dementia without the virus (1.9 percent hospitalized and 1.2 percent died). Likewise, Tahira, Verjovski-Almeida, and Ferreira (2021) explored the risk-factors associated with COVID-19 related mortality and dementia patients. Age could easily be a potential confounding variable in the mortality rates of those with COVID-19, and specifically dementia patients with COVID-19. However, upon univariable analysis with death as a dependent variable, this study suggests that age is an independent factor in COVID-19 mortality among populations with dementia. Further, all-cause dementia and Alzheimer's disease remained strongly associated with a higher possibility of COVID-19-related death (Tahira, Verjovski-Almeida, and Ferreira, 2021). Thus, the results of the aforementioned studies support the hypothesis of a highly impactful relationship between COVID-19 and dementia populations' mortality levels.

CAREGIVER BURDEN

Another noteworthy aspect mentioned in several of the discussed studies was the increase of caregiver burden throughout the COVID-19 lockdown. Tspanou et al. (2021) highlighted the responses of 204 caregivers of patients with dementia/mild cognitive impairment and found that 64.7 percent felt an increase in physical burden and around 80 percent felt an increase in psychological burden. It may be inferred that the presence of familial support played a role in the caregiver responses, since only about 40 percent reported feeling a sense of support. Likewise, Rainero et al. (2021) reported similar findings in caregiver responses. Out of 4913 caregiver responses, results signified a 45.9 percent increase in anxiety and an 18.6 percent increase in depression. Similarly, results from Capozzo (et al. 2020 as cited in Bianchetti et al. 2022) indicated a correlation between caregiver's stress levels and the severity of the patient's condition. This correlation is also observed within Borges-Machado (et al. 2020), where caregivers (around 50 percent) reported an increase of physical and emotional exhaustion as their patient's condition worsened. Overall, there was a significant increase in caregiver burden as patients psychological and cognitive health declined.

RESULTS AND DISCUSSION

The research publications featured in the present study support the argument that COVID-19 impacted the emotional, cognitive, and physical health of elderly individuals with cognitive disabilities. The results of the 20 studies reviewed within the present chapter were each supported by data analysis and or review of previous literature, with methods including self-report questionnaires, interviews, observational studies, retrospective studies, and or pre and post-test analyses. Of the seven studies which showcased a decline in emotional well-being, each reported an increase in identification of negative emotions, most notably anxiety, depression, and apathy, within patients presenting with dementia, Alzheimer's, or mild cognitive impairment (MCI). It may also be inferred that isolation was a key factor in the increase of negative emotions, as the findings of a few studies, (Farhang et al. (2021), Manca et al. (2020), Goodman-Casanova, et al. (2020), Simonetti et al., (2020)) reported that loneliness and other isolation-related factors had a strong negative influence.

Results of studies from Ismail, Kamel, Al-hashel, (2021), Borges-Machado (et al., 2020), Tondo et al. (2021), and Rainero (2021) each support the hypothesis that COVID-19 led to cognitive changes in patients and led to greater cognitive decline. A common symptom reported within these studies was memory decline or forgetfulness. Those with cognitive disabilities heavily benefit from structure within day-to-day activities, an aspect that COVID-19 isolation made almost impossible. Though the cause of cognitive decline as seen through forgetfulness is not exact, it is possible that the disruption in consistent structure of daily living due to isolation, was largely associated with cognitive decline.

Through exploration of COVID-19 and mortality of elderly patients with cognitive disabilities, it may be inferred that those with various forms of dementia, mild cognitive impairment, or Alzheimer's would be more vulnerable. As supported through previous research studies, these populations indeed face a higher risk of a negative impact from illness or infection, even in the absence of COVID- 19. The aggressive nature of the virus in combination with these patients' pre-existing declines in health increases their possibilities for hospitalization or death, as supported through statistical data and results from Bianchetti (2022), Hariyanto (2021), Caratozzolo (2020), and Tahira, Verjovski-Almeida, and Ferreira (2021).

CONCLUSION

The gathered research identified three key themes regarding COVID-19's impact on the lives of elderly populations with dementia, Alzheimer's disease, Parkinson's disease, and those with mild cognitive impairment (MCI): shifts in psychological (emotional and behavioral) symptoms, declines in cognitive symptoms, and the impact on mortality rates. The twenty publications discussed in this review confirm the hypothesis that COVID-19 had a negative impact on the lives of elderly individuals with cognitive disabilities and led to an increase in negative psychological symptoms, significant cognitive declines, and more COVID-19 related deaths. Overall, the results of these studies emphasize the particular vulnerability of elderly populations with cognitive disabilities to the effects of prolonged isolation due to the COVID-19 virus. Additionally, a number of studies point to the significant physical and psychological burden on those caring for elderly individuals with cognitive disabilities, as well. As we continue to deepen our understanding of the various implications of COVID-19 and elderly populations with cognitive disabilities, we can better provide adequate care to ensure this vulnerable population is prioritized.

FUTURE DIRECTIONS

Several of the studies in this publication were conducted during a time of heightened COVID-19 lockdown from March to July of 2020. The results of the compiled studies indicated notable changes in the lives of elderly patients with cognitive disabilities, ranging from the early stages of lockdown to a year after the pandemic. Shifts in psychological symptoms was a theme identified within the literature and many studies utilized pre and post-test analyses to gather results. For future research within this area, it would be valuable to conduct further pre-post-test analyses to compare the shifts between early pandemic emotional and behavioral changes with post-pandemic psychological states. In so doing, researchers would gather further information on the pandemic's effect on the psychological states of elderly populations with cognitive disabilities and discern whether the mental health effects from COVID-19-induced isolation were long-term. Similarly, these studies revealed significant shifts in cognition of elderly populations with cognitive disabilities throughout lockdown and the following months. It would be valuable to continue exploring the factors associated with rapid cognitive decline while in isolation. This could help enhance understanding around the needs of these populations while possibly providing helpful feedback in the development of new approaches to prolong inevitable cognitive decline.

At the present time of this research review, COVID-19 has now been in existence for two full years. Even though time has passed since its initial development, research is still needed in several areas. A limitation of this research was the amount and depth of prior research to draw upon. Time and further research are needed to develop a more thorough and comprehensive understanding of COVID-19's impact on each of the three discussed areas, psychological effects (emotional and behavioral), cognitive effects, and mortality rates. The public emergence of the COVID-19 vaccinations in January of 2021 substantially impacted the overall mortality rate of all populations and reduced the number of COVID-19 deaths. However, it is still unclear how the virus and its many variants will impact the physical health of individuals long-term, and further research is necessary to understand the entirety of the virus' impact on elderly populations with cognitive disabilities, more specifically.

Future studies may also examine which practices by family members, caregivers, hospital staff members and other pertinent personnel may have served as a protective factor for the adverse psychological and cognitive impact of COVID-19 on elderly individuals with dementia and other forms of cognitive decline. Whether it be creative uses of technology or other practices that proved to be particularly beneficial for this vulnerable population at the time; knowledge of these practices would be highly useful for those currently contending with COVID-19 and for those who may encounter a lockdown, quarantine or pandemic in the future. If we can best address the needs of the most vulnerable to the COVID-19 virus and the accompanying effects of the quarantine and lockdown, we can be even more confident when tackling the needs of those less at-risk.

REFERENCES

Bianchetti, A., Rozzini, R., Bianchetti, L., Coccia, F., Guerini, F., & Trabucchi, M. (2022). Dementia Clinical Care in Relation to COVID-19. *Current Treatment Options in Neurology*, *24*(1), 1–15. Advance online publication. doi:10.100711940-022-00706-7 PMID:35221646

Borges-Machado, F., Barros, D., Ribeiro, Ó., & Carvalho, J. (2020). The Effects of COVID-19 Home Confinement in Dementia Care: Physical and Cognitive Decline, Severe Neuropsychiatric Symptoms and Increased Caregiving Burden. *American Journal of Alzheimer's Disease and Other Dementias*, *35*(January). Advance online publication. doi:10.1177/1533317520976720 PMID:33295781

Caratozzolo, S., Zucchelli, A., Turla, M., Cotelli, M. S., Fascendini, S., Zanni, M., Bianchetti, A., Psy, M. P., Rozzini, R., Boffelli, S., Cappuccio, M., Psy, F. G., Psy, C. V., Bellandi, D., Caminati, C., Gentile, S., Psy, E. L., Di Fazio, I., Psy, M. Z., ... Padovani, A. (2020). The impact of COVID-19 on health status of home-dwelling elderly patients with dementia in East Lombardy, Italy: Results from COVIDEM network. *Aging Clinical and Experimental Research*, *32*(10), 2133–2140. doi:10.100740520-020-01676-z PMID:32918696

El Haj, M., Altintas, E., Chapelet, G., Kapogiannis, D., & Gallouj, K. (2020). High depression and anxiety in people with Alzheimer's disease living in retirement homes during the covid-19 crisis. *Psychiatry Research*, *291*, 113294. doi:10.1016/j.psychres.2020.113294 PMID:32763552

Farhang, M., Miranda-Castillo, C., Behrens, M., Castillo, E., Mosquera, S., & Rojas, G. (2021) Impact of social isolation and coping strategies in older adults with mild cognitive impairment during the covid-19 pandemic: A qualitative study. *Aging & Mental Health*. https://www.tandfonline.com/doi/full/10.1080/13607863.2021.1958145 doi:10.1080/13607863.2021.1958145

Goodman-Casanova, J., Dura-Perez, E., Guzman-Parra, J., Cuesta-Vargas, A., & Mayoral-Cleries, F. (n.d.). *Telehealth Home Support During COVID-19 Confinement for Community-Dwelling Older Adults With Mild Cognitive Impairment or Mild Dementia: Survey Study*. Academic Press.

Goodman-Casanova, J. M., Dura-Perez, E., Guzman-Parra, J., Cuesta-Vargas, A., & Mayoral-Cleries, F. (2020). Telehealth Home Support During COVID-19 Confinement for Community-Dwelling Older Adults With Mild Cognitive Impairment or Mild Dementia: Survey Study. *Journal of Medical Internet Research*, *22*(5), e19434. doi:10.2196/19434 PMID:32401215

Hariyanto, T.I., Putri, C., & Situmeang, R.F.V. (2020). Dementia is a predictor for mortality outcome from coronavirus disease 2019 (COVID-19) infection. *Eur Arch Psychiatry Clin Neurosci*, *271*, 393–395. doi:10.1007/s00406-020-01205-z

Hariyanto, T.I., Putri, C., Arisa, J., Fransisca, Situmeang, R.F., & Kurniawan, A. (2021). Dementia and outcomes from coronavirus disease 2019 (COVID-19) pneumonia: A systematic review and meta-analysis. *Archives of Gerontology and Geriatrics, 93*. https://www.sciencedirect.com/science/article/pii/S016749432030296X

Ismail, I. I., Kamel, W. A., & Al-Hashel, J. Y. (2021). Association of COVID-19 Pandemic and Rate of Cognitive Decline in Patients with Dementia and Mild Cognitive Impairment: A Cross-sectional Study. *Gerontology and Geriatric Medicine*. https://journals.sagepub.com/doi/full/10.1177/23337214211005223 doi:10.1177/23337214211005223

Miyashita, S., Yamada, T., Mikami, T., Miyashita, H., Chopra, N., & Rizk, D. (2020). Impact of dementia on clinical outcomes in elderly patients with coronavirus 2019 (COVID-19): An experience in New York. *Geriatrics & Gerontology International*, *20*(7), 732–734. doi:10.1111/ggi.13942 PMID:32691924

Nanyang, L., Jiahui, S., Xiyuan, W., Ming, Z., Qianqian, H., & Hao, L. (2020). The Impact of Dementia on the Clinical Outcome of COVID-19: A Systematic review and Meta-Analysis. *Journal of Alzheimer's Disease*, *78*(4), 1775–1782. https://content.iospress.com/articles/journal-of-alzheimers-disease/jad201016

Rainero, I., Bruni, A. C., Marra, C., Cagin, A., Bonanni, L., Cupidi, C., Laganà, V., Rubino, E., Vacca, A., Di Lorenzo, R., Provero, P., Isella, V., Vanacore, N., Agosta, F., Appollonio, I., Caffarra, P., Bussè, C., Sambati, R., Quaranta, D., Guglielmi, V., … Ferrarese, C. (2021). The Impact of COVID-19 Quarantine on Patients With Dementia and Family Caregivers: A Nation-Wide Survey. *Front. Aging Neurosci., 12*. https://www.frontiersin.org/articles/10.3389/fnagi.2020.625781/full

Riccardo, M., Matteo, D. M., & Annalena, V. (2020). The Impact of COVID-19 Infection and Enforced Prolonged Social Isolation on Neuropsychiatric Symptoms in Older Adults With and Without Dementia: A Review. *Frontiers in Psychiatry, 11*. https://www.frontiersin.org/article/10.3389/fpsyt.2020.585540 doi:10.3389/fpsyt.2020.585540

Roberta, B., Antonina, L., Alessandra, N., Maria, C., Edoardo, C. C., D'Agate, C., Lucia, D. G., Giuseppe, L. B., Tiziana, L. C., Mario, Z., & Roberto, M. (2020). Changes in Motor, Cognitive, and Behavioral Symptoms in Parkinson's Disease and Mild Cognitive Impairment During the COVID-19 Lockdown. *Frontiers in Psychiatry, 11*. https://www.frontiersin.org/article/10.3389/fpsyt.2020.590134

Ryoo, N., Pyun, J.-M., Baek, M. J., Suh, J., Kang, M.-J., Wang, M.-J., Youn, Y., Yang, D.-W., Kim, S.-Y., Park, Y.-H., & Kim, S.-Y. (2020). Coping With Dementia in the Middle of the COVID- 19 Pandemic. *Journal of Korean Medical Science, 35*(42), e383.

Simonetti, A., Pais, C., Jones, M., Cipriani, M. C., Janiri, D., Monti, L., Landi, F., Bernabei, R., Liperoti, R., & Sani, G. (2020). Neuropsychiatric Symptoms in Elderly With Dementia During COVID-19 Pandemic: Definition, Treatment, and Future Directions. *Front. Psychiatry, 11*. https://www.frontiersin.org/articles/10.3389/fpsyt.2020.579842/full

Suárez-González, A., Rajagopalan, J., Livingston, G., & Alladi, S. (2021). The effect of COVID-19 isolation measures on the cognition and mental health of people living with dementia: A rapid systematic review of one year of quantitative evidence. *EClinicalMedicine, 39*. https://www.sciencedirect.com/science/article/pii/S2589537021003278

Tahira, A. C., Verjovski-Almeida, S., & Ferreira, S. T. (2021). Dementia is an age-independent risk factor for severity and death in COVID-19 inpatients. *Alzheimer's & Dementia, 17*, 1818–1831. https://doi.org/10.100TT2/alz.12352

Tondo, G., Sarasso, B., Serra, P., Tesser, F., & Comi, C. (2021). The Impact of the COVID-19 Pandemic on the Cognition of People with Dementia. *International Journal of Environmental Research and Public Health, 18*(8), 4285.

Tsapanou, A., Papatriantafyllou, J. D., Yiannopoulou, K., Sali, D., Kalligerou, F., Ntanasi, E., Zoi, P., Margioti, E., Kamtsadeli, V., Hatzopoulou, M., Koustimpi, M., Zagka, A., Papageorgiou, S. G., & Sakka, P. (2021). The impact of COVID-19 pandemic on people with mild cognitive impairment/dementia and on their caregivers. *International Journal of Geriatric Psychiatry, 36*, 583–587. https://doi.org/10.1002/gps.5457

KEY TERMS AND DEFINITIONS

Alzheimer's Disease: Progressive mental deterioration that can occur in middle or old age, due to generalized degeneration of the brain. It is the most common cause of premature senility.

Apathy: Feeling indifferent or lacking emotion, often resulting in a lack of interest in activities.

Cognition: The mental action or process of acquiring knowledge and understanding through thought, experience, and the senses.

Delirium: A serious disturbance in mental abilities that results in confused thinking and reduced awareness of one's environment.

Dementia: A chronic and progressive syndrome that is characterized by cognitive impairment and loss of memory, orientation, comprehension, language, and judgment, and is accompanied by a decline in the ability to perform daily activities.

Mild Cognitive Impairment (MCI): The stage between the expected cognitive decline of normal aging and the more serious decline of dementia. It's characterized by problems with memory, language, thinking or judgment.

Mini-Mental State Examination (MMSE): The Mini-Mental State Exam (MMSE) is a widely used test of cognitive function among the elderly; it includes tests of orientation, attention, memory, language and visual-spatial skills.

Neuropsychological: The study of the relationship between behavior, emotion, and cognition on the one hand, and brain function on the other.

Parkinson's Disease (PD): Parkinson's disease is a progressive nervous system disorder that affects movement. Symptoms start gradually, sometimes starting with a barely noticeable tremor in just one hand. Tremors are common, but the disorder also commonly causes stiffness or slowing of movement.

Section 2

The Impact of COVID on Child Development, Education, and Media

Chapter 7
Assessing the Pandemic Impact on Students around Abuja, Nigeria

Uzoma Vincent Patrick Agulonye
https://orcid.org/0000-0003-2803-2218
Lisbon School of Economics and Management (ISEG), University of Lisbon, Portugal

Samaila Benedict Bahago
Veritas University, Nigeria

ABSTRACT

The lockdown occasioned by the COVID-19 pandemic impacted child development. Some states in Nigeria made efforts to carry out remote learning for senior secondary schools, leaving behind those in the basic education category, namely Primary 1 to Junior Secondary School Class 3 (Elementary 1 class to 9th grade). The impact of this is examined through surveys administered to students and teachers across all levels. Teachers were specifically interviewed across all levels (primary, secondary, and university) to reveal the impact of the lockdown on the students and the school system. The interviews revealed beyond expectation that the economic impact of the country's macroeconomic situation led to job losses that moved families into poverty and exposed many children to extreme childhood poverty. The hyper-inflation in the country made educating children more difficult for struggling households. The lengthy time spent at home impacted all students including those who learned remotely. Infrastructural gaps, economic conditions, and poor access to basic amenities made it difficult for many children to study remotely. The excitement that accompanied the resumption to school (from the lockdown) was more social than educational. The economic impact on households weighed heavily on students, hence the slow post-lockdown recovery. Two years later, the effect lingers.

DOI: 10.4018/978-1-6684-3484-0.ch007

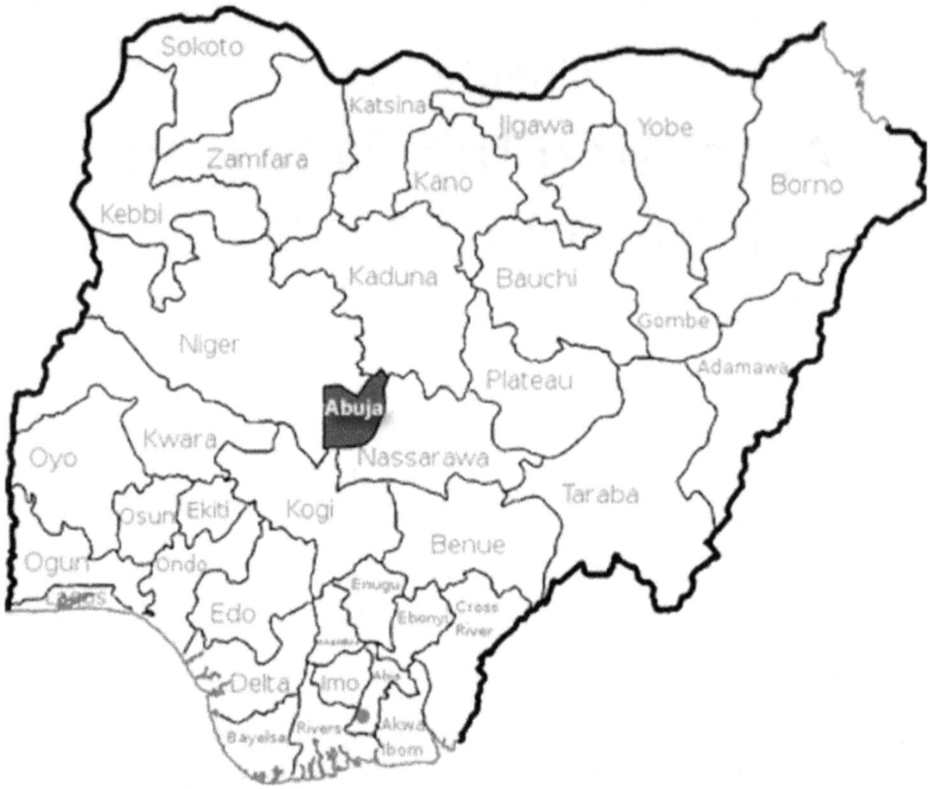

Figure 1. Map of Nigeria showing the Federal Capital Territory, Abuja
Source: UNIC Press, 2017

INTRODUCTION

The covid-19 virus took the world by storm since its discovery in December 2019 in Wuhan, China. The Chinese Government imposed a total lockdown on Wuhan and other cities in the Hubei region on the 23rd of January 2020 with only essential workers allowed to leave their homes. The spread and deaths in the country spurred the Italian Government to impose a lock-down in the Lombardy region on the 9th of March 2020- which was later made nation-wide to curtail the spread.

As of March 2020, the World Health Organization (W.H.O) confirmed that the virus had spread into many countries through infected travellers. Its bush fire-like spread prompted the WHO to classify it as a pandemic on the 11th of March 2020 (after initial reluctance to report it for a few months). This prompted preventive measures across the world. These measures included reduced social contacts through restrictions of human movement in public spaces which was climaxed with the total lockdown of districts, cities, states and in some cases whole countries by political leaders. These measures were introduced to curtail further spread and avert possible deaths.

The impact of such abrupt interruptions on the school curriculum and programme would need time to reconcile as the United Nations Educational, Scientific and Cultural Organization (UNESCO) stated that the closure of schools affected 862 million children globally, about half of the world's student population. UNESCO later reported that school closure in more than 188 countries directly affected over 1.5 billion children and adolescents globally (Segre, G. et al., 2021). The effects on the student's mental well-being, psychological, and social life manifested within a short time, equally taking its toll on child development. In Nigeria, the infection and death rate may not have been as high as in some other countries, but the lockdown in the country associated with the poor state of amenities and services would most likely affect its huge, young population. This chapter will therefore strive to answer the following questions: What are the effects of the lockdown on child and adolescent development and motivation? How does increased child poverty and decreased socioeconomic condition that accompanied the pandemic affect students? In what ways have the scheduled recovery efforts impacted the child?

These impacts are necessary to assess prior to prepare for subsequent waves of the Covid-19 pandemic and possible pandemics. Although, the casualties were less than expected in most African countries except for some African countries like South Africa, Morocco, and Tunisia, where cases were relatively high. Nigeria and some countries around it, had low cases. This chapter examines the efforts initiated by schools, teachers, ministries of education and parents to manage the impact on students.

SOME LOCKDOWNS IN HISTORY

Before recent epidemics, most governments had been reluctant to impose lockdowns due to Human Right infringement reasons. Except for the Chinese, who had done so thrice since 1901 (specifically during the Bubonic Plague re-emergence in 1901), the brief lockdown during the 2008 Sichuan earthquake and a brief lockdown during the Bubonic Plague resurgence in Gansu province in 2014. The Spanish government did not impose strict general lockdowns in 1901 during the Spanish Flu. The Bubonic Plague or Black Death Pandemic or the Pestilence of 1348-1352 forced lockdowns due to the severity of its spread and deaths. The 14th century pandemic forced lockdowns imposed by public leaders. The suffering was severe. By way of comparison, the Covid-19 pandemic with over four million deaths as of August 2021 has yet to come close to that pestilence which claimed over 200 million lives.

During the Ebola outbreak in 2014-15, reports of isolations and public preventive measures were recorded in West Africa where it occurred, yet there was no general lockdown in any city, suburb, village, state or country. The Coronavirus was the first in recent times, and the social condition in which the virus festered, occasioned a general lockdown in states and countries. The Ebola virus caused similar social conditions, but the governments and health departments of West African countries did not consider a lockdown. Whether a lockdown did not exist in the dictionary of health professionals in these countries or their value for the lives of the people was so low, remains a rhetorical question.

The Covid-19 pandemic occasioned by the novel Coronavirus, a respiratory disease, has prompted lockdowns across many countries on all the continents of the world to curb its spread. Since the initial lockdown of January 23, 2020, there have been similar preventive measures put in place to reduce human contact and spread, while managing the already infected. This measure came with the closure of schools, public institutions and spaces that subjected many to isolation; this triggered feelings of anger, anxiety, depression, fear, guilt, insomnia, loneliness, loss, sadness and suicidal-thoughts that had been experienced by people exposed to Ebola and Bird Flu (Wigg, *et al.*, 2021; Bailey, T., Hastings, R.P., & Totsika, V. 2021; Rajmil, L. *et al.* 2021) recently. The effects of the lockdowns on the mental health of youth has proven to be high, with cases of depression and anxiety in adolescent cohorts reportedly prevalent (Nearchou, F. *et al.*, 2021). This affected the motivation to return to school and normalcy after the lockdown.

PANDEMIC EFFECTS ON CHILDREN AND THE YOUNG

Previous research on the effects of epidemics on mental health revealed that Ebola and SARS (Severe Acute Respiratory Syndrome) Outbreaks had mental health effects on many, including young people. The Covid-19 pandemic had significant effects on the mental health of children, women, and adults. Prior to the Covid-19 pandemic, the Ebola epidemic had severe effects on the mental health of many survivors and relatives of victims (Rohweder, 2014; Bortel, *et al.* 2016; Jalloh, et al., 2018; James, *et al.*, 2019; Hall, 2019; O'Leary, *et al.*, 2020; Hallgarten, 2020; Bakrania, *et al.*, 2020; Kaputu-Kalala-Malu, *et al.*, 2021). The Covid-19 pandemic, with its preventive measures, especially the lockdowns that included the closure of schools in many countries, introduced as a containment measure, impacted the mental health of children and young people (Singh, *et al.*, 2020; Breaux, *et al.*, 2021; Chawla, *et al.*, 2021; Schnaiderman, *et al.*, 2021; Viner *et al.*, 2021; Waite, *et al.*, 2021).

Generally, the lockdown affected 91% of students globally. The prolonged lockdown had an emotional impact on the social behaviour of children. Their confinement at home caused children, with access to the internet, to spend more time on social media, thereby increasing tendencies and cases of bullying and abuse. School shutdowns during the height of the pandemic lockdown prevented around 2–4% of additional deaths less than other preventive measures (Singh, *et al.* 2020). Many children had experienced sleep disorders, nightmares, appetite issues, distress, distractions, and anxiety caused by isolation. A recent study showed that 96.3% of 267 parents studied confirmed emotional and behavioural change in their children during the lockdown (Schnaiderman, *et al.*, 2021). About 50% of the respondents, including children and adolescents, experienced boredom, frustration, irritation, reluctance, anger and anxiety. They argued with others more, as well.

Pizarro-Ruiz & Ordóñez-Camblor (2021) studied the effects of the lockdown on 788 minors with a complete response from 590 underage Spaniards (aged 8–18), who were not allowed to leave their homes between March 14 and April 26, 2020 except for very extenuating circumstances. The results showed that many children and adolescents exhibited emotional and behavioural changes during the six weeks long confinement. Ravens-Sieberer *et al.* (2021) studied 1586 German families and found that after the pandemic, more minors in these families exhibited mental health issues and poor life quality than they had before.

Abawi *et al.* (2021) studied the impact of the Covid-19 lockdown on lifestyle behaviours and the wellbeing of children with obesity. The study discovered that the lockdown impacted the eating habits, physical activity, screen time and quality of life (QoL) of children with severe obesity. This impact is not limited to obese children and adolescents. Most children have their impact level as well but physical habits and eating behaviours are cardinal to the wellbeing of obese children and adolescents. Though this study is not about the pandemic's impact on obese children or students body size.

METHODOLOGY

Primary data was sourced to discover the impact of the lockdown on children, students and the educational system in the specific geographical area of study. Available students and teachers were surveyed while in session, and an interview was conducted with some of the teachers. A limited number of responses were received due to the disparity in academic sessions between schools across levels in the capital city, Abuja and its suburbs which fall into three other states (namely, Kogi, Nasarawa, Niger). As a result of the lockdowns, resumption of school and school programmes varied across states and institutions. The data collected was from August 30 - September 8, from 19 teachers and school management staff, 70 students; 19 primary, 31 secondary and 20 university undergraduates. These 89 responses represent the population of students, teachers and school administrators in a population of 3.4 million city and suburb residents. Each of the surveys has four parts namely, respondent's brief lockdown location and study-impact, post-lockdown emotional and motivational impact, psychological and intellectual impact, and social behavioural impact. The survey questions were of four types administered to four groups, teachers and administrators, primary school students, secondary school students and university students.

Teachers and school administrators were sampled to understand the effects of school programme changes occasioned by the lockdown on students, parents and the system. The responses of these teachers and administrators were important in ascertaining the impact of the pandemic on adults in school management and their services. Since teachers and school administrators spend a minimum of eight hours daily with students, they can dictate and report behavioural changes and the motivational level of students. These changes and social behaviours are important to this study. They affect the motivation to return to school and normalcy after the lockdown.

Interviews were conducted after data collection, based on observations on the ground during data collection and the analysis of the data from the survey questions. Some of the teachers had reservations they could not explain in the survey questions, because those aspects were not mentioned, and there was no such opportunity. Ten teachers were interviewed and the data obtained were discussed after collecting the data from the survey. The interview was very revealing as the remote reasons behind the research questions, which were addressed at the peripheral level by the survey, were uncovered by the interview.

Data Analysis: Results

Since there are four surveys of data to be analysed, we grouped them into four: 1 for responses from primary school pupils, 2 for data from secondary school students, 3 for undergraduates and 4 from teachers and management staff.

Table 1. Responses from primary school pupils

Questions	Responses
Section A: Intro 1. What is your level of education? 2. Were you resident within your neighbourhood during the lockdown? 3. How did you study during the lockdown?	Primary (12), Secondary (6), University (1), None (1) Yes (15), No (4) Using a Computer (7), Not able to study (10), None (2)
Section B: Emotional & Motivational Impact 1. Did you enjoy resuming school after the lockdown? 2. Were you still interested in your favourite subjects? 3. Were your difficult subjects still difficult for you?	Yes (16), No (2) Not sure (1) Yes (16) No (3) Not sure (0). Yes (6) No (12), Maybe (1)
Section C: Psychological and Intellectual Impact 1. Did you feel like you were growing with your mates? 2. Were you able to solve more problems after the lockdown? 3. How fast was your recovery from the lockdown?	Yes (12) No (5) Maybe (2) Yes (10) No (9), Maybe (0) Quickly (4) Slowly (8) Averagely (7)
Section D: Social Behaviour 1. How was your interaction with your peers after the lockdown? 2. How was the school program after the lockdown? 3. Would you prefer to study from home or in school?	Easier (6) Normal (8) Difficult (5) Difficult (3) Long time (10) Easy (0), Interesting (6) From home (3), From school (12) Anywhere (4).

This table, in Section A, showcases responses from 19 primary school pupils, 12 (63.16%) of the pupils chose primary as their level of education. Eight (36.84%) of the primary school pupils chose secondary, one chose secondary and another none. This means that they have yet to fully understand what level of education they are at. Most (15, 78.95%) of them were within their residential area during the lockdown. During the lockdown (7 signifying 36.84%) were able to study with their computers and many (10 signifying 52.63%) of the students could not study during the lockdown and some (2 representing 10.53%) did not respond to the question. This section shows that most of the pupils were affected by the lockdown and were unable to study.

The emotional and motivational state of the students after the lockdown demonstrates that most (16 representing 84.21%) of the respondents enjoyed resuming school. However, two (representing 10.53%) students did not enjoy the resumption and only one (standing for 5.26%) offered an invalid response on this. Most (16 representing 84.21%) of the students still liked their favourite subject(s) pre-lockdown. Three students (which is 15.79% of the primary pupil's population) did not like their favourite subjects anymore. Some (6 that is 31.58%) of the primary pupils still had difficulties with their difficult subject(s). Surprisingly, 12 (that is 63.16%) of the students stated that their difficulty subjects were no longer difficult for them after the lockdown, and only one (representing 5.26%) of the pupils chose "maybe," indicating they are not sure

On child psychological and intellectual development, 12 (standing for 63.16%) of the pupils studied felt that they were growing with their mates. Five (that is 26.32%) of the pupils stated that they did not feel like they were growing with their mates and two (10.53%) chose maybe. On the ability to solve more problems post-lock down, ten (representing 52.63%) stated that they could still solve more after the lockdown and about half (which is 47.37%) of the pupils reported that they were unable to solve more problems post-lockdown. On an individual's recovery from the impacts of the lockdown, only four (standing for 21.05%) of the pupils admitted to a quick recovery, 7 (which is 36.84%) of the pupils reported an average level of recovery, and a majority (8 representing 42.11%) of the pupils indicated a slow recovery in school work after the lockdown.

Social behaviour after the lockdown revealed that most, eight (representing 42.11%) of the pupils stated that their interaction with their peers after the lockdown was normal. However, six (indicating 31.58%) of the pupils stated that their peer interaction was easier and a significant population, five (26.32%) of the pupils agreed that they had difficulties interacting with their peers. Regarding how they perceived the school session after the lockdown, a majority (10 standing for 52.63%) of the students perceived the usual school session as taking a long time. A significant p, six (31.58%) of the pupils perceived it as interesting and three (representing 15.79%) of the pupils perceived the school programme as difficult. In case of a future lockdown, most (12 which is 63.16%) of the students' population would still prefer to study in school. However, four (representing 21.05%) pupils were indifferent and could study anywhere. Only a small population, three (15.79%) of the students preferred to study at home.

Table 2. Responses from secondary/high school students

Questions	Responses
Section A: Intro 1. What is your level of education? 2. Did you reside within your neighbourhood during the lockdown? 3. How did you study during the lockdown?	Primary (0), Secondary (31), University (0), Yes (24), No (7) Using a Computer (2), Not able to study (29), None (0)
Section B: Emotional & Motivational Impact 1. Did you enjoy resuming school after the lockdown? 2. Were you still interested in your favourite subjects? 3. Were your difficult subjects still difficult for you?	Yes (31), No (0) Not sure (0) Yes (31), No (0) Not sure (0) Yes (13) No (15), Maybe (3)
Section C: Psychological and Intellectual Impact 1. Did you feel like you were growing with your mates? 2. Were you able to solve more problems after the lockdown? 3. How fast was your recovery from the lockdown?	Yes (22) No (9) Maybe (0) Yes (13) No (16), Maybe (2) Quickly (9) Slowly (13) Averagely (9)
Section D: Social Behaviour 1. How was your interaction with your peers after the lockdown? 2. How was the school program after the lockdown? 3. Would you prefer to study from home or in school?	Easier (5) Normal (21) Difficult (5) Difficult (4) Long time (4) Easy (6), Interesting (17) From home (0), From school (25) Anywhere (6).

Responses from secondary school students on table 2 above reveals that in section A, all the students fully understood their level of education as secondary hence the 100% choice of secondary. Most (24 standing for 77.42%) of them stated that they were within their residential area during the lockdown and seven (22.58%) were not. During the lockdown, only two (6.45%) of the students were able to study during the lockdown, while most (29 which is 93.55%) of them were not able to study during the lockdown.

The emotional and motivational impacts on the students after lockdown show that 100% of all the secondary school students enjoyed resuming school. Likewise, all the students agreed that they still found their favourite subjects interesting. This means that the pandemic lockdown did not affect their feelings toward education and their academic motivations. Surprisingly, the responses on their difficult subjects shows that while 13 (representing 41.94%) of them agreed that their difficult subjects were still difficult for them, many (15 accounting for 48.39%) of them stated that their difficult subjects were no longer difficult for them and three (that is 9.68%) of the students were not certain if they still had difficulties or not with their challenging subjects.

The students' psychological and intellectual development responses revealed that 22 (which is 70.97%) of the secondary school students studied felt that they were developing with their mates as they should. However, the remaining nine (standing for 29.03%) of the pupils stated that they did not feel like they were growing with their mates as they should. On problem solving competence, 13 (that is 41.94% of the population) of the students observed that they were still able to solve more problems while 16 (representing 51.61%) of the students noticed that they were no longer able to solve more problems and two (indicating 6.45%) of them are not sure if they could still solve more problems after the lockdown. The post lockdown recovery indicates that nine (accounting for 29.03% of the population) of the students stated that they had a quick recovery, many (13 amounting to 41.94%) of them said their recovery was slow and another nine (representing 29.03%) had an average recovery.

Social behaviour after the lockdown reveals that some (five students which is 16.13% of the population) of secondary school students agreed that they were able to interact with their peers easily after the lockdown. Many (21 representing 67.74%) of the population stated that their social interactions were normal and five (which is 16.13% of the population) expressed that they had difficulties in their social interactions after the lockdown. A post lockdown perception of the general school programme revealed that of the 31 secondary school students studied, four (which is 12.90%) perceived it as difficult, another four (standing for the same 12.90%) perceived the usual school programme as too lengthy, while six (representing 19.36%) perceived it as easy and as many as seventeen (54.84%) found it interesting. On study preferences, in the event of a future emergency situation, none of the respondents chose to study from home; rather most (representing 80.65% of the population) of the students preferred to study in school, and six (which is 19.35%) chose to study elsewhere.

Table 3. Responses from university undergraduates

Questions	Responses
Section A: Intro 1. What is your level of education? 2. Did you reside within your neighbourhood during the lockdown? 3. How did you study during the lockdown?	Primary (0), Secondary (0), University (20). Yes (14), No (2), Invalid (4) Using a Computer (11), Not able to study (6), None (3)
Section B: Emotional & Motivational Impact 1. Did you enjoy resuming school after the lockdown? 2. Were you still interested in your favourite subjects? 3. Were your difficult subjects still difficult for you?	Yes (10), No (3) Not sure (3), Invalid (4) Yes (10) No (4) Not sure (2), None (4) Yes (2) No (6), Maybe (6), Invalid (6)
Section C: Psychological and Intellectual Impact 1. Did you feel like you were growing with your mates? 2. Were you able to solve more problems after the lockdown? 3. How fast was your recovery from the lockdown?	Yes (12) No (1) Maybe (1), Invalid (6) Yes (7) No (3), Maybe (5), Invalid (5). Quickly (2) Slowly (6) Averagely (6), Invalid (6).
Section D: Social Behaviour 1. How was your interaction with your peers after the lockdown? 2. How was the school program after the lockdown? 3. Would you prefer to study from home or in school?	Easier (1) Normal (12) Difficult (0), Invalid (7) Difficult (6) Seemed to Last a Long time (4) Easy (1), Interesting (2), Invalid (7). From home (3), From school (11) Anywhere (0), Invalid 6.

University undergraduates' responses on the above table shows that in Section A, all the 20 (100% of the population of) undergraduates studied chose the proper level of education. Many (14, representing 70%) of the undergraduates were within their residences during the lockdown, only two (standing for 10%) of them were not within their residential area during the lockdown and six (which is 30%) of the respondents gave an invalid response, meaning that they were neither fully in their residential area nor fully out of it. Study during the lockdown shows that many (11 representing 55%) of the undergraduates studied remotely through their computers during the lockdown, six (that is 30%) of them were not able to study during the lockdown and three (accounting for 15%) of them were invalid because they partially studied remotely and were partially unable to study.

On the emotional and motivational condition of the students towards education after the lockdown shows that ten (that is 50%) of the undergraduates said they enjoyed resuming school. Three (representing 15% of the population) did not enjoy resuming school after the lockdown and four responses were invalid because they neither enjoyed nor did not enjoy resuming school. Another 10 (accounting for 50%

of the population) of undergraduates were still interested in their favourite courses. Four (standing for 20%) said they were no longer interested in their favourite courses after the lockdown, two (just 10%) were not sure of their interest after the lockdown and four (which is 20%) gave an invalid response. On their difficult courses after the lockdown, only two (10% of the population) agreed that their difficult courses were still difficult for them after the lockdown. Six (accounting for 30% of the population) stated that their difficult courses were no longer difficult for them after the lockdown; another six (30%) were not sure and six (30%) gave invalid responses.

The psychological and intellectual impacts revealed that twelve (that represents 60%) of the undergraduate population studied felt that they were growing with their mates as they should despite the lockdown. Only one (5%) of respondent agreed that they did not develop as they should have after the lockdown. Another one (5%) of the undergraduates, reported that he/she was not sure while six (that is 30%) gave invalid responses. The problem-solving abilities of the undergraduates revealed that seven (standing for 35%) of them indicated that they were still able to solve more problems after the lockdown. Only three (which is 15%) of them agreed that they were not able to solve more problems after the lockdown and five (25%) of them were not sure of their post-lockdown problem solving abilities while five (35%) gave invalid responses. The post lockdown recovery abilities reveal that only two (10%) of the undergraduates indicated a quick recovery, six (which is 30%) reported a slow recovery, another six (30%) said they had an average recovery and yet another six (30%) gave an invalid response.

Social behaviours after the lockdown show that only one (which is 5%) of the undergraduates admitted they've had easier peer interactions after the lockdown, while twelve (that is 60%) of them stated that they had normal peer interactions and none of them reported having difficulties with peer interactions. Yet seven (35%) invalid responses were received on this question. The perception of the general school programme after the lockdown shows that six (30%) perceived their usual school programme as difficult after the lockdown, four (20%) perceived it as taking a long time, only one (5%) saw it as easy while two (10%) saw it as interesting and seven (35%) gave an invalid response. The study preference revealed that three (15%) of the undergraduates preferred to study from home, eleven (55%) preferred to study in school and six (30%) gave an invalid response.

Table 4. Responses from teachers

Questions	Responses
Section A: Intro 1. What is your level of education? 2. Were you residing within your neighbourhood during the lockdown? 3. How did you teach during the lockdown?	Secondary (2), Tertiary (8), Graduate School (10). Yes (15), No (5). Using a Computer (7), Not able to study (10), None (3)
Section B: Emotional & Motivational Impact 1. Did your students enjoy resuming school after the lockdown? 2. Were they mostly interested in their favourite subjects? 3. Were their difficult subjects still difficult for them?	Yes (17), No (1), Not sure (2). Yes (13), No (6), Not sure (1). Yes (10), No (4), Maybe (6).
Section C: Psychological and Intellectual Impact 1. Did you notice their intellects developing as they should? 2. Were they able to solve more problems after the lockdown? 3. How fast was their recovery from the lockdown?	Yes (7), No (9), Maybe (3). Yes (6), No (11), Maybe (3). Quickly (2), Slowly (8), Normally (10).
Section D: Social Behaviour 1. How were most of their interactions with their peers after the lockdown? 2. What was their recovery of lost time like? 3. During a lockdown would you prefer they study remotely or in school?	Easier (0), Normal (13), Difficult (7). Difficult (9), Normal (6), Easy (4), Interesting (1). Remotely (3), From school (12) Anywhere (5).

The responses from teachers contained in the table above shows that the level of education of the teachers is composed of two (that is 10% of the population) teachers who studied with only a secondary education. Eight of the teachers (40%) have a tertiary or post-secondary education qualification that could be a bachelor or its equivalent, ten (50%) have a graduate degree which could be a master's degree or its equivalent. The place of residence during the lockdown indicates that 15 (75%) of the teachers resided within their residential area during the lockdown while five (25%) of the teachers resided elsewhere during the lockdown. Teaching medium during the lockdown shows that seven (which is 35%) of the teachers taught remotely, while ten (50%) of the teachers stated that they did not teach during the lockdown, and three (15% of the population) of the teachers gave no response.

Responses from the teachers on the emotional and motivational effects of the lockdown revealed that most (17 representing 85%) of the teachers stated that the students enjoyed resumption of school after the lockdown, and only three (which is 15%) noticed that some of the students did not enjoy the resumption. The students' interest in their favourite subjects shows that many (13 standing for 65%) of the teachers observed that the students were still interested in their favourite subjects while six (representing 30%) of the teachers noticed that the students were no longer interested in their favourite subjects after the lockdown, and one gave no response. The ability to solve their difficult subjects after the lockdown shows that ten (50% of the population) teachers agreed that the students were able to solve their difficult subjects after the lockdown while four (20%) of them agreed that the students were not able to solve their difficult subjects after the lockdown. Six (which is 30% of the teachers) were uncertain regarding the students post lockdown abilities.

The psychological and intellectual development of the students after the lockdown got this response from the teachers: seven (35%) of the teachers reported that their intellects developed as they should. However, nine (45%) of the teachers did not agree that their intellects developed as they should, while three (15%) were not certain about it. On their ability to solve problems after the lockdown, six (30%) of the teachers agreed that the students were able to solve more problems and eleven (55%) of the teachers noticed that the students were unable to solve more problems after the lockdown while three (15%) were not sure. Post lockdown recovery ability shows that only two (10%) of the teachers attested to a quick recovery. Eight (40%) of the teachers observed a slow recovery rate and ten (representing 50%) of the teachers noticed an average recovery.

The social behaviour of the students after the lockdown was observed by the teachers as 13 (standing for 65%) affirmed that they had normal peer interaction and seven (35%) of them observed difficulties in their peer interaction. The lost time recovery efforts were also observed by the teachers. Nine (45%) of the teachers stated that the students had difficulties with it. Although six (representing 30%) of the teachers noticed that it was a normal recovery, four (20%) observed that it was an easy recovery while one (which is 5%) observed that it was an interesting recovery. Subsequent lockdown study preference reveals that only three (15%) of the teachers preferred a remote teaching and learning method and twelve (standing for 60%) of the teachers preferred in school teaching and learning while five (25%) preferred anywhere.

Survey Discussion

The responses generated from the survey questions present some important discoveries. The fact that a few primary school teachers only have a secondary school certificate was a surprise. This prompted the quest for a further inquiry. On the contrary, there are some highly qualified teachers teaching in primary and secondary schools. This revealed a case of underemployment which is a common reality in the wider labour market. On residence during lockdown, it was discovered that while many lived within their neighbourhood during the lockdown, the few whose villages were nearby or a few kilometres away travelled home during the lockdown. Teaching during the lockdown presented difficult for teachers whose institutions initiated the process. For students across all levels, participation in remote learning was determined by socioeconomic factors, especially by the household's purchasing power.

In terms of motivation, the long lockdown of schools in Nigeria which was from March 20 to October 12 and November for primary schools in Abuja spurred the desire to return to school after it all. That motivation was not completely to study but to leave home, wear their uniforms, go to school, be with peers and enjoy the routine of going to school and returning home. The motivation behind the resumption was for more social than educational reasons. The students' poor academic performance and weaker intellect only reveal the effects of a long lockdown on child development. Although the students were generally still interested in their favourite subjects, their performance was lower than it had been before the general lockdown. Most of the students across levels were still having issues with their difficult subjects.

Psychological development across levels revealed that most of the students and teachers surveyed across levels attested to developing as they should, some of the teachers noticed that the children lagged behind psychologically after the lockdown. The development of the child or students can be noticed from their ability to solve problems as they should be solved. Although many claimed to still be able to solve more problems, some students and teachers boldly confirmed that they had issues solving more problems after the lockdown. In terms of their recovery rate, some revealed that they had made a quick recovery, a significant population of students and teachers stated that it was a normal recovery and a few stated that the recovery had been slow.

Socially, most of the responses received showed the social behaviours of the students after the lockdown were normal. A few students and teachers confirmed that the recovery has been slow. Some primary school pupils attest to the difficulty in the recovery to normalcy. Some secondary school students attest to the difficulties, as well. Many university undergraduates chose to describe the post lockdown school programme as difficult. Interestingly, most of the primary and secondary school students described the post lockdown school programme as taking a long time. This can be understood since they had spent months at home, without spending such a long time in the classroom. Despite the experiences, most of the students and teachers across levels preferred to study in school, rather than remotely, should there be another wave or a similar social situation of school closure.

Interview Discussion

Important factors affecting child development and the education system beginning with the socioeconomic condition of children and adolescent students to the managerial and political handling of child poverty, student's development, and education system in Nigeria are detailed here. Teachers were interviewed across various areas on remote factors associated with the same questions on the survey. These are their responses.

Teachers Qualification: Most of the teachers interviewed explained that some teachers are unable to further their education due to economic reasons. Some of them joined the profession because of their passion with the hope that things would improve and that it would give them an opportunity to further their education. Yet as days passed, tuition fees in private and public tertiary institutions were not more affordable, rather they were becoming more expensive, and the salary of teachers with lower qualifications were insufficient to pay tuition added to rent, basic bills, feeding and taking care of family needs and dependents. The teachers with higher education who had an interest in furthering their studies, were equally caught in the same web. There is no support system in place in the educational system at primary and secondary levels. The higher institutions have a government funded programme, introduced by the previous government, but today it has been highly politicized.

Lecturers in tertiary institutions stated that the programme is only accessible to those in public institutions that are close to highly placed public officials. Previously, it was granted to suitably qualified staff, according to seniority or those with admission who have resources to begin the programme so that when the funds are released, it would help them continue their studies. These days, it is only available to loyalists to the senior ruling party leaders or heads of departments and faculties. The University or Polytechnic are also forced to be loyal in order to get their appointments or renewals. The high rate of corruption in Nigeria today has corrupted the educational system so much that academics are made to be partisan to get anything from the state. One of the respondents reported that some lecturers in the Southwest part of the country rely on the connection of the governor or the national party leader who does not occupy a political position in the government to get a government scholarship. The lecturers in private tertiary institutions lamented that the difficult measures put in place makes the programme inaccessible to lecturers from private institutions.

Teaching and Learning During the Lockdown: Due to the duration of the lockdown, schools and the ministry of education devised learning alternatives. In the Federal Capital Territory, the Secondary Education Board (FCTSSEB), which is responsible for managing education at the senior secondary 1 – 3 (or 10th – 12th grade) levels, created a radio teaching programme. Another was created on the television station, and yet another was streamed through the internet to enhance remote learning at the senior secondary level. Due to an erratic power supply, the economic conditions of households and the high rate of childhood poverty, some students were unable to participate actively. The issues with participation made it difficult for many children to cope.

At the lower secondary and primary school levels, which are administered by the federal capital territory, the universal basic education board (FCTUBEB), the board was unable organize a learning platform, since its management of schools is funded by a counter-part funding system with the local government areas. Unlike its counterpart, the FCTSSEB, who were under the federal capital territory authority (FCTA), which gets its funding from it and has some level of autonomy. The FCTUBEB was unable to organize any remote learning activity, hence a dark age for public primary and junior secondary schools.

Private schools filled the gap created by the absence of a remote learning platform for children at that level. They taught remotely during the lockdown, but the parents and guardians were made to pay for the services. The programme enabled many children to learn remotely. Private schools are predominantly for average and struggling families, yet the economic impact of the lockdown which affected many household incomes impacted the ability of students to study remotely because it required the purchase of laptops, internet data plans and generators to power their generators. Some struggling households without a computer had to buy used desktops or laptops for the kids to share. This required that the children use it, one person at a time. Households that could afford it bought more depending on the number of children. Some homes had to buy a router and data plan for WIFI services to enable their child's study. They still had to subscribe and pay the school for the online learning service.

Economic factors played a major role in the remote learning programme since many students could not participate. Due to power cuts, the unavailability of a computer to learn remotely, family poverty made it impossible for parents to purchase internet data plans, generators and fuel for alternative electricity and personal computers. To add insult to injury, many private school teachers were not paid during the lockdown. Some had their salaries slashed. Some private schools had to downsize, and some teachers lost their jobs. There were job losses that exacerbated the economic conditions of educated people in a profession with poor remuneration. Many private school teachers started searching for a means of survival. Some started hawking food stuff during the pandemic since foodstuffs were in high demand during the lockdown.

After the lockdown, the teachers all affirmed that the students were happy and willing to return to school after an eight-month long lockdown (from March 20 – early November 2020). The resumption was set for October 12, 2020, but there was a primary school teachers' strike in the federal capital territory (FCT) that lasted until early November. Most of the students were excited and happy to meet their friends again. They were still interested in their favourite subjects, but due to economic reasons their interest dwindled. In fact, the public-school students had forgotten most of what was taught before the lockdown because they had no way to study. Private school teachers also complained of the same issue that at the commencement of remote learning, they faced the same challenges and had to start from foundational levels with two or three letter word explanations to enhance understanding. After the lockdown, they still were unable to completely catch up with their pre-lockdown performance. Most schools, especially public schools, had to operate two sessions to enhance population control and to avert a possible Covid-19 spread, should any of the students encounter a Covid-19 carrier or infected person.

Upon the resumption of studies, schools in the FCT had to first review the previous lessons taught to refresh the minds of the students. Afterwards, they cancelled the third term which ideally concludes the session with a promotional exam. In this case, there was no promotional examination held. Schools simply started a new session. All the students were moved along to the new class since there was no promotional examination. Despite this, the students still had challenges catching up with their studies, especially challenges in problem solving. The impact of the pandemic would be long-lasting in the intellectual development of the students, said one of the teachers.

At the tertiary level, most students could not study remotely for various reasons. A key factor was that tertiary institutions in Nigeria do not have the same calendar. The unharmonized calendar of Public tertiary institutions in Nigeria is caused by frequent trade union strikes of its academic and non-academic staff and the post-strike recovery programmes of each individual institution. Private institutions operate independently and may or may not run the conventional fall or autumn to summer academic programme. Although private tertiary institutions operate a more uninterrupted academic programme, the pandemic broke the jinx for most of them. Only Veritas University in Abuja was said to have studied remotely during the lockdown. This could be due to institutional factors since it is a Catholic university and Catholic institutions are known for their discipline and quality.

Motivation to study was generally marred by the socioeconomic realities beyond the classroom. Most of the teachers interviewed confirmed that the general economic ecology in the country moved more households into poverty and exposed child poverty even more. One of the respondents, a school head, stated that he was surprised to see some of his students hawking (peddling) during the lockdown. These were students from average families. Another teacher reported instances after the lockdown when her pupils would be crying from stomach pains two hours into the day. As an experienced teacher she would ask them what they ate before school only to discover that the child had not eaten since the night before. In some cases, she would notice that a child was dull or inactive upon inquiry, she would discover that the child was just hungry. Another teacher reported the case of a student who fell in class after standing for some time. Upon inquiry, it was discovered that the student had not had good food for days and had not eaten since the previous day's lunch.

Many private school teachers were not paid during the lockdown, hence many of them migrated to hawking food stuff which were the goods on demand that day. Many teachers lost their jobs, since schools were not able to keep up with their staff population. Many private school teachers left their jobs for good. Many students were withdrawn from private schools for economic reasons and enrolled in public schools after the lockdown. The economic troubles that affected students across the country after the lockdown offered poor motivation to learn. Many students stopped coming to school. The government noticed that students were not coming to school for economic reasons. In January of 2021, the government introduced a school feeding programme and stopped in July 2021, for no reason. The vendors stopped cooking because they were not paid by the government. The government propaganda stated that it feeds students every day. In actuality, they feed them for only one month in a term of three months. When they began, they were providing an egg twice a week and meat once a week to the students.

The school feeding programme is a welcome initiative, but its inconsistency makes it look like political propaganda. At the beginning the quality of the food was good, but it later declined. The feeding programme gave only lunch to the students and featured a weekly menu like this.

Monday – Rice, no meat

Tuesday – Yam porridge and vegetables, no meat

Wednesday – Beans and bread

Thursday – Potato porridge & vegetables; no meat

Friday – Rice, beans and Meat (tiny sized).

Despite the government's magnanimity, there was no food for the teachers, no lockdown incentive, no salary increment, no hazard or hardship allowance. In spite of the rising cost of living, many teachers had to struggle with a static salary that did not reflect the realities of the day with a high inflation rate. The political class received a hardship allowance despite their huge incomes, yet those who educate the future of society had no premium placed on their welfare. Teachers in public schools still received the same salary with no allowance or assistance to alleviate their sufferings. Those in private schools were worse off. This led to professional migration, since many could not watch their families starve. They would rather scout for a living elsewhere.

The economic cost of the resumption of studies dawned on parents as the economic challenge of an increment in school (or tuition) fees came as a surprise. Even the more affordable public schools to which many had moved their children, also increased their fees. For example, the school fees for senior secondary (boarding) schools that was N14,000 increased to N25,000. Junior secondary school registration fee that was N16,000 increased to N25-26,000. All of these increased the cost of schooling and affected the motivation (academic interest and performance) of the students. Aside for tuition, other areas witnessed increased cost. School uniforms which parents used to get in the market for N300 -N350 per trouser length increased to N600-N700 per trouser length. Since most of the children had grown within the period of the lockdown, many parents had to buy new uniforms for their children, and those who changed schools also had to get the new school's uniform. Sportswear that was N1,200 increased to about N2,000. Sportswear for private school students that was N2,000 was now N4,000. White Socks that students wore to school that were N100, were now N200. School sandals that were N600 now go for N1,200 – N1,300.

In the event of a future lockdown occasioned by an epidemic, a pandemic or any other factor, all of the teachers interviewed stated that due to the high level of poverty and basic high cost of accessing basic needs, they would prefer classroom teaching and learning methods to remote learning. They stated that the infrastructural and economic ecology now in Nigeria would not allow Nigeria and Nigerian children to learn remotely. This shows that the government needs to do more for the Nigerian child. In some other countries, governments have had to purchase laptops and provided the necessities for their children to learn remotely.

Strengths and Weaknesses

Personal details that contribute to overall academic and social performance such as sleep time and duration during and after the lockdown, quality of rest, screen time (the amount of time spent before the television at home or elsewhere), feeding patterns and timing during and after the lockdown were not included in studying the population sampled for this chapter. The chapter is focused on the impact of the pandemic on the educational system that includes the students, teachers, non-teaching staff, among others. The individual development of the student, which is part of the focus of this chapter, is attended to through their post pandemic performance and direct inquiry.

Observations made during and after data collection were used to strengthen the position of this thesis through the data obtained. It is difficult to properly estimate the total number of students in the city of Abuja and its suburbs. Hence, a rough estimate was made using this representational data to represent the population of students in and around the city. The effects of the lockdown on The Nigerian educational system is an area that requires much time and data collection, hence the choice of limiting this study to only some of the suburbs and parts of the city. The primary school available for study during data collection was in a separate location from that of the secondary school. The university sampled is in a separate location in the capital city. The figures of the unsampled population are unavailable but we estimate them to be about seven hundred thousand students from primary through tertiary institutions in and around Nigeria's capital.

Findings

The result of this study reveals the effects of social economic pressure on parents, homes and children occasioned by the lockdown. The motivation to study has declined considerably. For about a year since the resumption of classes, recovery is still at a slow rate. Aside from the economic effects of the lockdown, the psychological effect reflects the impact of a combination of stressors: the lockdown and the economic pressure with the reduction in social activities. Many children were happy to return to school to socialize more than to study. The recovery path has been slow. The teachers had to lower standards to enhance understanding. The impact on many teachers interviewed attests that it would take a long time to recover if they all would.

Fluctuating commodity prices, a huge infrastructural gap, an abysmal absence compared to developed countries and political irresponsibility to the needs of the Nigerian child all create a disastrous ecology for the Nigerian child to grow and thrive in a healthy manner. Despite the efforts of parents, these social dilemmas keep the Nigerian child in a state of constant mental and social stress. The persistent insecurity and kidnapping of students further in other parts of the state and other northern states in the country increases these mental and social stressors. It has depressed teachers, school managers and owners into fear, never knowing what would next befall them. This study observed the increased fear of suspicious movements in schools during the field study. The reality is that at the point of a possible attack, no one can save you. The security agents have never completely foiled any attack even the ones carried on its premises.

Nigeria's poorer situation occasioned by the fluctuation in commodity prices affects the macroeconomic condition of the country which has a direct impact on individual households at the micro level. This has narrowed the social sphere of individuals. It has limited household incomes and increased child poverty at a rate never seen in this generation. This has affected the development, academic performance and motivation of students across all levels, especially at primary and secondary school levels (i.e. 3 – 17 years old). Cases of self-withdrawal were observed among a few children from economically affected homes. Low performance has been recorded across all levels as some students from much more affected households were noted to self-detach after the resumption of classes, but some teachers were able to relate to them more to ameliorate their feelings.

The chapter revealed that the teachers and school administrators were not left out of this social situation as the general economic condition of the country has been far-reaching and abysmal. The motivation to work is also affected by this social condition. In addition, occupational stress has increased due the management's quest to meet up with the already distorted school programme and curriculum. The disparity in schooling programmes and schedules amidst increased pressure with hyper-inflation, offering the same salary and a delay in payments caused low work motivation and increased mental and social stress. All of these factors put the teacher in a helpless condition with her highly impacted students. The already stunted development of the child is a serious concern for the teachers especially those in public schools whose students (particularly those in basic school, Primary 1 – Junior Secondary School 3) were unable to study during the lockdown.

CONCLUSION

The effects of the Covid-19 pandemic on child development and the school system were enormous. The long duration (March 20 – October 12, 2020) of the pandemic lockdown in Abuja affected the mental and social state of young people. The academic performance of young people across all levels declined considerably after a long stay at home. Teachers had to teach using basic words and language explanations to enhance understanding. In Abuja, where this study is focused, the state had to cancel an entire term of three to four months and move into a new session. This administrative decision did not consider the psychological and intellectual impact of the pandemic on the students. The teachers were left with the burden of teaching a new curriculum that the teachers were not yet mentally prepared for amidst the impact. This also impacted the entire school system, as well.

A greater consequence of the pandemic is one that focuses on social and economic impacts of the pandemic; the macroeconomic ecologic disasters had direct impacts on households and individuals. The fall in commodity prices during the pandemic reflected that commodity dependent countries experienced economic difficulties. Firms and businesses experienced cash-crunch, households suffered meagre incomes and individuals became poorer. Many children in the suburbs of Abuja that we studied belonged to average and lower-class families where the impact has been high and more new cases of child poverty exist. Many children in these neighbourhoods did not have the opportunity to study remotely because of the socioeconomic conditions they live in. There is need to consider such people when decisions are made like a lockdown because it could impact them even more. Assistance in providing basic necessities or alternatives to encourage remote learning and a consistent, honest and altruistic effort from the political class for its people is a necessity to alleviate the sufferings of these people.

REFERENCES

Abawi, O. (2021). Impacts of the Covid-19 Lockdown and Relevant Vulnerabilities on Capability Well-being, Mental Health and Social Support: An Austrian Survey Study. *Journal of the Endocrine Society*, *5*(1). Advance online publication. doi:10.1210/jendso/bvab048.702

Bailey, T., Hastings, R. P., & Totsika, V. (2021). Covid-19 impact on Psychological Outcomes of Parents, Siblings and Children with Intellectual Disability: Longitudinal Before and During Lockdown Design. *Journal of Intellectual Disability Research*, *65*(5), 397–404. doi:10.1111/jir.12818 PMID:33634520

Bao, Y., Sun, Y., Meng, S., Shi, J., & Lu, L. (2020). 2019-nCoV Epidemic: Address Mental Health Care to Empower Society. *Lancet*, *395*(10224), e37–e38. doi:10.1016/S0140-6736(20)30309-3 PMID:32043982

Breaux, R., Dvorsky, M. R., Marsh, N. P., Green, C. D., Cash, A. R., Shroff, D. M., Buchen, N., Langberg, J. M., & Becker, S. P. (2021). Prospective impact of COVID-19 on mental health functioning in adolescents with and without ADHD: Protective role of emotion regulation abilities. *Journal of Child Psychology and Psychiatry, and Allied Disciplines*, *62*(9), 1132–1139. doi:10.1111/jcpp.13382 PMID:33543486

Cachón-Zagalaz, J. (2021). Systematic Review of the Literature About the Effects of the COVID-19 Pandemic on the Lives of School Children. *Frontiers in Psychology: Educational Psychology.* doi:10.3389/fpsyg.2020.569348

Chawla, N., & Tom, A. (2021). Psychological Impact of Covid-19 on Children and Adolescents: A Systematic Review. *Indian Journal of Psychological Medicine*, *43*(4), 294–299.

Cielo, F., Ulberg, R., & Giacomo, D. D. (2021). Psychological Impact of the Covid-19 Outbreak on Mental Health Outcomes among Youth: A Rapid Narrative Review. *International Journal of Environmental Research and Public Health*, *18*(6067), 1–15. doi:10.3390/ijerph18116067

Davico, C. (2021). Psychological Impact of the COVID-19 Pandemic on Adults and Their Children in Italy. *Frontiers in Psychiatry: Psychopathology.* doi:10.3389/fpsyt.2021.572997

Demaria, F. & Vicari, S. (2021). Covid 19 Quarantine: Psychological Impact and Support for Children and Parents. *Italian Journal of Paediatrics, 14*(58).

Fegert, J. M., & Schulze, U. M. E. (2020). Covid-19 and Impact on Child and Adolescent Psychiatry – a German and Personal Perspective. *Irish Journal of Psychological Medicine*, *37*(3), 234–245. doi:10.1017/ipm.2020.43 PMID:32404219

Hamoda, H.M. (2021). Addressing the Consequences of the COVID-19 Lockdown for Children's Mental Health: Investing in School Mental Health Programs. *Psychiatric Services, 202*(1), 729-731. . doi:10.1176/appi.ps.202000597

Jalloh, F. M., Li, W., Bunnell, R. E., Ethier, K. A., O'Leary, A., Hageman, K. M., Sengeh, P., Jalloh, M. B., Morgan, O., Hersey, S., Marston, B. J., Dafae, F., & Redd, J. T. (2018). Impact of Ebola Experiences and Risk Perceptions on Mental Health in Sierra Leone, July 2015. *BMJ Global Health*, *3*(2), e000471. doi:10.1136/bmjgh-2017-000471 PMID:29607096

Jalongo, R. M. (2021). The Effects of COVID 19 on Early Childhood Education and Care: Research and Resources for Children, Families, Teachers and Teacher Educators. *Early Childhood Education Journal*, *49*(5), 763–774. doi:10.100710643-021-01208-y PMID:34054286

James, P. B., Wardle, J., Steel, A., & Adams, J. (2019). Post-Ebola Psychosocial Experiences and Coping Mechanism among Ebola Survivors: A Systematic Review. *Tropical Medicine & International Health*, *24*(6), 671–691. doi:10.1111/tmi.13226 PMID:30843627

Janssen, L.H.C. (2020). Does the Covid-19 Pandemic impact parents' and adolescents' well-being? An EMA-study on daily effect and parenting. *Plus One.* doi:10.1371/journal.pone.0240962

Kaputu-Kala-Malu, C. (2021). PTSD, Depression and Anxiety in Ebola Virus Disease Survivors in Beni Town, Democratic Republic of Congo. *BMC Psychiatry*, *21*(342). PMID:34238249

Morelli, M., Cattelino, E., Baiocco, R., Trumello, C., Babore, A., Candelori, C., & Chirumbolo, A. (2020). Parents and Children During the Covid-19 Lockdown: The Influence of Parenting Distress and Parenting Self Efficacy on Children's Emotional Well-Being. *Health Psychology*, *11*, 584645. Advance online publication. doi:10.3389/fpsyg.2020.584645 PMID:33123063

Morgül, E., Kallitsoglou, A. & Essau, A.C. (2020). Psychological Effects of Covid-19 lockdown on Children and Families in the UK. *Revista de Psicología Clínica con Niños y Adolescentes*, *7*(3), 42–48. doi:10.21134/rpcna.2020.mon.2049

Nearchou, F., Flinn, C., Niland, R., Subramaniam, S. S., & Hennessy, E. (2020). Exploring the Impact of Covid-19 on Mental Health Outcomes in Children and Adolescents: A Systematic Review. *International Journal of Environmental Research and Public Health, 17*(22), 1–19. doi:10.3390/ijerph17228479 PMID:33207689

OECD. (2020). Combatting Covid-19's Effect on Children. *OECD Policy Responses to Coronavirus (COVID-19).* https://www.oecd.org/coronavirus/policy-responses/combatting-covid-19-s-effect-on-children-2e1f3b2f/

Pizarro-Ruiz, J. P., & Ordóñez-Camblor, N. (2021). Effects of Covid-19 Confinement on the Mental Health of Children and Adolescents in Spain. *Scientific Reports, 11*(11713), 11713. Advance online publication. doi:10.103841598-021-91299-9 PMID:34083653

Ravens-Sieberer, U., Kaman, A., Erhart, M., Devine, J., Schlack, R., & Otto, C. (2021). Impact of the COVID-19 Pandemic on Quality of Life and Mental Health in Children and Adolescents in Germany. *European Child & Adolescent Psychiatry, 1*, 3. doi:10.100700787-021-01726-5 PMID:33492480

Rodrigues, J. V. S. & Lins, A.C.A. (2020). Possible Impacts Caused by the Covid-19 Pandemic on Children's Mental Health and the Role of Parents in this Scenario. *Research, Society & Development, 9*(8).

Rohwerder, B. (2014). *Impact and Implications of the Ebola Crisis.* Applied Knowledge Services GSDRC Helpdesk Research Report 1177.

Schmidt, S., Barblan, L. P., Lory, I., & Landolt, M. A. (2021). Age-related effects of the COVID-19 pandemic on mental health of child8ren and adolescents. *European Journal of Psychotraumatology, 12*(1), 1–17. doi:10.1080/20008198.2021.1901407 PMID:34912501

Schnaiderman, D. (2021). Psychological impact of COVID-19 lockdown in children and adolescents from San Carlos de Bariloche, Argentina: Parents' perspective. *Archivos Argentinos de Pediatria, 119*(3), 170–176. PMID:34033416

Serge. (2021). Interviewing children: The impact of the COVID-19 quarantine on children's perceived Psychological distress and changes in routine. *BMC Pediatrics, 21*(231), 1–11. doi:10.118612887-021-02704-1 PMID:33985448

Shen, J. (2020). *Impact of the Covid-19 Pandemic on Children, Youth and Families.* A brief produced by the Evidence-Based Policy Institute.

Simon, J., Helter, T. M., White, R. G., van der Boor, C., & Łaszewska, A. (2021). Impacts of the Covid-19 Lockdown and Relevant Vulnerabilities on Capability Well- being, Mental Health and Social Support: An Austrian Survey Study. *BMC Public Health, 21*(314), 314. doi:10.118612889-021-10351-5 PMID:33557816

Singh, S. (2020). Impact of COVID-19 and lockdown on mental health of children and adolescents: A narrative review with recommendations. *Psychiatry Res, 293.* . doi:10.1016/j.psychres.2020.113429

Spiteri, J. (2021). The impact of the COVID-19 Pandemic on Children's Mental Health and Wellbeing, and Beyond: A Scoping Review. *Journal of Childhood, Education & Society, 2*(2), 126–138. doi:10.37291/2717638X.20212294

Sundarasen, S., Chinna, K., Kamaludin, K., Nurunnabi, M., Baloch, G. M., Khoshaim, H. B., Hossain, S. F. A., & Sukayt, A. (2020). Psychological Impact of COVID-19 and Lockdown among University Students in Malaysia: Implications and Policy Recommendation. *International Journal of Environmental Research and Public Health, 17*(6206), 1–13. doi:10.3390/ijerph17176206 PMID:32867024

UN. (2020). *The Impact of Covid-19 on Children.* Policy Brief. United Nations. https://unsdg.un.org/sites/default/files/2020-04/160420_Covid_Children_Policy_Brief.pdf

UNIC Press. (2017). *Nigeria: Southern Leaders Insist on New Constitution.* UNIC Press. https://unicpress.com/2017/09/07/nigeria-southern-leaders-insist-new-constitution/

Vardi, N. (2021). COVID-19 pandemic: Impacts on mothers' and infants' mental health during pregnancy and shortly thereafter. *Clinical Child Psychology and Psychiatry.* Advance online publication. doi:10.1177/13591045211009297 PMID:33855857

Viner, R. (2021). *Impacts of school closures on physical and mental health of children and young people: a systematic review.* MedReview., doi:10.1101/2021.02.10.21251526

Waite, P., Pearcey, S., Shum, A., Raw, J. A. L., Patalay, P., & Creswell, C. (2021). How did the mental health symptoms of children and adolescents change over early lockdown during the COVID-19 pandemic in the UK? *JCPP Advances: Child and Adolescent Mental Health, 1*(1), 1–10. doi:10.1111/jcv2.12009 PMID:34485988

Wigg, C. D. M., Coutinho, I. M. F. A., Silva, I. C., & Lopes, L. B. (2020). The Mental Health of Children and Adolescents During the Covid-19 Pandemic: A Narrative Review. *Research, Society and Development, 9*(9), 1–31. doi:10.33448/rsd-v9i9.7687

KEY TERMS AND DEFINITIONS

Adolescents: This refers to young person(s) growing into adulthood. It is the age of transition from being a child to being an adult (some posit that it is between 10 – 19 others opine that it is 13 - 19) and it comes with biological, mental, physical, and social changes. This chapter considers 13 – 19 as the age of adolescence.

Commodity Prices: This refers to the price of items or products like petroleum, cash crops and other commodities. The price of each at each point in time. The price of these items at the international market determines their prices.

COVID-19: The short form of the Coronavirus disease is an infectious disease caused by the SARS-CoV-2 virus. It is a highly contagious respiratory disease first discovered at the end of 2019 in Wuhan, China. Its symptoms include mild respiratory ailment, mild fever, or loss of sense of taste. It is spread through droplets and responsible for hundreds of thousands of deaths and millions of infections in many countries during its earliest waves.

Economic Ecology: This refers to the environment in which an economy exists and functions. The economic ecology could include the abstract and concrete environment with a geographical space. In the context used in this text, it covers the entire economic activities carried out within a geographical and political territory.

Fluctuations: This refers to unstable conditions. In the context in which it was used in this chapter, it means an unstable movement.

Obese: The word is from obesity which is used to refer to overweight. In the context in which it is used in this text, it refers to young overweight persons.

Psychological Behaviour: This has to do with mental attitude. It refers to the thoughts and the actions that follows. In the text, it refers to all actions connected to a mental perception, thought process and pattern of thoughts and actions.

Social Behaviour: This has to do with the person to person behaviour or interpersonal pattern of action and inaction. In the context of this chapter it refers to the interpersonal relationship exhibited by the subjects, students.

Chapter 8
The Effects of COVID-19-Imposed School Closures on Children

Ingrid Carla Brussier
The New School for Social Research, USA

ABSTRACT

This literature review investigates the numerous ways COVID-19-imposed school closures have impacted children, primarily in the United States. The pandemic forced schools to abruptly switch classes from an in-person to a remote-learning format. Remote learning, which is primarily conducted online, is predicted to significantly impact children's academic learning. In addition, this literature review considers the mental health implications of school closures in conjunction with pandemic-related stressors. Research across the world suggests that lockdowns and stressors caused by COVID-19 may lead to an increased risk of developing mood disorders among children. Also investigated are school closures, which have also disproportionately affected children from financially disadvantaged families. The impact of school closures on children's physical health is discussed since it has been predicted to raise childhood obesity. The adversities teachers encountered during this abrupt switch to online teaching and implications on their mental health are also investigated.

INTRODUCTION

The novel COVID-19 coronavirus has led to a worldwide health crisis which at the time of this review is responsible for a little over 570.000 deaths in the United States (CDC, 2021). The spread of this novel virus dramatically started in March

DOI: 10.4018/978-1-6684-3484-0.ch008

of 2020. At the end of March and the start of April of that year, approximately 1.5 billion learners worldwide, across 169 countries, were affected by school closures (Buonsenso, Roland, De Rose, Vásquez-Hoyos, Ramly, Chakakala-Chaziya, ... & González-Dambrauskas, S. 2021, p. 4). Remote learning was implemented as a tool to hinder the spread of the novel coronavirus. These global school closures led to an abrupt switch from in-person to remote online-learning. While researchers have now found that children were not "super-spreaders," the return back to in-person learning has been slow (Buonsenso et al., 2021).

This literature review will investigate the numerous ways in which school closures and the distress associated with a global pandemic has had on children. While research has shown that online schooling can be effective when planned accordingly, an abrupt switch has been found to have a negative impact on children's learning (Muller & Goldenberg, 2020). It is estimated that kindergarten-aged children will have lost approximately 67% of their average literacy gain during remote education between April 2020 and the end of that year's summer (Bao et al., 2020). These findings support that significant learning losses could come out of a short period of school closures. For this reason, it is essential to look at possible ways to mitigate these losses as schools reopen. This review also investigates the importance of parental academic and emotional support to help children navigate the stressors of online schooling and fears related to the ongoing health crisis.

Research overwhelmingly indicates that children living in poverty have been disproportionately affected by school closures. Statistical findings in the United States show that schools in poor areas were more likely to close and stay remote longer than those in wealthier neighborhoods (Parolin & Lee 2021). These differences in school closure rates indicate that the pandemic will most likely widen the already existing educational gap between economic classes. In addition, a lack of financial resources may impact children's ability to access necessary technological tools to appropriately participate in online learning (Lancker and Parolin, 2020). School closures have also exacerbated the difficulties faced by food-insecure children by making school-provided lunches challenging to access (Masonbrink & Hurley, 2020).

This review will also investigate the current projections of the effect of school closures on childhood obesity and weight gain in the United States. School closures have led to higher daily screen time and lower rates of daily physical activity. Findings suggest that children living in apartments are at particular risk for weight gain since they have the least amount of access to outdoor activities during lockdowns (Rundle, Park, Herbstman, Kinseym, & Wang, 2020). Before the pandemic, the U.S was already facing a childhood obesity crisis (Centre for Disease Control and Prevention, 2016). A simulation study found that the pandemic may result in an 11% rise in childhood obesity following school closure (Viner, Russell, Saulle, Croker, Stansfield, Packer, ... & Minozzi, 2021, p.9). This review will look at the health risks associated with childhood obesity and some of the actions taken by schools to help children engage in physical activities during remote learning. While these techniques may marginally help, the educational system must pursue strategies to mitigate the effects of school closures on children's health once classes are back to an in-person format.

The COVID-19 pandemic has also led to a mental health crisis worldwide, impacting both children and adults. The novel coronavirus has led to stress associated with fear of infections, social isolation, and financial insecurity (Brown, Doom, Lechuga-Peña, Lechuga-Peñ & Koppels, 2020). While this review does not investigate the rise of childhood maltreatment during COVID-19 lockdowns, it is essential to note that social isolation places children at a disproportionate risk of being maltreated. Brown et al. (2020) found that increased parental stress is linked to harsher parenting and a higher risk of maltreatment. The pandemic was a highly stressful time for many, suggesting that childhood maltreatment may have risen during 2020. The social isolation that comes with school closure also creates obstacles for school workers to notice signs of maltreatment, placing the safety of many children at risk. In addition, children are psychologically vulnerable to the stressors caused by the pandemic and to school closures (Imran, Zeshan, & Pervaiz, 2020). Some children may develop lasting mood or traumatic disorders due to their distress from lockdowns (Phelps & Sperry, 2020). This review investigates some of the covert signs of mental distress in young children and some tools that can be used to navigate pandemic-related stressors appropriately.

This review will also examine the effects of school closures on children with Attention Deficit-Hyperactivity Disorder (ADHD). Research suggests that school achievement and attitude towards schools have negatively impacted children with ADHD during remote learning (Kladias, 2021). Access to pharmaceutical treatment has been difficult during the lockdowns, leading to a worsening of ADHD symptoms (Cortese, Asherson, Sonuga-Barke, Banaschewski, Brandeis, Buitelaar, ... & Simonoff 2020). Lastly, this review will look at the effect of school closures on teaching and teachers' mental health. While the pandemic has led to an increase in children's mental distress, it has also dramatically affected teachers. Teachers are at particular risk for developing secondary traumatic stress, which occurs when witnessing others in distress while also wanting to help them (Muller & Goldenberg, 2020). Findings from the same researchers suggest that most teachers in the United States are not trained in supportive strategies to help children experiencing these novel traumatic experiences. A nationwide training of teachers in supportive techniques could make a significant difference in children with lasting effects of the mental distress caused by the pandemic.

ACADEMIC LOSSES

While most K-12 schools have reopened throughout the United States in 2021, the effects of school closures and remote learning on children's academic achievement remain unclear. It can be difficult to accurately assess the possible academic losses due to the recent occurrence of school closures. Some researchers have attempted to determine the potential adverse effects of momentary learning halts by looking at the impact of summer breaks, weather school closures, and student absenteeism (Kuhfeld, Soland, Tarasawa, Johnson, Liu, 2020, p.550). According to Kuhfeld et al. (2020), children lose, on average, a month of learning over a summer break. They also found that children seem to lose more mathematical knowledge than reading when classes are not in session. Kuhfeld et al. (2020) estimate that children who spent their spring semester learning remotely will lose between 32 and 37% of reading gains and 50 to 63% of mathematical gains compared to their peers who are learning in-person (p.549). They also note that socioeconomic status (SES) plays a significant role in assessing the effects of remote education and that lower SES may lead to more substantial losses in learning gains.

Bao et al. (2020) argue that Kuhfleld et al. (2020) underestimated the effectiveness of remote learning since they did not account for parental support. While virtual learning comes with numerous setbacks, Bao et al. (2020) suggest that spending more time with family could counter some educational losses linked to remote learning. They found that the lockdowns have led many parents to work from home while their child is learning remotely. While Bao et al. (2020) and Kuhfeld (2020) may have different outlooks on remote education, they agree that a significant loss in literacy will be linked to school closures. Bao et al. (2020) predict that kindergarten-aged children will lose up to 67% of literacy gains during remote learning over the spring and summer of 2020. These predictions are much more significant than Kuhfeld et al. (2020), probably because Kuhlfed et al. projected their findings on a broader range of school-aged children than Bao et al.'s (2020) focus on kindergarten-aged children.

Leppänen (2006) assessed kindergarten and school-aged children's development of literacy in Finland. She discovered that children who come across obstacles in their literacy learning process during the aforementioned ages will "fall behind in their reading skill development" (p11). Some of the challenges listed include a decrease in reading and practice. While remote learning creates a literacy obstacle for kindergarten-aged children, there may be ways to help mitigate these losses. Bao et al. (2020) suggest that a daily book-reading session between a child and their parent may help counteract the prediction of a 67% literacy loss by 31%. Bao et al.'s (2020) findings show that offering simple daily literacy exercises to children may significantly improve their learning gains during remote learning. While current research remains unclear of the possible lasting effects of school closures on literacy learning in children, it is essential to note that parental support, guidance, and supervision can make a tremendous difference in a child's experience with remote learning.

PARENTAL SUPPORT

Educational support through reading exercises and homework from parental presence can help mitigate some of the adverse effects of online learning. However, many families have to navigate a long list of pandemic-related stressors while also supervising their children's education at home, making parental support difficult for many. Gabe, Ogulu, Logan, and Cook (2020) conducted a study investigating the experience of a sample of 122, primarily upper-middle-class, parents. They found that the most commonly reported struggle was balancing work time and the monitoring of their child's remote learning. Many reported feeling guilty for choosing between their child's education and their employment (p.51). Another common problem encountered by the parents was their lack of "personal balance," meaning their ability to have personal time outside of work hours and parenting (p.51). Participants noted that they were overwhelmed by the number of responsibilities that came with supporting their children through remote learning while also working remotely themselves. These obstacles found by Gabe et al. (2020) may suggest that overwhelmed parents could be less likely to take the extra time to read a book with their child or help them with additional school work at the end of the day to help mitigate the adverse effects of remote learning. Gabe et al.'s (2020) study is limited by its poor diversity in participant's socioeconomic status (SES). Families from lower SES have to face a broader range of obstacles: employment insecurity, unstable financial resources, lack of internet access, and the inability to stay at home while their children are doing remote learning. While the middle-class demographic assessed by Gabe et al. (2020) has faced difficulties during the quarantine of the first wave, families from lower SES have had to face many more obstacles during lockdowns.

CHILDREN FROM FINANCIALLY DISADVANTAGED ENVIRONMENTS

School closures have affected children living under the poverty line in a multitude of ways. The pandemic caused 30 million people to lose their employment between March and May 2020 in the U.S, which placed many families in an unstable financial situation (Azevedo, Hasan, Goldemberg, Iqbal, and Geven, 2020, p. 623). Financial difficulties that come with unemployment, such as the inability to pay bills, rent, or to have adequate food, can negatively impact a child's remote learning (Azevedo et al., 2020). In addition to these obstacles, Masonbrink and Hurley (2020) found that 35 million children in the United States relied on nutrition programs typically offered by schools for food access. As a result of school closures during the spring semester of 2020, those children lost their access to a secure daily meal. Masonbrink and Hurley (2020) also found that in April 2020, 35% of households with children under eighteen were food insecure (p.4). Eleven percent of those families reported not being able to access take-home lunches offered by schools. While these problems may not directly influence children's academics, food insecurity is a grave problem, and school closures created a major obstacle for children living with hunger.

Children in financially disadvantaged families were also disproportionately affected by school closures due to their lack of resources. Those who did not have internet access, an appropriate learning environment, or faced homelessness were greatly impaired in their ability to participate in remote learning. These issues have impacted children worldwide. According to Lancker and Parolin (2020), 5% of European children did not live in a home appropriate for remote learning, 5% could not access books at their reading level, and 6 to 9% did not have access to the internet. These findings suggest that financially disadvantaged European children may have suffered significant learning losses due to their inability to follow classes appropriately while their schooling was remote. While Lancker and Parolin (2020) do not touch on the possible ways of rectifying these disparities, Azevedo et al. (2020) investigated the steps taken by the U.S education system to help children during school closures. Schools were able to buy and distribute laptops and wifi-hotspots through the CARES Act Grants and budgetary changes. While many rural areas provided technological support to their students, urban areas such as Cleveland had a more difficult time due its high density of population living under the poverty line. According to Salvin and Storey (2020), the city could only distribute supporting materials to 25% of their students in need. They also found that 40% of the most impoverished U.S children only accessed online classes once a week (p.623). These statistics highlight that even with financial help and a large-scale aid plan, certain school districts could not offer the necessary resources to their students. Those students who could not access regular online classes are most likely to fall behind in their learning and may have long-lasting learning losses as a result (Salvin and Storey, 2020).

School closures have also disproportionately negatively affected healthcare access for children in poverty (Masonbrink and Hurley, 2020). Masonbrink and Hurley (2020) have found that six million students in the United States rely uniquely on school health services for primary and preventive care (p. 5). While some school-based healthcare services switched to telehealth practice, children lacking technological resources may have been unable to access these services. Telehealth does not offer complete health screenings adequate for children, which is problematic. Masonbrink and Hurley (2020) suggest that schools should reach out and provide technological support to children and their families (p.5). However, as seen above, it can be difficult for schools in urban areas with dense poverty rates to help all children in need.

Children from a low socioeconomic status will be disproportionately affected by the financial impact of COVID-19 and school closures. Sadly, those children have had to face school closures the most throughout this pandemic (Parolin & Lee 2021). Parolin and Lee (2021) investigated an extensive data analysis of school closure rates in the United States from April to December 2020. They found that schools that scored the lowest in 3rd-grade math performance were 15% more likely to close between September and December 2020 than those who scored average on those tests. In conjunction with these results, they found that children from racial and ethnic minorities and those who experience homelessness were the most likely to experience school closures during the Fall semester. Seventy percent of schools with the lowest rate of white students were closed during the latter half of the year, while only 35% of primarily white schools were closed. Lastly, schools with the highest rate of free or reduced-price lunches were the most likely to close. These results suggest that the pandemic will widen the educational and health disparities between privileged and underprivileged backgrounds.

MENTAL HEALTH

The COVID-19 pandemic has led to a worldwide mental health crisis, which has impacted both adults and children. The isolation that comes with national and regional sporadic lockdowns can be challenging to navigate for both parents and children (Gabe et al., 2020). According to research conducted in China, 30% of children who experienced isolation from parents during the COVID-19 quarantine fit the clinical diagnostic criteria for post-traumatic stress disorder (Liu et al., 2020). In addition to these findings, research suggests that children who had gone through quarantine (not necessarily isolated from their parents) were four times more likely to develop Post-Traumatic Stress Disorder (PTSD) symptoms than children who were never quarantined (Imran, Zeshan, & Pervaiz, 2020). Liu et al. (2020) also found that those children were at a higher risk of developing mood disorders and psychosis, which is why taking active steps to help children cope with the psychological stress of isolation is critical.

The pandemic has affected children beyond the impact of remote learning on their education. Children have had to navigate disease, parental stress, and social isolation during lockdowns and school closures (Imran, Zeshan, & Pervaiz, 2020). These stressors are anxiety-inducing, and it can be difficult for parents to understand the depth of a child's distress due to a possible lack of communication. According to Imran et al. (2020), clinginess, distraction, and irritability are among the most common behavioral signs of mental distress in younger children. Often, these behavioral issues can be mistaken for temper tantrums or misbehavior (Imran et al., 2020), which can mislead parents into taking the wrong measures while attempting to resolve the child's conduct. Regressive behaviors and clinginess are also frequent signs of mental distress in a child and should be taken seriously.

Those suffering from pre-existing mental conditions such as anxiety, depression, and obsessive-compulsive disorder (OCD) are the most at risk for severe mental distress in response to pandemic-related stressors (Imran et al. 2020). Imran et al. (2020) proposed a list of ways to mitigate the effects of the pandemic on children's mental health. Setting up a daily routine, increased parental physical and verbal affection, and avoidance of pandemic-related topics are some of the interventions proposed by the researchers to help ease distress in younger children. School closures brought children home into a completely new academic environment in which they did not have a routine. Creating a structure around play, work, and meal times reinforces a sense of security and normalcy. Lastly, while avoiding conversations around the pandemic can be helpful, it is crucial to allow open communication on the crisis at hand. To create safe communication, Imran et al. (2020) note that parents should speak with developmentally appropriate words to avoid further confusion and stress. While staying realistic on the possibility of future illness in the family, reassuring them that everything will be okay is essential. In conclusion, parents must be aware of the covert behavioral signs of mental distress in younger children and the parenting techniques that can help their children mentally cope with some of the COVID-19 stressors.

EFFECTS ON HEALTH

School closures have significantly impacted children's ability to exercise. Remote learning has dramatically increased daily rates of screen time and has forced children to stay in their homes throughout most of the day. A Spanish investigation of the effects of lockdowns found that children's frequency of screen time use had risen by 2.9 hours, a 245% increase from the preceding year (Viner., Russell, Saulle, Croker, Stansfield, Packer, ... & Minozzi, 2021, p.9). Children living in urban areas, who live in apartment buildings and have limited access to the outdoors, are at a higher risk for decline in their mental and physical health (Rundle, Park, Herbstman, Kinseym, & Wang, 2020). Rundle et al. (2020) investigated the risk of weight gain due to school closures and found that high rates of daily screen time are correlated with childhood obesity. Online schooling has led to children spending more time viewing screens throughout the day, which could consequently lead to a higher risk for weight gain and childhood obesity. In conjunction with the lack of access to safe outdoor space in cities, these findings suggest that children living in urban areas are at a much greater risk for weight gain during school closures. Rundle et al. (2020) also note that families throughout the United States stocked up on highly processed, calorie-dense, shelf-stable foods in the early months of the pandemic. These findings may indicate that many children ate a high-calorie diet during lockdown with little to no daily exercise, leading to a possible unhealthy weight gain. As noted earlier, 35% of families with children under eighteen were food insecure in April 2020. Rundle et al. (2020) mentioned in their research that food insecurity is linked to childhood obesity, placing children living in poverty at a further disproportionate risk for weight gain due to the pandemic.

Viner et al. (2021) note in their systematic review that a microsimulation study suggested that two months of school closures in the United States would raise childhood obesity by 11.1% percent (p.9). These findings are alarming since the United States was already experiencing a childhood obesity crisis prior to the pandemic (CDC, 2021). According to the Center for Disease Control (CDC) (2021), 19.3% of children and adolescents between the ages of 2 and 19 were obese in 2017-2018. Some of the physical risk factors of childhood obesity are high blood pressure, diabetes, breathing problems, and fatty liver disease (CDC, 2021), which are serious health conditions. If Viner et al.'s (2021) findings are correct, school closures will have played a significant role in the rise of childhood obesity in the United States. Some schools around the country have taken the initiative to send exercise plans to their students and move physical education classes to an online format (Rundle et al., 2020). Strategies like these could make an impactful difference by offering structured directions to their students, motivating them to move around in their homes. Although these initiatives can help mitigate some physical activity losses, it is essential to keep in mind that there are limitations to their effectiveness, especially in children living in small apartments where indoor exercises can be challenging. The consequences of school closures on the increased prevalence of childhood obesity in the U.S. remains unclear as school re-openings have only recently begun. Extending physical education class hours once the pandemic is under control could help mitigate the negative impact of school closures on the rise of childhood obesity.

TEACHING REMOTELY AND MENTAL HEALTH IMPLICATIONS ON TEACHERS

The school closures around the United States forced teachers to switch their teaching methods from in-person classes to an online format. According to Muller and

Goldenberg (2020), remote learning can be effective in many situations, especially when the courses are designed and planned to be taught online. However, during the abrupt switch to remote learning, teachers around the country had to quickly transfer their lesson plan into an online format. Muller and Goldenberg (2020) found through a literature review that teachers used strategies that have been shown to have a high remote learning efficacy. Some of those tactics were: "peer marking, live discussion content, and sharing models of good work" (p.16). In addition to these strategies, teachers who offered clear explanations of their expectations through checklists to their students were much more effective during remote learning. On the other hand, self-quizzing and computer-generated instructions were found to be less effective during remote teaching (Muller & Goldenberg, 2020, p.16).

In addition to the logistical issues faced when abruptly changing teaching formats, teachers also had to navigate both their own and their student's pandemic-induced stress. Muller and Goldenberg (2020) found that although teachers generally have a good understanding of their students' needs and well-being, they are not prepared to support students during traumatic events (p.22). The study in question looked at teachers' abilities to help a child experiencing grief since they had never gone through any training for such situations. Results indicated that most teachers did not have the necessary tools to help a child in mental distress caused by trauma. Muller and Goldenberg (2020) believe that teacher's unpreparedness to help children through traumatic events can be applied to the COVID-19 health crisis. Children across the U.S have had to face the traumatic experience of the pandemic and, for some, the death of family members. As those students return to school, many could still be in mental distress from stressors caused by the pandemic. As noted earlier, children who have undergone quarantine are four times more likely to develop PTSD than those who have not (Imran et al.,2020). Many of those children will be returning to school; still struggling with their pandemic-related trauma. Offering teachers the ability to be trained in supportive approaches to help students in distress, could make a significant difference for children's transition back to in-person classes. According to Muller and Goldenberg (2020), there are five strategies that can help teachers support children in distress: "being attuned, converting positive regard, collaborating with families and professionals, supporting positive socio-emotional and communicative responses, and rethinking reactions to behavior" (p.23). A large-scale implementation of teacher training could offer educators the necessary tools to appropriately help students during these challenging times. While support within the family sphere is important, offering additional emotional support could make a significant difference. According to Muller and Goldenberg (2020), research suggests that trauma caused by disasters can have long-lasting effects on children's socio-emotional and academic development (p.6). For this reason, it is important to offer children the largest possible supportive network to help avoid lasting effects.

The impact of the pandemic on teachers' mental health is also a crucial topic to examine. According to Muller and Goldenberg (2020), teachers are at a risk for developing secondary traumatic stress as a result of the pandemic. Secondary traumatic stress occurs when one hears of someone else's traumatic experience and wants to help that person through his/her distress, also known as "compassion fatigue or vicarious traumatization" (Muller and Goldenberg, 2020, p. 26). Secondary traumatic stress has been associated with burnouts, emotional exhaustion, and an increased risk of tobacco and alcohol use. Burn outs are caused by long-lasting occupational stress, they manifest themselves through "feelings of fatigue, and feeling drained of emotional and physical resources" in addition to a depersonalization that can make teachers "negative, irritable, and cynical towards students" (Oberle & Schonert- Reichl, 2016, p.31). According to research conducted by Oberle & Schonert- Reichl (2016), burnout in teachers is linked to "stress contagion," which is an effect that occurs when one's stress can spread to others around them. After assessing 406 middle school teachers, they found that students of teachers with high burnout levels had the highest amount of salivary cortisol. High cortisol levels are linked to high stress, which indicates that a teacher's occupational stress may be "contagious" to others. While these findings are significant, Oberle and Schonert-Reichl (2016) note that there is a possibility that children's higher cortisol levels could be the reason for teacher's higher occupational stress. In either case, it can be concluded that stress in classrooms seems to be "contagious," which stresses the importance of training teachers in coping and supportive strategies. In addition, offering psychological support to teachers within the education system is important for their own well-being and for the well-being of their students.

CHILDREN WITH ATTENTION DEFICIT HYPERACTIVITY DISORDER

Attention Deficit-Hyperactivity Disorder (ADHD) is a neurodevelopmental disorder that affects approximately 6.1 million, or 9.4% of children between the ages of 2 and 17 in the United States, according to a 2016 survey (Center for Disease Control and Prevention, 2016) (Kladias, 2021). The fifth edition of the Diagnostic and Statistical Manual of Mental Disorders (American Psychiatric Association, 2013) lists ADHD's first diagnostic criteria as "a persistent pattern of inattention and/or hyperactivity-impulsivity that interferes with functioning or development" (p.59). Some common symptoms are difficulty paying attention to conversations, tasks, homework, details, and the inability to calmly stay put during long periods of time (p. 59-60). Physical restlessness, which manifests itself through inappropriate running and fidgeting, is also a common symptom of ADHD.

The symptomatology of ADHD could create obstacles in effectively navigating a remote educational format. The DSM V states that ADHD symptoms interfere with social, academic, and occupational functioning (p.60), which could all be exacerbated by online schooling and social distancing. According to Kladias's (2021) research on the impact of the COVID-19 pandemic on children with ADHD, online learning may exacerbate or initiate a dislike for school. Parental reports indicated that the academic achievement of children with ADHD lowered during remote learning. Kladias (2020) notes that remote learning can be effective with children diagnosed with ADHD if parents can offer resources and support during at-home schooling. Some parents may not have the time or the financial ability to provide adequate assistance to their children daily, which could also exacerbate the negative impact of online schooling on their child's academic achievement. Kladias (2021) also found that a parent-child perceived emotional closeness positively affects ADHD diagnosed children's attitude and achievement during traditional schooling. On the other hand, his findings suggest that perceived emotional closeness does not have an impact on the academic achievements of children with ADHD in the context of remote learning. Kladias (2021) notes that his results could indicate that emotional closeness between parents and their children does not have a mitigating effect on the negative impact of online schooling.

Cortese et al. (2020) suggest a list of guidelines that could help parents and children with an ADHD diagnosis during the trying times caused by the COVID-19 pandemic. They found that prescribed medication should be taken as prescribed and to avoid antipsychotic medication since doing the opposite could exacerbate the stress of confinement (paragraph 5). Cortese et al. (2020) also note that children who were newly diagnosed with ADHD before the pandemic could face difficulties starting a pharmacological treatment due to a lack of healthcare access caused by lockdown measures. This obstacle to treatment could worsen the negative effects of school closures and social isolation. A study conducted in China by Zhang, Shuai, Yu, Wang, Qiu, Lu, & Chen, R (2020) discovered that parents who had difficulty accessing psychiatric medication for their children, showing that countries worldwide have had similar issues. Maintaining a routine, and more specifically, a set sleep schedule, is helpful in such conditions since it helps create a sense of structure and mitigates some of the symptoms associated with ADHD (Cassoff, Wiebe, & Gruber, R, 2012). In addition, offering parents supportive strategies for their children to increase their child's wellbeing through telehealth training programs could be an effective way to lower the negative impact of the COVID-19 lockdowns (Pecor, Barbyannis, Yang, Johnson, Materasso, Borda, ... & Ming, 2021).

While parental support can play a crucial role in helping children with ADHD during the pandemic, schools can also help them through their services. A report of the U.S educational response to COVID-19 by Storey and Slavin (2020) states that some schools have had difficulties providing the aids and assistance needed for children with disabilities. Those services are required to be offered by schools under the Individuals with Disabilities Act (Salvin & Storey, 2020, p.621). As a response to these adversities, the education system employed special education teachers to virtually help parents in need by teaching them practices that could aid their children. In addition, many students were offered the ability to use technological aids through access to screen-reading software (Salvin & Storey, 2020, p.622). Support from the educational system has allowed many children with learning disabilities, such as ADHD, to navigate online learning obstacles.

In conclusion, the isolation, remote learning, and health stressors caused by the pandemic could worsen ADHD symptoms as well as their academic achievements. While it may seem that mitigating these effects is difficult, making sure that children have the appropriate pharmaceutical treatment, a regular sleep schedule, and support are essential.

DISCUSSION

Since the COVID-19 pandemic has affected 89% of learners around the world through school closures and delays, it is critical to take a close look at its impact on academic learning and mental health (Buonsenso et al., 2021). While it is too soon to know the full extent of school closures' effects, we know that some will be long-lasting for some children. As noted earlier, the anticipated literacy losses in kindergarten-aged children are significant enough to have a lasting negative impact on future literacy learning (Leppänen, 2006) (Bao et al., 2020). In addition to these losses, children have had to face particularly distressing times due to pandemic-related stressors. Researchers found that children who had experienced lockdowns were four times more likely to develop PTSD symptoms than those who had not (Imran et al., 2020). Imran et al. (2020) also showed that children with pre-existing mood disorders were at a greater risk for severe mental distress due to pandemic-related stressors. These findings indicate a great risk for long-lasting psychological effects in children, which is why it is essential to take protective steps when coming back into in-person schooling. Both teachers and parents should be given the necessary tools through training to help their children navigate their feelings of distress. As discussed in this literature review, parents can be taught ways to help their children if they are in distress through telehealth training from professional counselors (Pecor et al., 2021). Training can teach teachers emotional support strategies for children in significant distress, which can help the reintegration process into in-person learning.

Weight gain and childhood obesity are also possible long-lasting effects of the pandemic on children's wellbeing. A simulation study found that childhood obesity would rise by 11.1% following two months of remote schooling (Viner et al., 2020, p.9). If these predictions are correct, this sharp rise will be a consequence of a lack of physical activity, increased daily hours of screen time, and a rise in food insecurity primarily linked to school closures and nationwide lockdowns (Rundle et al. 2020). Schools can attempt to counter this rise in weight gain by offering home exercise plans, highly nutritional school lunches, and additional physical education classes once schools are fully open.

Research has also shown that children with ADHD and their parents have had difficulty navigating the switch from in-person to remote learning. Online schooling seems to negatively impact children's academic achievements as well as their attitudes toward school. When coming back into in-person learning, these effects might dissipate over time; however, it is essential to give those children adequate academic support if they have experienced significant learning losses.

Finally, children living in poverty are by far the most negatively impacted by the school closures. Financial difficulties caused by the rise in unemployment throughout the United States due to the pandemic have placed children in a difficult position (Azevedo et al., 2020). Parents struggling with unemployment or who were essential workers at the peak of the pandemic may not have had the time to offer necessary academic and emotional support during remote learning. Many children did not have internet access or the technological tools necessary for appropriate online schooling (Salvin & Storey, 2020). Even with the help of schools through the distribution of laptops and wifi-hotspots, all children in need were not able to access those resources (Salvin & Storey, 2020). Food-insecure children are also at a higher risk of developing childhood obesity. School closures and the loss of school-supplied lunches could place them at a disproportionate risk of weight gain than food-secure children (Rundle et al., 2020). School closures in less privileged communities will most likely lead to a widening of the educational gap between economic classes (Parolin & Lee 2021). The U.S education system needs to place the needs of schools from those who are financially disadvantaged at the forefront of their attempt to minimize the losses from online schooling.

FUTURE DIRECTIONS

The COVID-19 pandemic has had a negative impact on children in numerous ways. Future research should be aimed at assessing the extent of school closure's effect on mental and physical health, as well as on their academic achievements. Longitudinal studies investigating the disparities between children who have never experienced emergency remote learning and those who have, would allow us to better understand the impact of school closures. The alarming findings from Bao et al. (2020) predict that kindergarten children will have lost approximately 67% of their expected literacy gains due to school closures. It would be interesting to look at the actual losses and how they affected further literacy learning in the following year.

REFERENCES

American Psychiatric Association. (2013). *Diagnostic and statistical manual of mental disorders* (5th ed.). Author.

Azevedo, J. P., Hasan, A., Goldemberg, D., Iqbal, S. A., & Geven, K. (2020). *Simulating the potential impacts of COVID-19 school closures on schooling and learning outcomes: A set of global estimates*. The World Bank.

Bao, X., Qu, H., Zhang, R., & Hogan, T. P. (2020). *Literacy Loss in Kindergarten Children during COVID-19 School Closures*. Academic Press.

Brown, S. M., Doom, J. R., Lechuga-Peña, S., Watamura, S. E., & Koppels, T. (2020). Stress and parenting during the global COVID-19 pandemic. *Child Abuse & Neglect*, *110*, 104699. doi:10.1016/j.chiabu.2020.104699 PMID:32859394

Cassoff, J., Wiebe, S. T., & Gruber, R. (2012). Sleep patterns and the risk for ADHD: A review. *Nature and Science of Sleep*, *4*, 73. PMID:23620680

Centers for Disease Control and Prevention. (2020, November 16). *Data and Statistics About ADHD*. Centers for Disease Control and Prevention. https://www.cdc.gov/ncbddd/adhd/data.html

Centers for Disease Control and Prevention. (2021, April 5). *Childhood Obesity Facts*. Centers for Disease Control and Prevention. https://www.cdc.gov/obesity/data/childhood.html

Cortese, S., Asherson, P., Sonuga-Barke, E., Banaschewski, T., Brandeis, D., Buitelaar, J., Coghill, D., Daley, D., Danckaerts, M., Dittmann, R. W., Doepfner, M., Ferrin, M., Hollis, C., Holtmann, M., Konofal, E., Lecendreux, M., Santosh, P., Rothenberger, A., Soutullo, C., ... Simonoff, E. (2020). ADHD management during the COVID-19 pandemic: Guidance from the European ADHD Guidelines Group. *The Lancet. Child & Adolescent Health*, *4*(6), 412–414. doi:10.1016/S2352-4642(20)30110-3 PMID:32311314

Garbe, A., Ogurlu, U., Logan, N., & Cook, P. (2020). Parents' experiences with remote education during COVID-19 school closures. *American Journal of Qualitative Research*, *4*(3), 45–65.

Imran, N., Zeshan, M., & Pervaiz, Z. (2020). Mental health considerations for children & adolescents in COVID-19 Pandemic. *Pakistan Journal of Medical Sciences, 36*(S4), S67.

Kladias, A. (2021). *Parent-Child Relationships and Student Outcomes in Children: A Comparison Before and During the COVID-19 Pandemic* (Doctoral dissertation). Otterbein University.

Kuhfeld, M., Soland, J., Tarasawa, B., Johnson, A., Ruzek, E., & Liu, J. (2020). Projecting the potential impact of COVID-19 school closures on academic achievement. *Educational Researcher, 49*(8), 549–565. doi:10.3102/0013189X20965918

Leppänen, U. (2006). *Development of literacy in kindergarten and primary school* (No. 289). Jyväskylän yliopisto.

Liu, J. J., Bao, Y., Huang, X., Shi, J., & Lu, L. (2020). Mental health considerations for children quarantined because of COVID-19. *The Lancet. Child & Adolescent Health, 4*(5), 347–349. doi:10.1016/S2352-4642(20)30096-1 PMID:32224303

Masonbrink, A. R., & Hurley, E. (2020). Advocating for children during the COVID-19 school closures. *Pediatrics, 146*(3), e20201440. doi:10.1542/peds.2020-1440 PMID:32554517

Müller, L. M., & Goldenberg, G. (2020). *Education in times of crisis: The potential implications of school closures for teachers and students. A review of research evidence on school closures and international approaches to education during the COVID-19 pandemic*. Chartered College of Teaching.

N., & González-Dambrauskas, S. (2021). Schools closures during the covid-19 pandemic: a catastrophic global situation. *The Pediatric Infectious Disease Journal, 40*(4), e146-e150.

Oberle, E., & Schonert-Reichl, K. A. (2016). Stress contagion in the classroom? The link between classroom teacher burnout and morning cortisol in elementary school students. *Social Science & Medicine, 159*, 30–33. doi:10.1016/j.socscimed.2016.04.031 PMID:27156042

Parolin, Z., & Lee, E. K. (2021). Large socio-economic, geographic and demographic disparities exist in exposure to school closures. *Nature Human Behaviour, 5*(4), 522–528. doi:10.103841562-021-01087-8 PMID:33737734

Pecor, K. W., Barbyannis, G., Yang, M., Johnson, J., Materasso, S., Borda, M., ... Ming, X. (2021). Quality of Life Changes during the COVID-19 Pandemic for Caregivers of Children with ADHD and/or ASD. *International Journal of Environmental Research and Public Health, 18*(7), 3667. doi:10.3390/ijerph18073667 PMID:33915884

Phelps, C., & Sperry, L. L. (2020). Children and the COVID-19 pandemic. *Psychological Trauma: Theory, Research, Practice, and Policy, 12*(S1), S73–S75. doi:10.1037/tra0000861 PMID:32525366

Rundle, A. G., Park, Y., Herbstman, J. B., Kinsey, E. W., & Wang, Y. C. (2020). COVID-19–related school closings and risk of weight gain among children. *Obesity (Silver Spring, Md.), 28*(6), 1008–1009. doi:10.1002/oby.22813 PMID:32227671

Slavin, R. E., & Storey, N. (2020). The US educational response to the COVID-19 pandemic. *Best Evid Chin Edu, 5*(2), 617–633. doi:10.15354/bece.20.or027

Van Lancker, W., & Parolin, Z. (2020). COVID-19, school closures, and child poverty: A social crisis in the making. *The Lancet. Public Health, 5*(5), e243–e244. doi:10.1016/S2468-2667(20)30084-0 PMID:32275858

Viner, R. M., Russell, S., Saulle, R., Croker, H., Stansfield, C., Packer, J., & Minozzi, S. (2021). *Impacts of school closures on physical and mental health of children and young people: a systematic review*. MedRxiv., doi:10.1101/2021.02.10.21251526

Zhang, J., Shuai, L., Yu, H., Wang, Z., Qiu, M., Lu, L., Cao, X., Xia, W., Wang, Y., & Chen, R. (2020). Acute stress, behavioural symptoms and mood states among school-age children with attention-deficit/hyperactive disorder during the COVID-19 outbreak. *Asian Journal of Psychiatry, 51*, 102077. doi:10.1016/j.ajp.2020.102077 PMID:32315967

Chapter 9
Erikson's Stages:
The Impact COVID-19 Has Had on Childhood Develeopment

Ariana Lopez
Marymount Manhattan College, USA

ABSTRACT

This chapter will take a closer look at the COVID-19 pandemic and its underlying effects on human development in relation to Erik Erikson's psychosocial stages of development. Erikson developed his eight stages of psychosocial development in 1950, and they have been used as development benchmarks ever since. The authors look at trust vs. mistrust and the inability of some parents to adequately care for their children in the current climate, followed by autonomy vs. shame and doubt and the lack of independence children may have been able to experience. Thirdly is initiative vs. guilt and the inability children had to develop curiosity about the world. The final stage of childhood, industry vs. inferiority, has been affected by the restriction of social interaction. The fifth stage is identity vs. role confusion, which is a time that has been plagued by an onset of increased substance use and abuse. We then see the first stage of adulthood, intimacy and solidarity vs. isolation, in which many have been unable to marry or start families. This continues into middle adulthood, generativity vs. self-absorption or stagnation, during which many have been either unable to start a family or have suddenly been unable to care for their families. The final stage in late adulthood, integrity vs. despair, has been impacted by isolated seniors forced into retirement or isolation in homes. Despite each developmental stage being affected by this pandemic, the authors are hopeful that by educating ourselves about our own development and our immediate environments, we will be able to nurture its continuing growth.

DOI: 10.4018/978-1-6684-3484-0.ch009

INTRODUCTION

For psychoanalyst Erik Erikson, the area of most interest was the human brain and its development from fetus to adulthood. Erikson drew from neurologist Sigmund Freud's Theory of Psychosexual Development and expanded childhood stages to four, which incorporated the influence of the social environment surrounding each respective stage, as well as the psychosocial developmental path to adulthood. The end result was eight chronological stages which encompass one's biological, psychological, and social influences throughout development.

The first stage is infancy, followed by early childhood as Stage Two; then comes the play age, Stage Three, and Stage Four: the school age. Afterwards, the child continues into young adolescence with Stage Five and young adulthood as Stage Six. At this point, the person reaches Stage Seven, adulthood, and finally, old age, Stage Eight. Each stage is accompanied by a series of developmental milestones that are expected to occur at that said time, based on years of research on the interactions between biological and social influences. However, what happens when society as we know it is drastically altered? Society has been changed several times in the last hundred years, including the Second World War, the end of segregation, and the Women's Rights Movement. However, nothing was quite as universally impactful as the Coronavirus Pandemic of 2020. It was felt nearly all at once globally, equalizing the experience for all humanity. The COVID-19 pandemic is believed to have begun in late 2019 in Wuhan, China, and to this day remains one of the most impactful events in society. The uncontrollable spread of the coronavirus has infected over 153 million people and has killed over 3.2 million as of this writing (Centers for Disease Control and Prevention, 2021) so far, making it the deadliest virus since the influenza pandemic of the late 1960s. This, of course, caused mass hysteria in countries all over the world, landing society in global quarantines or a "pause," during which billions of people were asked to stay in their homes, to leave only when absolutely necessary and to wear a face covering and remain six feet away from all other people when they must go into public space. This was a significant culture shock, since it drastically changed everyday life nearly overnight. It kept people working from home and spending all of their time in their homes, rarely interacting with anyone in person. While the effects on mental health were commonly discussed, the developmental effects this would cause on the population, received less consideration. Most theories like Erikson's are based on a "normally" functioning society, similar to the world before the pandemic. What happens to these developmental changes and milestone stages when the society and the environment change overnight?

STAGE 1: TRUST VERSUS MISTRUST

In order to begin exploring the impact the COVID-19 pandemic had on human development, it is significant to take a look at Erikson's first stage, Trust vs. Mistrust, which occurs during infancy and continues until about 18 months old. This is considered to be the most crucial stage, since it sets the child's personality and views of the surrounding world. During this time, children are completely dependent on their caregivers to supply them with everything they need, including being fed, washed, and loved. Receiving these things builds trust in those caregivers, as well as a feeling of safety and security. On the other hand, not having their needs met by caregivers can result in distrust of them, and subsequently, distrust of the world. This differentiation is generally where people are able to predict if a child will be capable of forming trusting relationships throughout his/her life. While this stage primarily involves a child's immediate caretakers rather than the surrounding society, it would appear as if development in this stage would be very mildly affected by the pandemic. In recent research looking specifically into developmental disruptions during these trying times, scientists are able to discern that the pandemic has actually brought about more factors than ever that could affect this developmental milestone (Rafanelli, 2019).

For one, there is the working parent, who normally would have outside assistance in childcare while he/she was at work, something which, for most people, did not pause but simply readjusted. The inability to have additional caregivers for a child could significantly impact the frequency of one-on-one interactions, care, and the ability to meet urgent needs. Additionally, there are the emotional and physical effects the virus could cause parents to consider, including fear or anxiety about the pandemic, causing parents to become depressed or anxious to the point of an inability to function. This could also mean having to care for family or friends who have contracted the illness, such as grandparents, and having to choose between caring for dying relatives and putting their children at risk. This could also come about if one of the parents becomes sick inside the home: how that affects the other parent, if there is one, and the child, having half the usual number of caregivers. Of course, one would hope these situations could be limited, but the reality is that its unpredictability has exposed many issues for which parents were not prepared, at the very least, causing immense life stress, which can also affect the child. The literature suggests that the developmental outcome will have effects similar to those noted from previous outbreaks such as SARS and H1N1. Children born and developing at the time showed less than optimal adjustment and struggled with anxiety, depression, and PTSD (Sprang, 2013). COVID-19, as with previous pandemics, has also left a substantial economic downfall in its wake, which also correlates with child development. Financial difficulties have been linked to a series of problems for children, including behavioral problems during infancy, self-efficacy, and confidence issues (Benner et al., 2020). The first eighteen months of life, during which children are the most dependent, is also arguably the most difficult time for parents, as well. Couple that with the mental and financial difficulties of a global pandemic, and it could become a very challenging situation for a caregiver. The inability to care can directly impact the baby and could leave the baby feeling uncared for, leading to long-term behavioral issues. In a recent study conducted during the COVID-19 pandemic, researchers found that over 32% of adults were overweight and 34% were obese, in a sample of 7,753 adults. In addition, anxiety scores increased by 8.78% during the pandemic (Flanagan et al., 2020). Statistics of declining physical and mental health in adults are concerning at best, but when in tandem with worldwide seclusion, we can only assume how the effects are trickling down into children's well-being and development.

STAGE 2: AUTONOMY VERSUS SHAME

The next stage, early childhood, is the period during which the child learns Autonomy vs. Shame and Doubt; it occurs from eighteen months until approximately three years of age. During this stage, a child begins to learn independence, such as walking, talking, feeding, and using the restroom by him or herself. This gives a child a sense of autonomy when he or she is able to complete these tasks successfully, with the assistance of their caregivers. However, if they are shamed when they are unable to complete a task, they develop a greater sense of shame and doubt rather than developing autonomy and a greater sense of self. This is arguably one of the periods most easily impacted by the COVID-19 pandemic. In previous literature, it can be seen that some of the most important things caregivers can do is not to do anything. During this stage, it is crucial that toddlers are given the opportunity to try—and fail—without immediate assistance but rather, with support. Self-help opportunities that allow children to practice tasks without it being done for them are the best ways to ensure safety as well as developmental success (Miller, 2021).

However, the pandemic has altered many caregiver perceptions of self-help; many have noticed regressions in their children's development during these times. This can occur for many reasons, the first being the parents' inability to separate themselves. Normally, children will have moments when they're being watched by additional caregivers apart from their normal ones or when they are left alone in a crib or playpen while a parent completes other tasks. However, with the pandemic making the parents or caregivers unable to leave, they have had no reason to separate from their children, and in some ways, they have not allowed their children to become independent. Stress could be another reason for the perceived regression or hindrance to development. While it may be hard to believe that a toddler experiences stress, toddlers often can be more overwhelmed by stress than adults, because they cannot communicate feelings of stress, nor do they understand it. Observing stress and stressful behaviors in caregivers is one reason that the child may be less likely to want to branch out and be independent, especially if the caregiver is performing all of the tasks without attempting to allow the child to do them him or herself. Studies conducted during the COVID-19 pandemic show that one of the most important tools learned during this stage, self-sufficiency in feeding ourselves, has also been impacted by stay-at-home measures. A total of 498 parents completed an online survey on their children's food-related behaviors. The results indicated that there were significant changes in eating behaviors during the lockdown, including changes in appetite, food enjoyment, and emotional overeating (Philippe et al., 2021). The majority of these changes were attributed to boredom and greater access to food, in addition to less supervision. The problem arises where, as adults, we have previously learned behaviors to understand normal food behaviors. However, for children experiencing autonomy for the first time, these will be the only behaviors surrounding food that they know. For many, this could lead to a long-term unhealthy relationship with food, such as using food for coping, not knowing the difference between hunger and boredom, or experiencing weight gain due to overeating. This is a further concern due to the stay-at-home measures providing little opportunity for exercise, and the combination could result in lifelong behavioral and health issues.

STAGE 3: INITIATIVE VERSUS GUILT

Erikson's third stage is that of the play age period, during which time the child learns Initiative vs. Guilt, generally between the ages of three and five years old. During this time, children learn the basic strength of purpose and take initiative in playing games that mimic real-life situations, such as chefs or cleaners or play with dolls. The subconscious goal here is to explore the *whys* of the world and to play roles and imagine what it is like to be an adult, essentially to identify one's role in the world. If children struggle with this, they will easily experience guilt for their inability to understand their role and purpose. This is a very internalized stage, when after years of playing with family and friends, playing house and playing with dolls, the process of initiating it out of one's own curiosity is something difficult to force a child to do. Recent research takes a closer look at what some of the various forms and scenarios could be, and it investigates ways play can be used to subconsciously work through understanding life's purpose. The researchers describe play initially as object manipulation, such as practicing control, and later as replicating activities needed to survive, like how playing house replicates cooking, cleaning, and caretaking. Finally, it helps children practice skills and behaviors that are required in society, like social interaction and working with others. Since this is such a self-directed stage, meaning it is not something that a caregiver can initiate in a child; it is one of the stages in which the child is less likely to be affected compared to the first two stages. However, since the majority of play involves mimicking previously witnessed scenarios, a lack of exposure could certainly lead to delays in the playing of social scenarios (Bergan, 2020). For example, in previous conditions, a child would accompany a caregiver on trips to the store, to visit other family and friends, and to the doctor's office. But since families were unable to have these social interactions during the Pandemic, there were no scenarios to mimic. This could be most consequential in the development of a child's socialization and curiosity about the surrounding world. It could also be detrimental in terms of causing anxiety and confusion when society returns to normal and the child is observing interactions he or she has never seen before. Additional research investigated the play patterns of 1,472 children during the current global pandemic. The results indicated that only 4.7% (2.8% girls and 6.5% boys) were getting the suggested amount of physical movement. These children showed less time participating in physical activities, greater time participating in sedentary behaviors, and less time outside, as compared to pre-pandemic behaviors (Moore et al., 2020). The greatest concern is the decreased amount of playtime, likely replaced by gaming or media consumption, which in turn decreases curiosity about the surrounding world and one's purpose. If the stay-at-home measures were to remain through the play age and into school age, these children would likely have little desire to investigate or learn, since their curiosity about the world would have been replaced by non-interactive forms of play.

STAGE 4: INDUSTRY VERSUS INFERIORITY

The fourth and final stage of childhood is school age, which is when children are expected to learn about Industry vs. Inferiority. This stage generally occurs between the ages of six to 12. This is when children are fully capable of learning and creating, which, therefore, makes this an ideal time to use tools to accomplish and understand new skills and knowledge, creating a sense of industry. As these skills develop, so do social development and understanding, which can lead to a sense of inferiority if a child feels inadequate compared to his or her peers. As if this age were not difficult enough, during this development stage people cultivate either good or bad self-esteem, something they will carry throughout the rest of their lives. During this time, children also begin growing independently of their parents and continue their development mostly through school and peer interactions. Unfortunately, one of the greatest areas in which our youth has been affected by the pandemic is the social restrictions that have been put in place as a consequence of not being able to physically interact with people outside of the home. Previous literature discusses how critical the late childhood stage really is. Researcher Dr. Learmonth stated,

In late childhood and adolescence, children start to strike out on their own. ... Friendships become more complex and more about shared interests. This is when children try out the things that will make their adult friendships work, or not. (Campbell, 2020)

Learmonth continued by mentioning how, at this age, people begin to venture into friendships by seeking and providing support, they learn that trust and betrayal can result from it. For these reasons, Dr. Learmonth agreed that long-term social isolation would likely have the most negative impact on children and adolescents in this stage. The lack of personal interaction, touch, and excitement is being replaced by electronic interactions, which do not have the same beneficial effects on development. The overall separation from peers would result in inferiority over industry, since they will never be able to feel adequate if they are never given the opportunity to do so amongst peers (Campbell, 2020). Additionally, current research surrounding the lack of social interaction studied 442 school-aged children and their feelings regarding perceived stress, instability at home, and their home-schooling experience. Results showed that 78% of children reported missing their friends, with 51% concerned about being infected or infecting others. The majority of children showed increased feelings of loneliness and difficulty concentrating. Children also exhibited a decrease in emotional reactions, but an increase in cognitive reactions (Larsen et al., 2021). The main issue surrounding the results of this data is the lack of social interaction as well as increased feelings of seclusion that are occurring at a vital time in one's social development. Additionally, becoming desensitized to emotional matters, likely because of daily discussions about death and illness, could also affect the development of empathy and compassion. Due to the late-breaking pandemic, long-term data is not yet available to measure the social and emotional well-being of children developing during these times; however, previous data seems to suggest that there could be long-term negative effects.

STAGE 5: IDENTITY VERSUS ROLE CONFUSION

The fifth stage is adolescence, occurring at ages 12–18. At this stage, the child begins to learn Identity vs. Role Confusion. This is the first stage that is dependent not on what is done to them but rather on what they choose to do. By this age, people are "tweens" or teenagers, neither child nor adult, leaving them in an uncomfortable stage in which they are trying to assess who they are and what their place is in the world. They are no longer solely members of their family, and it is their subconscious priority here to discover their place in society, as well as their stance on moral issues and situations they encounter. The negative side of this stage is the confusion and withdrawal from groups and responsibilities people feel. If the adolescent is unable to overcome this, they are left with role confusion. The pandemic has had both positive and negative effects on this stage for a multitude of reasons. On the one hand, there is no opportunity for interaction in a manner that allows a deeper understanding of one's place in the world. The pandemic has caused a pause that has prevented most people from moving forward with their lives. It can be emotionally distressing not to know or be confident about one's place in the world during a time when one cannot venture out and discover it. Additionally, role confusion can be amplified when responsibilities are put off due to drug use, which has spiked during the pandemic. In a recent study, it can be seen that alcohol use among teens increased over 2%, from 28.6% to 30.4%, in the short period that COVID-19 has affected our society. As an additional consequence, marijuana use among underage teens increased from 3.28 days per three weeks to 3.76 days per three weeks (Cenikor Foundation, 2020). While these numbers are not astronomical, they reveal a very vulnerable population. Allowing responsibilities and confrontation of issues to be pushed off through drug use only furthers role confusion into becoming a long-term issue. Since teens are highly isolated, it is likely that their drug and alcohol use is far greater and more frequent than reported and that the effects are greater. This could lead to long-term developmental delays, since pushing off role confirmation can result in a lessened desire to understand one's place, and, for many people who are entering COVID-19 as teenagers and leaving as adults, this could have serious consequences. In the literature previously mentioned, researchers investigated the relationship between substance use and mental illness during the pandemic. A total of 13,829 people were surveyed on their alcohol use before and during the COVID-19 pandemic, and they were also assessed on their mental health. The results indicated that one in five people were drinking more than they had been before the pandemic. There was also a correlation between the increase in alcohol consumption and the experience of having severe symptoms of anxiety or depression (Tran et al., 2020). Since anxiety affects more than 40 million people in the U.S. over the age of 18 alone (Anxiety and Depression Association of America, 2021), it can be assumed that the long-term impact of increased alcohol consumption caused by anxiety over the pandemic will result in severe long-term behavioral and health-related issues.

STAGE 6: INTIMACY AND SOLIDARITY VERSUS ISOLATION

The sixth stage, young adulthood, is the first of adulthood and occurs between the ages of 18–35, during which the development of Intimacy and Solidarity vs. Isolation occurs. This is the initial stage in which we take a deeper look into the way our developing romantic relationships affect our personal psychological and sociological development. As people enter adulthood, they begin to seek love and affection from romantic partners and generally negotiate their way into marriage and families. When young adults are able to have successful and meaningful romantic relationships, they are able to experience and understand intimacy. However, if they're unable to forge these relationships, social isolation may occur, leading to feeling distant and therefore superior to those peers who they blame for not connecting with them. In a recent study regarding the recent decline of marriages, we take a closer look at the way marriages and intimate relationships have been affected by the COVID-19 pandemic and its related social distancing measures. One statistic from this piece shows that as of July 2020, there were 23,627 fewer marriages recorded in Florida than in 2019, a significant 26% decrease (Wagner et al., 2020). This is significant because it is not solely the decrease in actual legal marriages but also the implied decline in people meeting and interacting, leading to marriage. One would assume we could achieve intimacy at any time; however, during the social isolation of a pandemic and, it is the exact opposite. The inability to interact socially has a direct correlation to the decrease in marriages and thus the inability to achieve intimacy, causing a feeling of isolation. This is likely to greatly delay the age at which someone is able to accomplish intimacy and is further likely to create a decrease in the birth rate around the world. Recent studies regarding the reproductive health of young adults during the pandemic reported that long-term consequences might result in altered sexual health care, including sexual disease care, contraceptives, abortions, and pre-natal care (Lindberg et al., 2020). While the majority of current research studies surrounding the topic of the Pandemic is concerned with the inability to socialize and create long-term intimate relationships, there is still also cause for concern as far as sexual health care goes. For many young adults, sexual education and healthcare are available through college or a doctor's office. However, since the pandemic has caused everyone to stay at home, access to these resources is limited, and for many, it is far from their minds. Since there are over 10 million new STD cases among young adults estimated per year (Centers for Disease Control and Prevention, 2021), people can only imagine what the data will look like after the pandemic, with the addition of those who could not access contraceptives such as condoms as well as those who were not previously exposed to the reality of sexual disease when they entered young adulthood during the pandemic. An additional noteworthy issue is the inability to receive non-essential healthcare, and in many areas, abortions were included in this, as well. Restriction from abortion procedures is likely to result in many unwanted pregnancies or a request for abortions that are not conducted by a medical provider.

STAGE 7: GENERATIVITY VERSUS SELF-ABSORPTION

The subsequent stage, middle adulthood, is the seventh stage, beginning at age 35 and continuing until age 55 or 65. In this stage, the most important aspects of one's life are, put simply, work and family, appropriate stressors leading to the conflict of Generativity vs. Self-absorption or Stagnation. Generally, this is when life's priority is creating a stable environment for one's family and teaching one's children sociality and cultural values. Bettering one's family and society through being productive and contributing will lead to a sense of generativity. However, when people's family members no longer rely on them or a people feel that they are not contributing to the environment around them, they strive to find a new purpose. If they are unsuccessful, they will develop a sense of self-absorption and stagnation. This is perhaps the stage that has been most discussed during the pandemic, since the inability to care for one's family has been a major consequence of the stay-at-home orders and resulting job loss. Recent research discusses the major inadequacy many parents and homemakers are feeling due to the pandemic and the mass layoffs that occurred because of it. Statistics state that over 20.5 million people have become unemployed during the COVID-19 pandemic, and as a result, millions have become unable to support their families. The research continues to discuss how the pandemic affects not only the financial aspect of the family but also the work–family interface, as parents who were previously happy and relaxed are now anxious and on edge. The psychological effects of feeling inadequate and unable to produce are likely to result in negative feelings of stagnation (Falk et al., 2021). Although it is possible that people may be able to recoup once work begins again, this negative effect still alters the normal way one would be developing socially and psychologically at this age. Stagnation is also cause for concern among adults who feel unimportant or undervalued during the pandemic. Additional research suggests that older adults who feel undervalued, as if they do not matter, can be especially impacted mentally and physically, and health-wise, as a result of confinement measures (Flett et al., 2020). Feeling unimportant is certainly not a novel concept, especially for older parents whose kids have grown out of living at home and have lives of their own. However, it is more frequently those without kids who experience illness issues related to these feelings. For adults who had still hoped to start families in their middle adult years, the pandemic may have caused complications in many ways, such as preventing them from meeting a spouse or the virus preventing a couple from having children.

Those who still had the desire to have children may develop increasingly painful feelings of unimportance and stagnation, since the virus is literally preventing them from making the necessary steps to move onto the next stage in their lives.

STAGE 8: INTEGRITY VERSUS DESPAIR

The eighth and final stage, late adulthood, can begin anywhere between the ages of 55 and 65, continuing until death. This is perhaps the most difficult stage, since all of the previous stages were preparing one for the next; however, this stage is more reflective of the past than looking into the future. At this point in life, one has completed all of life's great tasks, from social development and friendship to love and family; if these are completed to one's liking, one may feel content. The concept of knowing you contributed to the world and have created a meaningful life for yourself and those around you can produce a sense of integrity. However, if individuals feel that they did not accomplish what they wanted to in their younger years or did not make their mark on the world, they may feel a sense of despair. For these individuals, the concept of looming death produces a constant reminder that one did not succeed and cannot go back. Previous literature takes a look at the prioritization the world needs to take on not only the physical but also the mental health of the elderly during these unprecedented times. While COVID-19 has been found to most greatly affect the over-65 population, seniors have been placed in the strictest and longest isolation. While this is done with the good intentions of protecting our elderly from this deadly virus, it has created concerns over their mental health. This developmental period may often be overlooked, but it is just as valued as the rest, and for many seniors who previously had plans for the remainder of their lives, the pandemic has stripped this away from them. The article continues by saying that for some, losing a spouse during the pandemic has created a developmental sense of despair, since they had not yet completed all the things they wished to do with their partner, and they are looking back with regret. Others went into isolation, still working and participating daily in society, but due to the pandemic, they have either chosen or have been forced to retire, generally sooner than they had planned (Lee et al., 2020). Recent studies conducted during the pandemic gathered information on 3,421 adults over the age of 60 and looked into their interaction with social media during the pandemic. Results showed that the use of social media during these trying times led to increased anxiety and lower social trust; however, it did not help improve the adoption of COVID-safe behaviors (Wong et al., 2021). The adoption of social media by the older generation is slowly becoming widespread, with over 62% of Americans over the age of 70 owning smartphones and participating in social media (Kakulla, 2020). The media, however, during the pandemic, has become a pandemic in its own way by promoting hysteria and inaccurate information. For older adults at this time, who are already on edge since they are the most high-risk group, meaning the most secluded, the addition of media hysteria has been devastating. Anxiety and paranoia have become increasingly common among senior adults due to the pandemic, leaving many unsure if they will ever be able to return to the way life was before. The pandemic has created a great sense of unease among the elderly community, it has displaced many of their future plans and desires, and with social media's influence, it has caused an entirely new series of issues for a group, who were ready for retirement and grandchildren.

FUTURE DIRECTION

As we move into the future, we can only hope for a speedy end to this virus that has ravaged the world. However, whether it ends tomorrow or in a year, the developmental delays which occurred during the pandemic will continue to ripple throughout everyone's lives. What we can do is to be more aware of the development we are progressing through each day and attempt to be conscious of the ways we can influence it. For parents of infants, perhaps we can seek additional childcare from vaccinated family members or friends or partake in free online therapy to calm ourselves over being the sole provider of a child's well-being. During the stage of independence, "self-sufficient" games could be created to perhaps provide respite to the caregiver, as well as offer the child an opportunity to be productively sufficient. As children move into the play age, making a conscious effort to pull children away from their games and into nature could have a long-term beneficial impact. While school-aged children may not be able to socialize closely, the introduction of outdoor, socially distanced sports games may help. As children move into the teenage years, inclusion in the discussion of the negative effects of substance use and abuse may help in deterring them from experimenting in the first place. For those entering adulthood, the most valuable advice to support them may simply be to remember that there is no timeline on life and that they have plenty of time. The same can be said for those experiencing insufficiency in middle adulthood, who perhaps just need a reminder that there is more time to complete the things they desire. For those entering or living in their senior years, usage of virtual social gatherings may be beneficial for providing a sense of comfort to combat loneliness. While life is not without its challenges, it is human nature to adapt, and because of this, there is hope for the future.

CONCLUSION

When Erikson created his eight stages of development in 1950, it is likely that he never imagined a world where socialization would come to a complete halt, creating an invisible crease in human development. While some age groups can perhaps be affected more substantially than others by the pandemic, it is safe to say that every individual's development was paused or altered in one way or another. In 2021, the global population is still under the influence of this deadly virus, and so it is unknown how these delays will affect the future. What is clear is the underlying psychosocial development, that we often take for granted, was substantially impacted by the COVID-19 pandemic.

REFERENCES

Anxiety and Depression Association of America. (2021). *Facts & Statistics: Anxiety and Depression Association of America*. https://adaa.org/understanding-anxiety/facts-statistics

Benner, A. D., & Mistry, R. S. (2020). Child development during the COVID-19 pandemic through a life course theory lens. *Child Development Perspectives*, *14*(4), 236–243. doi:10.1111/cdep.12387 PMID:33230400

Bergan, D. (2020). *Psychological approaches to the study of play*. doi:10.31838/jcr.07.01.38

Blustein, D. L., Duffy, R., Ferreira, J. A., Cohen-Scali, V., Cinamon, R. G., & Allan, B. A. (2020, June). Unemployment in the time of COVID-19: A research agenda. *Journal of Vocational Behavior*. https://www.ncbi.nlm.nih.gov/pmc/articles/PMC7206417/

Campbell, L. (2020). How COVID-19 could affect kids' long-term social development. *Healthline*. https://www.healthline.com/health-news/social-distancing-effects-on-social-development

Cenikor Foundation. (2020, October 26). *Mental health and substance abuse is on the rise for teens because of COVID-19*. https://www.cenikor.org/mental-health-and-substance-abuse-is-on-the-rise-for-teens-because-of-covid-19/

Centers for Disease Control and Prevention. (2021). *COVID-19 data tracker weekly review*. https://www.cdc.gov/coronavirus/2019-ncov/covid-data/covidview/index.html

Falk, G. (2021). *Unemployment rates during the COVID-19 pandemic: In brief.* Congressional Research Service. https://fas.org/sgp/crs/misc/R46554.pdf

Flanagan, E. W., Beyl, R. A., Fearnbach, S. N., Altazan, A. D., Martin, C. K., & Redman, L. M. (2020). The impact of COVID-19 stay-at-home orders on health behaviors in adults. *Obesity (Silver Spring, Md.)*, *29*(2), 438–445. doi:10.1002/oby.23066 PMID:33043562

Flett, G. L., & Heisel, M. J. (2020, June 15). Aging and feeling valued versus expendable during the COVID-19 pandemic and beyond: A review and commentary of why mattering is fundamental to the health and well-being of older adults. *International Journal of Mental Health and Addiction*. https://link.springer.com/article/10.1007/s11469-020-00339-4

Kakulla, B. N. (2020, January 1). *2020 tech trends of the 50+*. AARP. https://www.aarp.org/research/topics/technology/info-2019/2020-technology-trends-older-americans.html

Larsen, L., Helland, M. S., & Holt, T. (2021, March 26). The impact of school closure and social isolation on children in vulnerable families during COVID-19: a focus on children's reactions. *European Child & Adolescent Psychiatry*. https://link.springer.com/article/10.1007/s00787-021-01758-x

Lee, K., Jeong, G.-C., & Yim, J. E. (2020, November 3). Consideration of the psychological and mental health of the elderly during COVID-19: A theoretical review. *International Journal of Environmental Research and Public Health*. https://www.ncbi.nlm.nih.gov/pmc/articles/PMC7663449/

Lindberg, L. (2020). The sexual and reproductive health of adolescents and young adults during the COVID-19 pandemic. *Perspectives on Sexual and Reproductive Health*. https://pubmed.ncbi.nlm.nih.gov/32537858/

Miller, S. (n.d.). *Ages and stages: Nurturing young children's independence*. Scholastic. https://www.scholastic.com/teachers/articles/teaching-content/ages-stages-nuturing-young-childrens-independence/

Moore, S. A., Faulkner, G., Rhodes, R. E., Brussoni, M., Chulak-Bozzer, T., Ferguson, L. J., Mitra, R., O'Reilly, N., Spence, J. C., Vanderloo, L. M., & Tremblay, M. S. (2020, July 6). Impact of the COVID-19 virus outbreak on movement and play behaviours of Canadian children and youth: A national survey. *International Journal of Behavioral Nutrition and Physical Activity*. https://ijbnpa.biomedcentral.com/articles/10.1186/s12966-020-00987-8

Orenstein, G. A., & Lewis, L. (2020). *Erikson's stages of psychosocial development.* StatPearls. https://www.ncbi.nlm.nih.gov/books/NBK556096/

Philippe, K., Chabanet, C., Issanchou, S., & Monnery-Patris, S. (2021, January 23). Child eating behaviors, parental feeding practices and food shopping motivations during the COVID-19 lockdown in France: (How) did they change? *Appetite.* https://www.sciencedirect.com/science/article/pii/S0195666321000404

Rafanelli, A. (2021, July 22). *Growing up in a pandemic: How covid is affecting children's development.* Direct Relief. Retrieved March 29, 2022, from https://www.directrelief.org/2021/01/growing-up-in-the-midst-of-a-pandemic-how-covid-is-affecting-childrens-development/

Sprang, G., & Silman, M. (2013, April 25). *Posttraumatic stress disorder in parents and youth after health-related disasters: Disaster Medicine and Public Health Preparedness.* Cambridge Core. Retrieved March 29, 2022, from https://www.cambridge.org/core/journals/disaster-medicine-and-public-health-preparedness/article/abs/posttraumatic-stress-disorder-in-parents-and-youth-after-healthrelated-disasters/4F3E4300F74CEEAFA8EE95E490944888

Tran, T. D., Hammarberg, K., Kirkman, M., Nguyen, H. T. M., & Fisher, J. (2020, December 1). Alcohol use and mental health status during the first months of COVID-19 pandemic in Australia. *Journal of Affective Disorders.* https://www.ncbi.nlm.nih.gov/pmc/articles/PMC7476559/

Wagner, B. (2020). *Decline in marriage associated with the COVID-19 pandemic in the United States.* https://journals.sagepub.com/doi/full/10.1177/2378023120980328

Wong, F. H., Liu, T., Leung, D. K., Zhang, A. Y., Au, W. S., Kwok, W. W., Shum, A. K., Wong, G. H., & Lum, T. Y.-S. (2021). Consuming information related to COVID-19 on social media among older adults and its association with anxiety, social trust in information, and COVID-safe behaviors: Cross-sectional telephone survey (preprint). doi:10.2196/preprints.26570

KEY TERMS AND DEFINITIONS

Autonomy: The capacity to self-govern.

Milestone: A marker signifying change.

Pandemic: An epidemic or outbreak that is widespread across a population.

Role Confusion: To be uncertain about oneself and one's place in various social settings.

SARS: A disease encompassing symptoms such as fever, cough, and headache, which is caused by a coronavirus.

Self-Absorption: To be consumed with oneself or one's own priorities.

Solidarity: To have a feeling of unity amongst a group with common interests or goals.

Stagnation: The lack of movement.

Chapter 10 The Changing Landscape of Children's Media During the Pandemic

Regina Colie
Marymount Manhattan College, USA

ABSTRACT

This chapter discusses the evolution of children's media, particularly throughout the COVID-19 pandemic. The last two years have been filled with drastic changes and unexpected challenges, so adaptability has been essential in continuing to produce children's content. This chapter will begin with the early versions of children's television with the release of Sesame Street in 1969. Then it will transition to the present day, with the beginning of the pandemic, which resulted in global lockdowns that caused school closures. From March 2020 to the present day, Zoom became the norm for children and their families. Teachers taught their students through computer screens, and parents held virtual meetings to maintain contact with their colleagues. Finally, the chapter will conclude with how entertainment companies had to provide TV shows and films from home. This chapter is a testament to the transitional and adaptive techniques of children's networks, such as television shows and schools, used throughout this pandemic to maintain stability.

INTRODUCTION

When describing television, Paddy Chayefsky, a famous American novelist and playwright, once said, "Television is the menace that everyone loves to hate but can't seem to live without." Television holds the entertainment that we enjoy through shows

DOI: 10.4018/978-1-6684-3484-0.ch010

and movies. Television broadcasts news we watch flash by our screens- the news that describes the current climate in our society. And most importantly, television fuels the uproar of media that we consume daily. Parents and children alike are glued to their televisions and screens now more than ever, with the shifting dynamic of the pandemic playing out each day. When we look back on how children's television began, could we ever have predicted that children's media would never be the same? Could we have done things differently with the knowledge that we have now? This chapter will explore how the past and the present will affect how children's media has been and will be effective in affecting a child's future.

HISTORY OF CHILDREN'S TELEVISION

The incorporation of educational topics on children's television began in 1969 when the Children's Television Workshop announced they were releasing a show that would provide children with educational resources. During the late 1960s and early 1970s, many low-income children were not attending school, and as a result, they were not receiving an academic education. "After all, only 19 percent of 4-year-olds were in preschool in 1970 - a reality that Morris points out in the first sentence of his 4,000-word essay (Wong, 2015)." When *Sesame Street* aired on November 10, 1969, a cultural shift occurred. However, *Sesame Street* did not place all children on an equal playing field towards receiving an education due to their varied home environments or levels of accessibility. The Educational Testing Service (ETS) studies showed that *Sesame Street* would prevail in the entertainment industry while promoting both engagement and enrichment of their young audience. It would be a powerful medium through which to enrich the world of children's television.

In 1970, one year after *Sesame Street* premiered, Samuel Ball and Gerry Ann Bogatz performed a research study involving U.S. children from advantaged suburban areas and disadvantaged inner-city areas. The children were divided into four groups, based on the range of how often they watched the show, from "Infrequently" or "Not at All" to "Multiple Times Per Week." The results indicated that children between the ages of three to five, from different backgrounds, could develop complex cognitive skills (Ball & Bogatz, 1970). Today, *Sesame Street* continues to play a significant role in educating children. The show has incorporated societal concepts, which are critical for child development, in an enjoyable and kid-friendly way and encourages other networks to promote learning through children's television shows, as well.

Research has shown that engaging in educational programming at an early age affords enhanced benefits for children's social and mental development as they progress through school. However, networks have had problems getting this message across to their viewers. Thus, to address this issue, the 1990 Children's Television

Act, or CTA, was born. Through the Federal Communications Commission (FCC), this act allowed broadcasters to create and produce educational television programs for children that would "further the child's positive development in any respect, including the child's cognitive, intellectual or social-emotional needs" (Calvert & Kotler, 2003). However, significant criticisms emerged after this act was enacted, since broadcasters were not following the specific guidelines that the Federal Communications Commission (FCC) set out. "For example, the license renewal form for WDIV-TV in Detroit, MI, listed *GI Joe*, a violent action-adventure cartoon, as an educational and informational television program (Calvert, Kotler, 2003)." Once researchers continued to raise issues regarding the CTA, the FCC improved their guidelines and implemented the "Three-Hour Rule" in 1997.

The "Three-Hour Rule"' required programs to meet the educational needs of children (16 and under) and mandated that the hours of airtime be between 7 AM and 10 PM. It also prescribed that programs should be 30 minutes in length and scheduled weekly. The implementation of straightforward guidelines gave broadcasters a better picture of what they needed to create, which ultimately paved the way for the improved children's television shows that we know today. And yet, as Hayes states in her article, "The future of the Children's Television Act remains uncertain (Hayes, 1994)." While the children's television industry has changed dramatically since the 1990s, we've seen the benefits of how this act has shaped television networks such as *PBS* and *Nickelodeon* to create fun and appropriate content for children.

CHILDREN'S LEARNING DURING QUARANTINE

The outbreak of the SARS-CoV2 virus, commonly known as COVID-19, resulted in a catastrophe unlike anything imaginable. Emerging from Wuhan, China, in the early weeks of 2020, this virus quickly and silently spread worldwide, resulting in thousands of cases and deaths. The disturbing and drastic rise in the death toll prompted the World Health Organization to declare that the COVID-19 outbreak was a global pandemic. To avoid spreading the virus further, national lockdowns began a few days after this announcement. All non-essential businesses closed their doors and mandated that families should not leave their homes unless there was an emergency. Children were no longer allowed to attend school in-person and were forced to switch to online learning using social platforms, such as *Zoom*. With this unexpected new mode of education, the question on the minds of many was: How will this impact our children?

For starters, children from low-income neighborhoods often have no accessibility to computers or the Internet. "If certain students are prevented from learning online either due to limited access or because online learning does not benefit them, then they may fall behind academically". (Frenette et al., 2020). Researchers may not understand the depths to which children's learning will be affected due to this pandemic at this current moment. However, there is a wide gap in the discrepancy between what children can learn and attain in an in-person classroom setting compared to absorbing information via a virtual application.

Although many children returned to school in-person at various points throughout 2020, 2021, and 2022, immediate closures due to spikes in cases took a toll on children's learning. Teachers had to use their creativity in virtual classroom settings. Children's media played a vital role in these scenarios, as teachers incorporated videos from YouTube, television shows, and movies into their lesson plans. However, better education systems must be implemented for children living in low-income neighborhoods or struggling with learning disabilities to structure their pedagogy. In particular, families need to have more access to technology, specifically for children of parents who work from home. There need to be partnerships between the government and school systems to provide students with computers and Internet access (Goldschmidt, 2020). Despite the economic hardships companies have faced throughout the pandemic, future collaborations should serve low-income neighborhoods with free Internet and computers. They should also provide training sessions to families who may not be well-acquainted with the applications and devices offered. The tools that children use to access their media have been compromised due to either inefficiency or inaccessibility. This needs to change in order for children to have a valuable learning experience from now into the future.

LACK OF PHYSICAL ACTIVITY FOR CHILDREN

The rate of obesity in children has been a significant public health crisis in the U.S. for decades. However, its prevalence has dramatically increased as a result of the pandemic. Despite the overwhelming demands and advice that healthcare professionals offer to families, these words of wisdom may fall on deaf ears until the health and safety of others are under control. "Health guidelines recommend that children achieve 60 min of moderate-to-vigorous physical activity (MVPA) daily or approximately 12,000 steps to ensure healthy development. Unfortunately, 18%-20% of U.S. children aged 2-19 years are classified as obese (Tulchin-Frances et al., 2020)." Since many families have continued to stay home well after quarantine has ended, the window for children to gain accessibility to exercise outside the confinement of their homes is very limiting. Indoors, kids are more likely to maintain unhealthy eating habits. They also express more interest in staying connected to their phones, tablets, and computer screens rather than being energetic and participating in physical activities and events with their family and friends. However, the result of this increase could be due in part to other risk factors; such as socioeconomic status, living conditions, genetic makeup, and food availability. Once schools begin to open up again and students can return to the classroom, how will a year and a half without adequate physical activity be dealt with in an institutional setting?

Kristen Tulchin-Francis and her fellow researchers (2021) designed a survey to answer some of these puzzling questions. The survey was developed in Texas and spread across various social media platforms, such as Twitter and Facebook. The survey was active between April and June of 2020, which was the critical time in which families were in quarantine, and the responses were anonymous. The 1,310 surveys collected revealed that children experienced less physical activity due to social distancing and limited interactions with others. Based on the results, schools and families should improve physical activities in children through continuing physical education classes and maintaining physical activities in children's free time (Tulchin-Francis et al., 2021). As discussed, the issues at hand relating to exercise and dieting need further research as we move towards a healthier and brighter future, with the assistance of the COVID-vaccine. In many areas, the necessary precautions were taken to help prevent the further spread of this deadly virus. More than ever, public health officials must take a closer look at how their lack of addressing these other diseases that emerge from unstable lifestyle choices can affect families and their children for years to come.

CONCERNS SURROUNDING CHILDREN'S AWARENESS OF SOCIAL MEDIA

Due to the unexpected isolation and the massive strain working from home has had on families, they have steadily increased their reliance on technology. Social media has become the gateway for people throughout the pandemic, especially for kids who seek connectivity with their friends, whom they could not connect with in-person. Although this form of media can help inform us of the latest news and help us maintain relationships with family and friends, social media can also be hazardous. Since parents are working from home, they have less accessibility and time to see what their children are watching. Because of this, the risks of them being exposed to explicit and violent content are high. For example, a popular social media platform like Twitter, where users have access to news and scope worldwide, has become quite popular within the last few years. Specific social media platforms take the initiative of restricting viewers from seeing inappropriate or sensitive content and only allow people aged 13 years or older to sign up for an account. However, there are ways to manipulate the system. For example, without parents' viewership, children can change their birthdays to access these social media accounts. As such, their exposure to violence in the news can steadily change their behaviors, with additional hardships faced throughout the pandemic. Even if children are not directly targeted online, the risks of them being exposed to public content that is either abusive or negative between users can be harmful for their well-being. (Babvey et al. 3).

While some may argue that the outpouring of survivor stories is empowering and brave, they may also be considered harmful to children who may or may not be experiencing abuse in their lives. Especially now, with several anti-Asian hate crimes occurring due to the pandemic, children are now becoming more cognizant of some harmful aspects of the world, especially at ages where they may not understand why this type of behavior is wrong. Children are silent observers who pick up on almost everything that happens in their environment. Their behaviors are reflective of what they have been exposed to from their parents, siblings, and peers. They also can learn to model what they have seen on a TV show or through a news outlet. Their actions can be a direct reflection of the normalizing of violent or innate behaviors. The argument is that increased exposure to social media involving violence may cause children to develop violent tendencies and behaviors.

TELEVISION NETWORKS ADDRESSING COVID-19

Due to the impact COVID-19 on families, television networks created informational TV events educating families about celebrity appearances and famous cartoon characters. Two networks that used this to their advantage were Nickelodeon and the Disney Channel. Last year, Nickelodeon hosted an hour-long show lead by Kristen Bell called *#KidsTogether: The Nickelodeon Town Hall.* The special featured celebrities like Alicia Keys, Chari D'Amelio, Josh Gad, Kenan Thompson; clips from shows such as *SpongeBob SquarePants* and *Henry Danger;* and two experts in the medical field, Dr. Nadine Burke Harris and Dr. Vivek H. Murthy. The TV special was intended to address concerns children had regarding the virus, providing tips from medical experts on how to stay healthy, and accounts from families globally on their experiences during quarantine. (Haring, 2020).

The Disney Channel also followed a similar pattern, with their series entitled, *We're All In This Together (#WAITT),* that featured personalized messages from Disney Channel actors and actresses to kids (between the ages of 6 to 14) to help reassure children and families, who were experiencing the severity of the pandemic. "The series includes over 35 Disney Channel stars who each filmed their message from their homes and around their neighborhood, sharing how they stay positive, active and, with the help of parents and family members, navigate through this uncertain time." (Haring, 2020). With the familiarity of celebrities that kids recognize and their presence in some of their favorite TV shows, these television series influenced how kids view the pandemic and stay happy while being at home.

GEN C

Since quarantine began, the new generation of children is dubbed "Gen C," also known as "Generation COVID," due to the wearing of masks in public with their parents and their inability to engage in activities with their friends. Although the vaccines have had promising results, the increase in cases due to emerging variants has resulted in more school closures, increased rates of testing, and increased isolation and loneliness. Because of this, children have spent more time at home on their devices. "As a result, children and families have become increasingly reliant on screens for online learning, entertainment, and social interaction (e.g., Zoom meetings, Google Hangouts, FaceTime, and Houseparty App) (Vanderloo et.al, 335)." Since both parents and children suffer from incredibly strained schedules, how do parents appropriately manage children's screen-time? Is there a way to prevent increasing hours of screen exposure without removing children's access to media completely?

EFFECTIVE WAYS OF MANAGING CHILDREN'S SCREEN-TIME

Parents can use a few harm-reduction principles to help manage and possibly reduce the amount of technology their children use. For example, a harm-reduction principle called "humane values" uses negotiation and compassion to manage screen usage. This principle recognizes why parents need to use technology more while limiting their children's hours on-screens outside of school time. Other principles could constitute significant steps in the right direction for parents struggling to manage their children's technology usage. Parents could also introduce some techniques while working or facilitating school from home, such as having screen-time focusing on phone call conversations with family and friends and initiating more hands-on playtime without using screens. Also, there should be more parental monitoring of children's viewing and prioritizing screen-free moments during meals throughout the day and before going to sleep. Trying to manage how much children can use their screens can be challenging, especially when technology has become more heavily relied upon over the last year. However, with the right interventions introduced early on within a child's development, parents will better manage media use in their homes in the future.

CHILDREN WITH DISABILITIES DURING THE PANDEMIC

One of the greatest challenges that have emerged during the pandemic is how to best accommodate children with disabilities. Before the pandemic began, children who had disabilities such as ADHD, Autism, and Down syndrome went to school under their aides' watchful eye. They had a structured, individualized education plan (IEP) to ensure they would have a smooth and transitional academic experience. However, once schools shut down to help contain the virus' spread, the implications of the unexpected changes fell onto these families. "The implications of losing these in-person educational and medical supports are profound, adding substantially to caregiver burden and also compromising the child's overall health and well-being (Jeste et al., 2020)." These children particularly struggle when they are taken out of their typical routine. When you take these children out of a pattern that they are familiar with, then the accessibility and reliability they once had, is temporarily gone.

Jeste and her colleagues (2020) conducted a survey distributed to caregivers who have children with disabilities. They were able to share their experiences with losing educational and healthcare services during the pandemic. Within this survey, there were 818 responses from families both within and outside of the U.S. The results found that 75% of parents lost one form of therapy or educational service during the pandemic, 36% of parents no longer had access to a doctor, and 56% of parents were still eligible to receive accommodations through telehealth or online schooling (Jeste et al. 2020). This astronomical loss shows that the educational and medical system have needed to adapt to the lack of structure and address the problems associated with a lack of accessibility. The researchers noted that "The loss of critical services post-COVID-19 restrictions evidenced across the sample reinforces the need for close monitoring, creativity in the delivery of care, and optimization of strategies to improve the delivery of all resources that promote optional medical and developmental outcomes for children with syndromic intellectual and developmental disabilities (IDD's) during this pandemic." (Jeste et al. 2020). Now that the vaccine rollout has continued throughout the United States, the only hope is that children with disabilities who need this support can gain access again to schools with special programs once the pandemic draws to a close.

The other conflicting point of interest is the increased need for media use throughout the pandemic, particularly for children with disabilities. For parents trying to manage their busy schedules from home, the added necessity of working with a child with a disability can be difficult. However, with their classes being held online and limited interactions with others, there may be some benefits to giving a child more access to their screens. In her article, Mangaello (2020) discusses her experiences with her son, who has multiple disabilities, and the trials and tribulations that came with managing his screen time. For example, school hours were shortened since teachers and students were operating in the classroom remotely. Because of this, Manganello (2020) worked to find online programs that her son would not only enjoy but would afford him an organized structure throughout the week. "He took classes including cooking, and I was shocked by how much his skills improved. He is now able to cook a basic meal on his own and develop ideas for recipes (Manganello, 2020)." With this expanded opportunity to learn more, parents could find new and interactive ways to involve their children while staying at home. Another option that Manganello experienced during quarantine was allowing her son to play video games and watch new television shows. With video games, her son could participate in social interaction with others, gain conversational skills, and connect more with his older brother. And by exploring new outlets of television genres, her son developed what she calls "a more mature media diet" that he could discuss with friends and connect with others in fan clubs.

On the flip side, however, giving these children more screen access comes with the challenge of determining how to best manage their usage. "One child becomes very upset when watching shows that do not showcase social distancing. Some children are experiencing physical issues from extended screen time, such as eye strain. One mother wonders why her child becomes aggressive with some video games but not others (Manganello, 2020)." Although children with disabilities must rely on technology to participate in school, the implications may become more challenging for parents to manage once the pandemic subsides and children return to school. How will parents and schools separate children from their screens? Could technology be considered as more of a helpful tool for these children? While there need to be restrictions enforced on how much these children can access their devices, we must also consider that the way we live and work has drastically changed in the last year. As such, the way children and parents use media will become more integrated into how we operate than ever before. We must consider the harmful effects of increased screen time and the benefits of having screens that still provide us with the access we need to connect and collaborate.

THE CHALLENGES OF FILM PRODUCTION DURING QUARANTINE

With the mass closures of restaurants, businesses, studios, and companies with the goal of preventing the spread of COVID-19, the lockdown forced people to begin working from home and switching all of their work to remote work. The biggest challenges that came with the pandemic fell on entertainment and production companies that either worked to produce or had TV shows and films slated for 2020. Filmmakers and producers had to develop more creative approaches towards completing their movies while working from home. One of the many great examples of this creativity comes from the latest installment of the SpongeBob film saga, *Sponge On The Run.*

SpongeBob SquarePants first aired on May 1, 1999 on Nickelodeon and followed SpongeBob and his friends' comical adventures through the lens of their oceanic hometown, Bikini Bottom. Stephen Hillenberg, a marine science teacher turned comic animator, created the show and brought the story to life through his creativity and imagination. Since SpongeBob's first emergence on TV, the show has had continued success with many seasons, spin-off films, and even a Broadway musical. The show combines both childhood imagination with adult verbiage. Unfortunately, Hillenberg died on November 26, 2018, due to complications from ALS. However, his legacy continues to live on through the hearts and minds of SpongeBob fans. Fast-forward to the present day, and the movie has found success through various streaming platforms, including the release of Paramount Plus from Paramount Studios. However, the hard-working team behind this film had to make do with the limited resources they had while working from home.

One of the challenges the team faced was creating the film's musical score. Since musicians could not meet in recording studios, they had to find new ways to pull pieces together and hit the record button. "Instead, performers were instructed to individually record their parts for composer Hans Zimmer's soundtrack in their local studios. Then sound engineers overlaid those components with Zimmer's trademark synths to create the final product (De La Garza, 2020)." Despite the many obstacles, this experience opened their eyes to the fact that films could be made differently following the end of the pandemic. "If there is anything good that comes of this crisis for the movie-making business, it might be a decoupling of geographic proximity and production. Late-night storyboarding sessions in stuffy rooms may be gone for the time being, but what has replaced them is a newfound flexibility to collaborate with creators beyond the Hollywood Hills (De La Garza, 2020)." This discussion of this film's production reflects how much children's media has changed and adapted throughout this year. Despite the number of trials and tribulations that came off the heels of this pandemic, this creative team essentially proved that children's media could still be produced and released into the world for families to enjoy, no matter how far away everyone was from their local theatres.

Another film that received the COVID post-production treatment was the remake of *Tom & Jerry,* released on February 26, 2021. Due to the mass closures of studios, film teams needed to convert their on-site work to remote. As mentioned with *SpongeBob SquarePants'* origins, *Tom & Jerry* was created as a cartoon series by William Hanna and Joseph Barbera in 1940. The story focused on the rivalry between the two main characters; Tom, a housecat, and Jerry, a mouse. Between 1940 and 1958, the two directors created 114 shorts and several spin-offs years after. Because of the show's mass popularity with children and adults alike, the continuation of this saga unfolds even further, with the release of *Tom & Jerry,* directed by Tim Story.

This film narrowly escaped facing lockdown since the story incorporates both natural and animated characters, including Chloe Grace Moretz, Colin Josh, and Michael Pena. However, by the time quarantine took place, the film's live-action shots were already completed. The problem that the team faced afterward was completing post-production successfully and separately. The group initially wanted to complete this process in London, but stay-at-home orders prevented this possibility. "By the time production and their Framestore and Warnes partners ran the logistics and associated costs, the industry-wide shutdown was already underway, making *Tom & Jerry's* only option to break into a remote workflow with artists split between London and Montreal, story and editors were scattered throughout Europe, with an editor in Los Angeles (D' Alessandro 2020)." The scatterplot process was an extreme challenge for those working in the film industry. There was no easy way to connect with co-workers about splitting scenes, adding dialogue, and inserting music through a computer screen lens. However, this project's success came in February, with the film finally being released on popular streaming platforms. Despite the many challenges that this film went through during its final touch-ups, the quality of the film crew's creativity and hard work cannot be ignored, even after studios return to normal.

FUTURE DIRECTIONS

So, where do we go from here? What will children's media look like in the future? Can we continue to demonstrate effective use of technology as we adapt to a new "normal?" For some, children's memories will be filled with virtual learning and mask-wearing, with no recollection of the times before the pandemic. They will forever be changed by these last two years of their lives. Schools may continue to use virtual learning as a facet to optimize children's education. Their favorite television shows will always exist on their screens, so the playful adventures they seek can be reached from the comfort of their homes. The next generation of children will shape the future of media consumption. For others, however, children will absorb the media they've consumed and respond negatively to the effects of the pandemic. Their social development may be hampered due to their inability to connect with others as a result of lockdowns or school closures. Children could experience severe behavioral changes, either from the media they've consumed or from the stress and anxiety they've witnessed from their parents and have experienced themselves. There is no clear-cut way to determine the full psychological impact of the pandemic on children, but future research should focus on the influence of children's media.

CONCLUSION

Children's media has been and forever will be a stable feature of American television. Even now, as we emerge out of this pandemic, entertainment companies will return to their offices to continue to produce fun and interactive content for children and their families to enjoy at home. However, there is something to be said about how these networks will use the lessons taught to children over the last year and a half to create educational and informational programming to continue facilitating healthy practices. Social media platforms will also continue to produce news and facts from public health officials to showcase how we move away from quarantine and social distancing and resume everyday life. Additionally, parents themselves will be leaving their homes and returning to their offices. However, we will also still consider that children's media, and media in general, have dramatically transformed since the beginning of 2020. Children's media consumption will continue to increase as we slowly but surely reopen schools and continue to use online learning as a backup. The lack of parents' knowledge about what their children are watching will increase since they will no longer be home to monitor their children's content. Most importantly, researchers will begin to uncover the psychological and emotional effects this pandemic has had on children as they move through life. Until then, we must continue to protect children's health and safety and keep their media usage at bay so that they may continue to maintain social interactions with others, while also stimulating their imagination through presenting their favorite cartoons.

REFERENCES

Babvey, P., Capela, F., Cappa, C., Lipizzi, C., Petrowski, N., & Ramirez-Marquez, J. (2020). Using social media data for assessing children's exposure to violence during the COVID-19 pandemic. *Child Abuse & Neglect*, 1–12. https://www.sciencedirect.com/science/article/pii/S0145213420304026 PMID:33358281

Ball, S., & Bogatz, G. A. (1970). A Summary Of The Major Findings In "The First Year Of Sesame Street: An Evaluation." *Educational Teaching Service*, 3–15. https://eric.ed.gov/?id=ED122799

Calvert, S., & Kotler, J. (2003). Lessons from children's television: The impact of the Children's Television Act on children's learning. *Journal of Applied Developmental Psychology*, *24*(3), 277–282. doi:10.1016/S0193-3973(03)00060-1

D'Alessandro, A. (2020, May 8). *How Animated Pics Like 'Tom & Jerry', 'SpongeBob Movie', 'Sing 2', Skydance's 'Luck' & More Are Working Through The COVID-19 Crisis*. Deadline. https://deadline.com/2020/05/animated-movies-coronavirus-production-tom-and-jerry-spongebob-scoob-skydance-illumination-1202928961/

Frenette, M., Frank, K., & Deng, Z. (2020). School Closures and the Online Preparedness of Children during the COVID-19 Pandemic. *Economic Insights*, 1–6. https://files.eric.ed.gov/fulltext/ED605398.pdf

Garza, A. (2020, August 24). *How Paramount Animation Shifted to Remote Work—and Made a "Beautiful" SpongeBob Movie in the Process*. Time. https://time.com/5882272/spongebob-movie-coronavirus/

Goldschmidt, K. (2020). The COVID-19 Pandemic: Technology Use to Support the Wellbeing of Children. *Journal of Pediatric Nursing*, *53*, 88–90. doi:10.1016/j.pedn.2020.04.013 PMID:32317129

Haring, B. (2020, March 27). *Nickelodeon & Disney Channel Address Kids' Coronavirus Concerns While Maintaining Quarantine*. Deadline. https://deadline.com/2020/03/kidstogether-the-nickelodeon-town-hall-addresses-kid-coronavirus-concerns-1202893877/

Hayes, D. A. (1994). The Children's Hour Revisited: The Children's Television Act of 1990. *Federal Communications Law Journal*, *46*(2), 294–311. https://www.repository.law.indiana.edu/cgi/viewcontent.cgi?referer=https://scholar.google.com/scholar?hl=en&as_sdt=0%2C33&q=children's+television+act&btnG=&httpsredir=1&referer=&httpredir=1&article=1016&context=fclj

Jeste, S., Hyde, C., Distefano, C., Halladay, A., Ray, S., Porath, M., Wilson, R. B., & Thurm, A. (2020). Changes in access to educational and healthcare services for individuals with intellectual and developmental disabilities during COVID-19 restrictions. *Journal of Intellectual Disability Research*, *64*(11), 825–833. doi:10.1111/jir.12776 PMID:32939917

Manganello, J. (2020). Media use for children with disabilities in the United States during COVID-19. *Journal of Children and Media*, *15*(1), 29–32. doi:10.1080/17482798.2020.1857281

Tulchin-Francis, K., Stevens, W., Jr., Gu, X., Zhang, T., Roberts, H., Keller, J., Dempsey, D., Borchard, J., Jeans, K., & VanPelt, J. (2021). The impact of the coronavirus disease 2019 pandemic on physical activity in US children. *Journal of Sports and Health Science*, 1–10. https://reader.elsevier.com/reader/sd/pii/S2095254621000259?token=CA20D877B2AE88EDF759D7077742CCA3BAE816FCBBC709F360B40BC35A1049173DA8A15C17204192E366AAB188DA804A&originRegion=us-east-1&originCreation=20210406004449

Vanderloo, L., Carsley, S., Aglipay, M., Cost, K., Maguire, J., & Birken, C. (2020). Applying Harm Reduction Principles to Address Screen Time in Young Children Amidst the COVID-19 Pandemic. *Journal Of Development And Behavioral Pediatrics, 41*(5), 335–336. https://journals.lww.com/jrnldbp/Citation/2020/07000/Applying_Harm_Reduction_Principles_to_Address.1.aspx

Wong, A. (2015, July 16). *The 1960s 'Sesame Street' Revolution and the Persistence of America's Educational Problems.* The Atlantic. https://www.theatlantic.com/education/archive/2015/07/the-1960s-experiment-childrens-tv/398681/

Chapter 11
Mindset:
The Effect on College Student Adjustment to Remote Learning

Emily Angelillo
Marymount Manhattan College, USA

ABSTRACT

In March 2020, the COVID-19 pandemic changed lives throughout the world. The present study focused on the effect of these changes on college students in the U.S. Specifically, the study examined the relationship between students' 'mindsets' (i.e., attitudes toward the malleability of intelligence) and their adjustment to online schooling. Results indicated a strong positive correlation – the greater the belief in the potential growth of intelligence, the better the adjustment from in-person to virtual instruction.

INTRODUCTION

COVID-19 (coronavirus disease 2019), a disease caused by the virus SARS-CoV-2, was discovered in December 2019 in Wuhan, China. The disease is very contagious and quickly spread around the world (Centers for Disease Control and Prevention, 2021). The Centers for Disease Control (CDC) confirmed the first U.S. case on Jan. 21, 2020 and by the end of January, 2020, the World Health Organization (WHO) had declared a world-wide public health emergency (cdc.gov). In early March, 2020, the WHO declared COVID-19 a pandemic; on March 13, 2020, U.S. President Trump declared COVID-19 a national emergency and on March 19, 2020, California became the first U.S. state to issue a stay-at-home order, rapidly followed

DOI: 10.4018/978-1-6684-3484-0.ch011

by similar orders in other states, cities, and counties, although some parts of the country refused to follow suit.

At the time of the current study (April 2021), vaccines for COVID-19 had received emergency use authorization in the United States. Administration of the vaccines had begun in late December 2020, however, availability was limited, and eligibility was restricted to evolving lists of recipients, depending on age, occupation, and medical condition.

Throughout the country, most areas had closed schools, businesses, and public places. Transportation options were limited; many employees were working from home or had been terminated from employment; health care facilities were overwhelmed with cases of COVID-19, and the death rate and caseload remained high. The NY Times (nytimes.com) reported that new cases in the U.S. in mid-April totaled over 75,000. Effects of the long-lasting pandemic (and accompanying restrictions) included health challenges, economic challenges, loss of loved ones, isolation from the community, and considerable psychological stress.

Researchers (e.g., AlAzzam, 2021) noted the devastating effects on mental health. College students were among those facing numerous and overwhelming difficulties. Apart from their serious concern with physical health, many students had been forced to adjust to sudden and unanticipated changes in their lives. These included shifts in residence (parental homes replacing college dormitories), new modes of instruction (virtual/online instruction replacing in-person classes), loss of employment for parents and themselves, leading to financial hardships, and the social isolation of lockdown.

Shamblaw (2021) noted that the Coronavirus pandemic had "caused widespread detrimental effects on mental health and quality of life, yet little research (had) examined effective coping strategies to mitigate these negative effects'' (Shamblaw, 2021, p.1). The present study focused on one pandemic challenge, namely the shift to online instruction, and one potential predictor of response to the challenge, namely mindset. As described by Bernecker and Job (2019), Dweck's Mindset Theory proposes that "people hold different beliefs about the malleability of human attributes, such as intelligence and personality" (p. 1). The mindset continuum ranges from a growth mindset (growth and development are possible throughout the lifespan) to a fixed mindset (basic characteristics do not change).

Bernecker and Job (2019) proposed that a growth mindset is typically more "adaptive" (p. 1) than a fixed mindset. Other authors (e.g., Rege et al., 2020) have concurred. Based on this reasoning, the present author hypothesized that those with a stronger growth mindset would make a more successful transition to online learning. The author reasoned that those with a growth mindset would be positively affected by the belief that it is possible to adjust to difficult changes - adapting to circumstances and overcoming challenges.

METHOD

The participants included 50 college students from 13 different institutions across the East coast of the United States. They were students from freshman through senior year and all of the participants had taken one or more online classes during the pandemic.

Participants responded to an online survey. The survey included two measures created by the author: 1) Mindset Regarding Intelligence (11 items), and 2) Adjustment to Online Education (11 items). All items were rated by using 5-point (strongly disagree to strongly agree) rating scales. Both measures included positively-keyed and negatively-keyed items and the items were presented in an inter-mixed order.

RESULTS

An examination of the internal consistency of the measures indicated the following levels of Cronbach's alpha: .705 for mindset and .621 for adjustment.

A Pearson's r supported the hypothesis of a positive correlation between mindset and adjustment, $r(48) = .552$, $p < .001$. The more growth-oriented the participants, the more positively the participants perceived their adjustment to online learning.

DISCUSSION AND CONCLUSIONS

The data strongly supported the hypothesis that a growth-oriented mindset may facilitate adjustment to change (online learning in this case). The finding was consistent with other studies in similar and varying contexts (e.g., Rege et al., 2020).

The conclusion must be assessed with caution. The results are limited in external validity, given the study's correlational design, small and narrow sample, untested measures, and online data collection at a particular point in time. Future studies might validate the measures and broaden the sample. In addition, attention might be paid to such moderating variables as student status, type of institution, and demographic characteristics. Finally, attention might be shifted to effects of mindset and adjustment over time (and post-college).

Despite caveats, the overall conclusion that growth mindset facilitates adjustment has far-reaching implications for pre-college and college-level education. Moreover, the fact that some students and others will be in need of mental health and adjustment support as the pandemic (hopefully) winds down may dictate the design of institutions and services in the coming years.

March of 2020 marked the start of the Coronavirus pandemic for the United States and the start of adjustments to many new "normals." Some of these included changes in everyday safety procedures in our work and school environments, a new lack of social interaction, and for some, financial hardship. The pandemic has caused "widespread detrimental effects on mental health and quality of life, yet little research has examined effective coping strategies to mitigate these negative effects" (Shamblaw, 2021, p.1). This has left our society broken and struggling throughout all age groups. All of the changes that have occurred since the beginning of COVID-19 have been difficult and uncomfortable around the world but some individuals have adapted better than others. Many recent studies have focused on the "significant contribution of the COVID-19 pandemic on adolescents' mental health" (AlAzzam, 2021, p.5), specifically referring to students. These studies have justified that students have been hit with large increases in levels of anxiety and depression. Even though all types of students have been affected mentally, financially, and physically, it seems that college students have faced a heavier burden. College students have experienced online classes, financial hardships, and social isolation. Not only have they faced the concerns of adults but also the ones of younger students at the same time. All of these changes during early adulthood have caused detrimental effects in many ways, short-term and long.

Among one of the most difficult adjustments, the pandemic has forced most students to switch to attending college online. Some students have adapted better than others. After moving to online learning, those students maintained consistent grades and motivation, positive leaning mental health, and continued success throughout extracurriculars, if applicable.

The purpose of the present study was to determine whether students would have different outcomes when it came to their adjustment to online school because of their mindsets and attitudes. "Mindset Theory proposes that people hold different beliefs about the malleability of human attributes, such as intelligence and personality (Bernecker and Job, 2019, p.1)." Those who have more positive outlooks are more likely to have a growth mindset and believe that intelligence is malleable. Meanwhile, the people who have more negative outlooks are more likely to have a belief that these same things are fixed. Becknecker and Jobs (2019) in a previous study, concluded that "The belief that people can change is usually (but not always) more adaptive than the belief that human attributes are fixed (Bernecker and Job, 2019, p.1)." Considering the factors of mindset and adjustment in the present study, it can be hypothesized that there may be a connection between the two.

In the present study, data were collected from 50 college students across 13 institutions who were asked about their mindsets and how they felt about adjusting to taking classes online. Previous studies have stated that "the benefits of the growth mindset were apparent at the end" (Rege, 2020, p.3) of their studies, therefore connecting the idea that a growth mindset can lead to positive outcomes in the long run. In the present study assessing the connection between mindset and adjustment, it can be hypothesized that this study would have similar results. If students were to display a similar positive/growth mindset during the transition to online classes then, they would be more likely to adjust to these courses compared to a student with a negative mindset. Students with a positive mindset would believe that intelligence is malleable, enabling them to believe that the circumstances can be adapted to and overcome rather than seeing adaptation as impossible.

METHOD

Participants

The participants were 50 college students from 13 different institutions across the east coast of the United States. These institutions included Marymount Manhattan College, Adelphi University, Baruch College, Binghamton University, Coastal Carolina University, Farmingdale State College, John Jay College of Criminal Justice, Long Island University, Penn State University, Rensselaer Polytechnic Institute, Stony Brook University, Suffolk Community College, and SUNY Potsdam. All data were collected from the participants through an anonymous survey.

Type of Study

The study conducted was a correlational study. It took place through an online survey that was created with questions about mindsets about intelligence and questions about adjustment to online education.

Materials

The only materials needed for this study were a computer and access to the internet. The computer was used to create the survey, collect the responses, review previous literature, analyze data, and write the final research paper. The internet was needed to distribute the survey and search for other literature relating to the topic.

Development of Survey

The survey was created over a period of time, including many steps. First, I conducted research on previous studies that have assessed the variables which were mindset and adjustment. Then, I used this information to formulate questions that pertained to each of these topics. Following this, the survey was reviewed by peers and professors to gain a second opinion on what questions would be helpful for the survey. Lastly, the survey was revised and then distributed.

Survey Details

The survey included an informed consent statement, nine demographic questions, ten questions referring to mindset, and twelve questions referring to adjustment. The mindset questions were numbers 17, 19, 20, 21, 23, 24, 25, 26, 27, and 28. The adjustment questions were numbers 12, 13, 14, 15, 16, 18, 22, 29, 30, 31, 32, and 33. A 5 point Likert scale was used for the questions referring to mindset and adjustment. 1 being strongly disagree, 2 being slightly disagree, 3 being neither disagree nor agree, 4 being slightly agree, and 5 being strongly agree. Both positively and negatively keyed questions were included for each measure. Examples of mindset questions in the survey included "I am confident in my ability to succeed" and "If an individual struggles with a topic, they will never improve on it." Meanwhile, examples of adjustment questions included "I was able to connect with my peers while taking classes online" and "I never really understood the material from my online class".

Informed Consent

The focus of this study is to gather information on the experiences of college students taking online courses during the 2020 Coronavirus pandemic. This survey will take no more than 5 minutes and provides no potential risks. This survey is also anonymous.

You will be presented with questions about your gender, GPA, age, and other facts about yourself. These details, along with the rest of the survey, will remain completely confidential.

Your participation in this survey is completely voluntary, and you are free to withdraw at any time during the study without giving a reason and without prejudice. If you have any questions about the survey or you would like to withdraw, please feel free to contact the principal investigator. Please feel free to keep this consent page for your records. Thank you for your participation.

Measures

1) Do you wish to participate?
   Mark only one oval
   Yes
   No

2) Are you in college or were you in college during the Coronavirus pandemic?
Mark only one oval
Yes, I am currently enrolled.
No.
Yes, I was enrolled during the pandemic but I am not currently.
3) How old are you?
Mark only one oval
18
19
20
21
22
23
24
25+
4) What is your gender?
Mark only one oval
Female
Male
Prefer not to say
Other:____________
5) Where do you go to college?_________
6) What year of college are you in?
Mark only one oval
Freshman
Sophomore
Junior
Senior
7) What is your major?____________
8) What is your enrollment status?
Mark only one oval
Part-Time
Full-Time
9) How many semesters have you taken online during the pandemic?
Mark only one oval
1 semester
2 semesters
3 semesters
4 semesters

10) Did you take any pass/fail courses while taking classes online during the pandemic?
Mark only one oval
Yes
No
11) What is your current GPA?
Mark only one oval
1.0-2.0
2.1-2.9
3.0-2.5
3.6-4.0
12) I was comfortable with the idea of taking classes online.
13) I was able to connect with my peers while taking classes online.
14) I was able to form connections with my professors while taking classes online.
15) The amount of work I was given while attending virtual classes was fair.
16) I was able to concentrate while taking my classes virtually from another environment besides a school.
17) People can learn anything if they study enough.
18) I never really understood the material from my online classes.
19) I can learn from my mistakes and improve from them.
20) When I work harder, I am more pleased with my work.
21) I find myself having a hard time becoming motivated to complete my work.
22) I found a sense of routine and normalcy, eventually, in my online classes.
23) There is always something new to learn.
24) If individuals struggle with a particular topic, they can never improve in it.
25) I am confident in my ability to succeed.
26) When I choose to speak up in class, I am confident.
27) I am always too nervous to get an answer wrong when raising my hand in class.
28) The more you study material for a course, the better the grades that you get will be.
29) I contemplated taking some time off of school because virtual classes seemed difficult.
30) I retained significantly less information taking classes online compared to when I took classes in person.
31) I disliked sitting in front of a computer for long periods of time.
32) I would voluntarily take an online class again in the future.
33) I easily adjusted to online learning during the pandemic.

Procedure

After the development of the survey, it was distributed through a variety of mediums to gain data. The survey was posted on Snapchat, Instagram, and was also sent out as a link during two zoom classes at Marymount Manhattan College. Once the data were collected, it was analyzed for conclusions.

RESULTS

Data

Reliability (Cronbach's)

Table 1. Reliability Statistics for Adjustment

Cronbach's Alpha	N of Items
.621	11

Table 2. Reliability Statistics for Mindset

Cronbach's Alpha	N of Items
.705	11

Table 3. Item-Total Statistics For Adjustment

	Scale Mean if Item Deleted	Scale Variance if Item Deleted	Corrected Item-Total Correlation	Cronbach's Alpha if Item Deleted
VAR00001	24.6200	27.098	.611	.516
VAR00002	25.6000	30.776	.510	.558
VAR00003	25.0400	30.937	.419	.571
VAR00004	25.1600	30.709	.423	.569
VAR00005	25.6800	27.161	.663	.509
VAR00007	25.1400	40.653	-.320	.698
VAR00011	24.6000	28.122	.616	.524
VAR00018	24.8000	42.776	-.393	.743
VAR00019	25.6800	32.508	.244	.605
VAR00020	25.9000	33.765	.159	.622
VAR00021	24.7800	28.379	.525	.540

Table 4. Item-Total Statistics For Mindset

	Scale Mean if Item Deleted	Scale Variance if Item Deleted	Corrected Item-Total Correlation	Cronbach's Alpha if Item Deleted
VAR00006	32.3600	28.888	.534	.651
VAR00009	31.2000	33.673	.370	.685
VAR00008	31.3200	33.324	.409	.680
VAR00010	33.3000	28.214	.527	.651
VAR00013	34.2000	35.878	.159	.707
VAR00017	32.2000	32.490	.342	.686
VAR00016	33.5600	38.496	-.142	.758
VAR00014	31.4200	30.004	.586	.649
VAR00015	32.3200	28.793	.447	.668
VAR00012	31.1600	32.953	.431	.677
VAR00022	32.9600	31.019	.322	.692

Participants' Demographic Characteristics

Figure 1. Percentage of Students Current Year in College

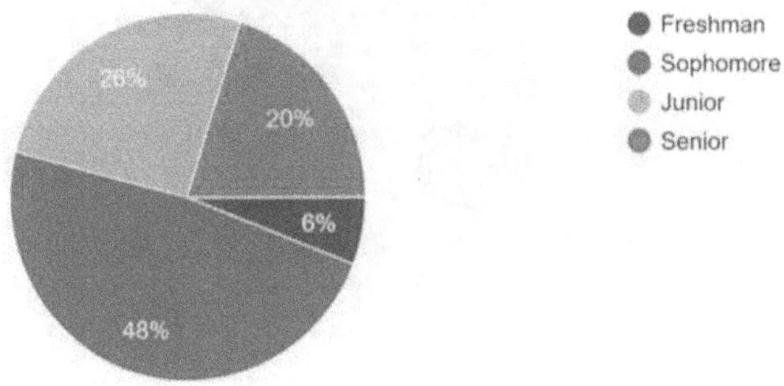

Figure 2. Percentage of Semesters that Students Took Online During the Pandemic

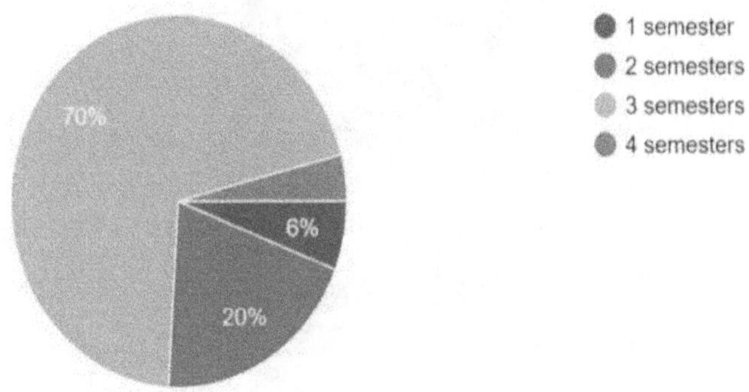

Figure 3. Percentage of Students that Took Pass/Fail Courses During the Pandemic

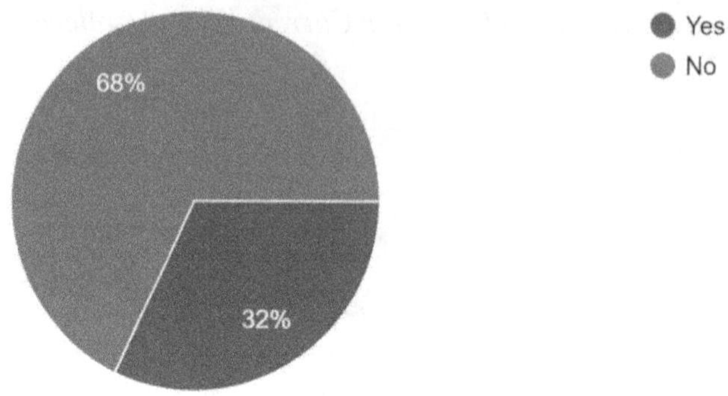

Figure 4. Percentage of Students Current GPAs

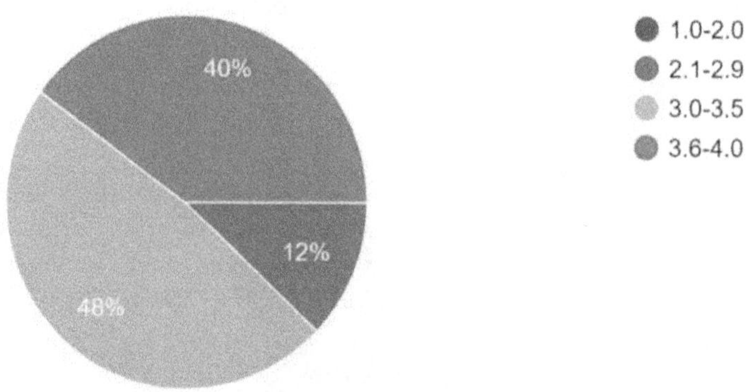

Correlation Between Mindset and Adjustment

Table 5. Correlations

		Adjustment	Mindset
Adjustment	Pearson Correlation	1	.552**
	Sig. (2-tailed)		.000
	N	50	50
Mindset	Pearson Correlation	.552**	1
	Sig. (2-tailed)	.000	
	N	50	50

**. Correlation is significant at the 0.01 level (2-tailed).

Summary

The study analyzed college students and the correlation between their mindset and their ability to adjust to online school during the Coronavirus pandemic. Tables 1-4 show Cronbach's alpha data for both mindset and adjustment, documenting the reliability within the data set. Specifically, in Tables 3 and 4, each question was given a different score to determine whether it should be removed from the data set to improve the results. This was done for both the mindset and adjustment questions in the survey. Following this, Figures 1, 2, 3, and 4 all include demographic responses from the survey. Lastly, Table 5 included the correlation between mindset and adjustment. The relationship between the variables was extremely significant with r=.552. Therefore, the hypothesis that there would be a positive correlation between college students' mindsets and their adjustment to online school was strongly supported by the data.

DISCUSSION

The survey data indicated that there was a strong correlation between college students' mindsets and how they adjusted to online school. Therefore, the data supported the original hypothesis of this study.

Despite the results, if the same study were to be conducted again, a few limitations should be considered beforehand. The responses were taken from a small sample (N=50) which may have skewed the data to not be completely representative of college students as a whole. Along with this, this study only included colleges and universities on the east coast of the United States, again which might have skewed the data. Students in a different area of the country that experience warmer weather for longer periods of time might claim to have more positive adjustments. It is also possible that the time of year in which the survey was conducted might have skewed the data. For instance, an individual who suffers from seasonal depression might respond differently in the summer than in the spring or winter. Also, it is possible that there may have been confounding or extraneous variables that the researcher did not take into consideration when creating the survey. For example, a student's home life could have affected his/her responses. Someone who was an only child and went home to a quiet house might have had a less frustrating experience than an individual who was from a chaotic home environment with three young siblings screaming and their dog barking.

After considering these factors, this study could be used to justify conducting more research related to this topic because the hypothesis was supported and the evidence was statistically significant. Further research might determine whether there is a link between personality type and mindset, whether individuals who adapt faster are more likely to have successful careers, or even whether children's upbringing might have an effect on their ability to adjust, therefore leading to further conclusions relating to the pandemic, adjustment, and mindset.

This study itself has practical implications. After analyzing the data as well as data from previous studies, it can be seen that a growth mindset facilitates adjustment. If a growth mindset were encouraged and maintained in a classroom setting throughout development, it might lead to more long-term success in students over time.

However, regardless of the conclusion of this research, the pandemic has been and continues to be a source of serious stress for college students. The challenge of the pandemic is far from over and future environmental challenges await the students of today. Hopefully, as these students further their education, they will continue to receive support and understanding to reach their goals and dreams.

ACKNOWLEDGMENT

I would like to express the deepest appreciation to Linda Z. Solomon, Ph.D., a Professor of Psychology at Marymount Manhattan College. She convincingly conveyed spirit in regard to research, scholarship, and teaching at all times. Without her guidance and persistent help with this research, it would have not been possible. Thank you.

REFERENCES

AlAzzam, M., Abuhammad, S., Abdalrahim, A., & Hamdan-Mansour, A. M. (2021). Predictors of Depression and Anxiety Among Senior High School Students During COVID-19 Pandemic: The Context of Home Quarantine and Online Education. *The Journal of School Nursing: the Official Publication of the National Association of School Nurses*, *37*(4), 241–248. Advance online publication. doi:10.1177/1059840520988548 PMID:33563066

Bernecker, K., & Job, V. (2019). Mindset theory. In Social Psychology in Action (pp. 179-191). Springer. https://file.zhisci.com/202005/2019-Social_Psychology_in_Action-Sassenberg-cn20200527173725.pdf#page=187

Rege, M., Hanselman, P., Solli, I. F., Dweck, C. S., Ludvigsen, S., Bettinger, E., Crosnoe, R., Muller, C., Walton, G., Duckworth, A., & Yeager, D. S. (2020). How can we inspire nations of learners? An investigation of growth mindset and challenge-seeking in two countries. *American Psychologist*. https://slb.mmm.edu:2208/10.1037/amp0000647.supp

Shamblaw, A. L., Rumas, R. L., & Best, M. W. (2021). Coping during the COVID-19 pandemic: Relations with mental health and quality of life. *Canadian Psychology*, *62*(1), 92–100. doi:10.1037/cap0000263

KEY TERMS AND DEFINITIONS

Coronavirus Disease (COVID-19): An infectious disease caused by the SARS-CoV-2 virus.

Correlational Study: A non-experimental research method that studies the relationship between two variables with the help of statistical analysis.

Cronbach's Alpha: A measure of internal consistency, that is, how closely related a set of items are as a group. It is considered to be a measure of scale reliability.

Isolation: The state of being in a place or situation that is separate from others.

Malleable: Having a capacity for adaptive change.

Mental Health: A person's condition with regard to his/her psychological and emotional well-being.

Mindset: The established set of attitudes held by someone.

Pearson's R: A type of correlation coefficient that represents the relationship between two variables that are measured on the same interval.

Compilation of References

Abawi, O. (2021). Impacts of the Covid-19 Lockdown and Relevant Vulnerabilities on Capability Well-being, Mental Health and Social Support: An Austrian Survey Study. *Journal of the Endocrine Society*, *5*(1). Advance online publication. doi:10.1210/jendso/bvab048.702

ADDitude Editors. (2021, January 19). *ADHD Brains Working at Home: A Beginner's Guide to Telecommuting*. ADDitude. https://www.additudemag.com/working-from-homeadhd/

Agyapong, V. I. O., Hrabok, M., Shalaby, R., Mrklas, K., Vuong, W., Gusnowski, A., Surood, S., Greenshaw, A. J., & Nkire, N. (2020). Closing the COVID-19 psychological treatment gap for cancer patients in Alberta: Protocol for the implementation and evaluation of Text4Hope-Cancer Care. *JMIR Research Protocols*, *9*(8), e20240. doi:10.2196/20240 PMID:32750012

AlAzzam, M., Abuhammad, S., Abdalrahim, A., & Hamdan-Mansour, A. M. (2021). Predictors of Depression and Anxiety Among Senior High School Students During COVID-19 Pandemic: The Context of Home Quarantine and Online Education. *The Journal of School Nursing: the Official Publication of the National Association of School Nurses*, *37*(4), 241–248. Advance online publication. doi:10.1177/1059840520988548 PMID:33563066

Al-Hanawi, M. K., Ahmad, K., Haque, R., & Keramat, S. A. (2021). Willingness to receive COVID-19 vaccination among adults with chronic diseases in the Kingdom of Saudi Arabia. *Journal of Infection and Public Health*, *14*(10), 1489–1496. doi:10.1016/j.jiph.2021.08.002 PMID:34417135

American Psychiatric Association. (2013). *Diagnostic and statistical manual of mental disorders* (5th ed.). doi:10.1176/appi.books.9780890425596

American Psychological Association. (2008). *Clinical health psychology*. https://www.apa.org/ed/graduate/specialize/health

American Psychological Association. (n.d.). Well-being. In *APA dictionary of psychology*. Retrieved October 20, 2021, from https://dictionary.apa.org/well-being

American Speech-Language-Hearing Association. (n.d.) *Types of Hearing Loss*. American Speech-Language-Hearing Association. https://www.asha.org/public/hearing/types-of-hearing-loss/

Ando, M., Takeda, T., & Kumagai, K. (2021). A qualitative study of impacts of the COVID-19 pandemic on lives in adults with attention deficit hyperactive disorder in Japan. *International Journal of Environmental Research and Public Health, 18*(4), 2090. doi:10.3390/ijerph18042090 PMID:33669970

Anxiety and Depression Association of America. (2021). *Facts & Statistics: Anxiety and Depression Association of America.* https://adaa.org/understanding-anxiety/facts-statistics

Apostolidis, S. A., Kakara, M., Painter, M. M., Goel, R. R., Mathew, D., Lenzi, K., ... Bar-Or, A. (2021). Cellular and humoral immune responses following SARS-CoV-2 mRNA vaccination in patients with multiple sclerosis on anti-CD20 therapy. *Nature Medicine*, 1–12. doi:10.103841591-021-01507-2 PMID:34522051

Archer, N., Keshavjee, K., Demers, C., & Lee, R. (2014). Online self-management interventions for chronically ill patients: Cognitive impairment and technology issues. *International Journal of Medical Informatics, 83*(4), 264–272. doi:10.1016/j.ijmedinf.2014.01.005 PMID:24507762

Aspinwall, L. G., & Taylor, S. E. (1997). A stitch in time: Self-regulation and proactive coping. *Psychological Bulletin, 121*(3), 417–436. doi:10.1037/0033-2909.121.3.417 PMID:9136643

Azevedo, J. P., Hasan, A., Goldemberg, D., Iqbal, S. A., & Geven, K. (2020). *Simulating the potential impacts of COVID-19 school closures on schooling and learning outcomes: A set of global estimates*. The World Bank.

Babvey, P., Capela, F., Cappa, C., Lipizzi, C., Petrowski, N., & Ramirez-Marquez, J. (2020). Using social media data for assessing children's exposure to violence during the COVID-19 pandemic. *Child Abuse & Neglect*, 1–12. https://www.sciencedirect.com/science/article/pii/S0145213420304026 PMID:33358281

Bailey, T., Hastings, R. P., & Totsika, V. (2021). Covid-19 impact on Psychological Outcomes of Parents, Siblings and Children with Intellectual Disability: Longitudinal Before and During Lockdown Design. *Journal of Intellectual Disability Research, 65*(5), 397–404. doi:10.1111/jir.12818 PMID:33634520

Ball, S., & Bogatz, G. A. (1970). A Summary Of The Major Findings In "The First Year Of Sesame Street: An Evaluation." *Educational Teaching Service*, 3–15. https://eric.ed.gov/?id=ED122799

Bao, X., Qu, H., Zhang, R., & Hogan, T. P. (2020). *Literacy Loss in Kindergarten Children during COVID-19 School Closures*. Academic Press.

Bao, Y., Sun, Y., Meng, S., Shi, J., & Lu, L. (2020). 2019-nCoV Epidemic: Address Mental Health Care to Empower Society. *Lancet, 395*(10224), e37–e38. doi:10.1016/S0140-6736(20)30309-3 PMID:32043982

Baron, E. J., Goldstein, E. G., & Wallace, C. T. (2020). Suffering in silence: How COVID-19 school closures inhibit the reporting of child maltreatment. *Journal of Public Economics, 190*, 104258. doi:10.1016/j.jpubeco.2020.104258 PMID:32863462

Basit, S. A., Mathews, N., & Kunik, M. E. (2020). Telemedicine interventions for medication adherence in mental illness: A systematic review. *General Hospital Psychiatry*, *62*, 28–36. doi:10.1016/j.genhosppsych.2019.11.004 PMID:31775066

Basner, M., Dinges, D. F., Mollicone, D. J., Savelev, I., Ecker, A. J., Di Antonio, A., . . . Sutton, J. P. (2014, March 27). *Psychological and behavioral changes during confinement in a 520-day simulated interplanetary mission to mars*. Retrieved from https://www.ncbi.nlm.nih.gov/pmc/articles/PMC3968121/

Battistin, T., Mercuriali, E., Zanardo, V., Gregori, D., Lorenzoni, G., Nasato, L., & Reffo, M. E. (2021). Distance support and online intervention to blind and visually impaired children during the pandemic COVID-19. *Research in Developmental Disabilities*, *108*, 103816. doi:10.1016/j.ridd.2020.103816 PMID:33271446

Bauman, S., & Pero, H. (2011). Bullying and Cyberbullying Among Deaf Students and Their Hearing Peers: An Exploratory Study. *Journal of Deaf Studies and Deaf Education*, *16*(2), 236–253. doi:10.1093/deafed/enq043 PMID:20855432

Beatty, L., & Lambert, S. (2013). A systematic review of internet-based self-help therapeutic interventions to improve distress and disease-control among adults with chronic health conditions. *Clinical Psychology Review*, *33*(4), 609–622. doi:10.1016/j.cpr.2013.03.004 PMID:23603521

Benatti, B., Albert, U., Maina, G., Fiorillo, A., Celebre, L., Girone, N., Fineberg, N., Bramante, S., Rigardetto, S., & Dell'Osso, B. (2020). What Happened to Patients with Obsessive Compulsive Disorder During the COVID-19 Pandemic? A Multicentre Report from Tertiary Clinics in Northern Italy. *Frontiers in Psychiatry*, *11*, 720. Advance online publication. doi:10.3389/fpsyt.2020.00720 PMID:32793008

Benner, A. D., & Mistry, R. S. (2020). Child development during the COVID-19 pandemic through a life course theory lens. *Child Development Perspectives*, *14*(4), 236–243. doi:10.1111/cdep.12387 PMID:33230400

Bergan, D. (2020). *Psychological approaches to the study of play*. doi:10.31838/jcr.07.01.38

Bernecker, K., & Job, V. (2019). Mindset theory. In Social Psychology in Action (pp. 179-191). Springer. https://file.zhisci.com/202005/2019-Social_Psychology_in_Action-Sassenberg-cn20200527173725.pdf#page=187

Bianchetti, A., Rozzini, R., Bianchetti, L., Coccia, F., Guerini, F., & Trabucchi, M. (2022). Dementia Clinical Care in Relation to COVID-19. *Current Treatment Options in Neurology*, *24*(1), 1–15. Advance online publication. doi:10.100711940-022-00706-7 PMID:35221646

Blustein, D. L., Duffy, R., Ferreira, J. A., Cohen-Scali, V., Cinamon, R. G., & Allan, B. A. (2020, June). Unemployment in the time of COVID-19: A research agenda. *Journal of Vocational Behavior*. https://www.ncbi.nlm.nih.gov/pmc/articles/PMC7206417/

Bobo, E., Lin, L., Acquaviva, E., Caci, H., Franc, N., Gamon, L., Picot, M. C., Pupier, F., Speranza, M., Falissard, B., & Purper-Ouakil, D. (2020). Comment les enfants et adolescents avec le trouble déficit d'attention/hyperactivité (TDAH) vivent-ils le confinement durant la pandémie COVID-19? [How do children and adolescents with Attention Deficit Hyperactivity Disorder (ADHD) experience lockdown during the COVID-19 outbreak?]. *L'Encéphale*, *46*(3, 3S), S85–S92. doi:10.1016/j.encep.2020.05.011 PMID:32522407

Bonavita, S., Sparaco, M., Russo, A., Borriello, G., & Lavorgna, L. (2021). Perceived stress and social support in a large population of people with multiple sclerosis recruited online through the COVID-19 pandemic. *European Journal of Neurology*, *28*(10), 3396–3402. doi:10.1111/ene.14697 PMID:33368849

Borges-Machado, F., Barros, D., Ribeiro, Ó., & Carvalho, J. (2020). The Effects of COVID-19 Home Confinement in Dementia Care: Physical and Cognitive Decline, Severe Neuropsychiatric Symptoms and Increased Caregiving Burden. *American Journal of Alzheimer's Disease and Other Dementias*, *35*(January). Advance online publication. doi:10.1177/1533317520976720 PMID:33295781

Bradbury, C., & Isham, L. (2020). *The pandemic paradox: The consequences of COVID-19 on domestic violence*. Academic Press.

Braga, D. T., Cordioli, A. V., Niederauer, K., & Manfro, G. G. (2005). Cognitive-behavioral group therapy for obsessive–compulsive disorder: A 1-year follow-up. *Acta Psychiatrica Scandinavica*, *112*(3), 180–186. doi:10.1111/j.1600-0447.2005.00559.x PMID:16095472

Brannon, L., & Feist, J. (2013). *Health Psychology: An Introduction to Behavior and Health* (9th ed.). Wadsworth.

Breaux, R., Dvorsky, M. R., Marsh, N. P., Green, C. D., Cash, A. R., Shroff, D. M., Buchen, N., Langberg, J. M., & Becker, S. P. (2021). Prospective impact of COVID-19 on mental health functioning in adolescents with and without ADHD: Protective role of emotion regulation abilities. *Journal of Child Psychology and Psychiatry, and Allied Disciplines*, *62*(9), 1132–1139. doi:10.1111/jcpp.13382 PMID:33543486

Brivio, E., Guiddi, P., Scotto, L., Giudice, A. V., Pettini, G., Busacchio, D., Didier, F., Mazzocco, K., & Pravettoni, G. (2021). Patients living with breast cancer during the coronavirus pandemic: The role of family resilience, coping flexibility, and locus of control on affective responses. *Frontiers in Psychology*, *11*, 3711. doi:10.3389/fpsyg.2020.567230 PMID:33519580

Brodziak, A., Sigorski, D., Osmola, M., Wilk, M., Gawlik-Urban, A., Kiszka, J., Machulska-Ciuraj, K., & Sobczuk, P. (2021). Attitudes of patients with cancer towards vaccinations—Results of online survey with special focus on the vaccination against COVID-19. *Vaccines*, *9*(5), 411. doi:10.3390/vaccines9050411 PMID:33919048

Brown, S. M., Doom, J. R., Lechuga-Peña, S., Watamura, S. E., & Koppels, T. (2020). Stress and parenting during the global COVID-19 pandemic. *Child Abuse & Neglect*, *110*(Pt 2), 104699. doi:10.1016/j.chiabu.2020.104699 PMID:32859394

Burker, E. J., Evon, D. M., Marroquin Loiselle, M., Finkel, J. B., & Mill, M. R. (2005). Coping predicts depression and disability in heart transplant candidates. *Journal of Psychosomatic Research*, *59*(4), 215–222. doi:10.1016/j.jpsychores.2005.06.055 PMID:16223624

Cachón-Zagalaz, J. (2021). Systematic Review of the Literature About the Effects of the COVID-19 Pandemic on the Lives of School Children. *Frontiers in Psychology: Educational Psychology*. doi:10.3389/fpsyg.2020.569348

Cacioppo, J. T., Hawkley, L. C., & Thisted, R. A. (2010, June). *Perceived social isolation makes me sad: 5-year cross-lagged analyses of loneliness and depressive symptomatology in the Chicago Health, Aging, and Social Relations Study*. Retrieved from https://www.ncbi.nlm.nih.gov/pmc/articles/PMC2922929/

Cacioppo, J. T., Hawkley, L. C., Norman, G. J., & Berntson, G. G. (2011, August). *Social isolation*. Retrieved from https://www.ncbi.nlm.nih.gov/pmc/articles/PMC3166409/

Calvert, S., & Kotler, J. (2003). Lessons from children's television: The impact of the Children's Television Act on children's learning. *Journal of Applied Developmental Psychology*, *24*(3), 277–282. doi:10.1016/S0193-3973(03)00060-1

Campbell, L. (2020). How COVID-19 could affect kids' long-term social development. *Healthline*. https://www.healthline.com/health-news/social-distancing-effects-on-social-development

Cannon, W. B. (1932). *The Wisdom of the Body*. Norton. doi:10.1097/00000441-193212000-00028

Capuano, R., Altieri, M., Bisecco, A., d'Ambrosio, A., Docimo, R., Buonanno, D., Matrone, F., Giuliano, F., Tedeschi, G., Santangelo, G., & Gallo, A. (2021). Psychological consequences of COVID-19 pandemic in Italian MS patients: Signs of resilience? *Journal of Neurology*, *268*(3), 743–750. doi:10.100700415-020-10099-9 PMID:32725312

Caratozzolo, S., Zucchelli, A., Turla, M., Cotelli, M. S., Fascendini, S., Zanni, M., Bianchetti, A., Psy, M. P., Rozzini, R., Boffelli, S., Cappuccio, M., Psy, F. G., Psy, C. V., Bellandi, D., Caminati, C., Gentile, S., Psy, E. L., Di Fazio, I., Psy, M. Z., ... Padovani, A. (2020). The impact of COVID-19 on health status of home-dwelling elderly patients with dementia in East Lombardy, Italy: Results from COVIDEM network. *Aging Clinical and Experimental Research*, *32*(10), 2133–2140. doi:10.100740520-020-01676-z PMID:32918696

Casanova, M., Bagliacca, E. P., Silva, M., Patriarca, C., Veneroni, L., Clerici, C. A., & .... (2020). How young patients with cancer perceive the Covid−19 (coronavirus) epidemic in Milan, Italy: Is there room for other fears? *Pediatric Blood & Cancer*, *67*(7), e28318. doi:10.1002/pbc.28318 PMID:32240567

Cassoff, J., Wiebe, S. T., & Gruber, R. (2012). Sleep patterns and the risk for ADHD: A review. *Nature and Science of Sleep*, *4*, 73. PMID:23620680

Cenikor Foundation. (2020, October 26). *Mental health and substance abuse is on the rise for teens because of COVID-19*. https://www.cenikor.org/mental-health-and-substance-abuse-is-on-the-rise-for-teens-because-of-covid-19/

Cennimo, D. J. (2021, April 30). *How did the coronavirus outbreak start?* Medscape. https://www.medscape.com/answers/ 2500114-197402/how-did-the-coronavirus-outbreak-start

Centers for Disease Control and Prevention. (2020, November 16). *Data and Statistics About ADHD*. Centers for Disease Control and Prevention. https://www.cdc.gov/ncbddd/adhd/data.html

Centers for Disease Control and Prevention. (2021). *COVID-19 data tracker weekly review*. https://www.cdc.gov/coronavirus/2019-ncov/covid-data/covidview/index.html

Centers for Disease Control and Prevention. (2021, April 5). *Childhood Obesity Facts*. Centers for Disease Control and Prevention. https://www.cdc.gov/obesity/data/childhood.html

Centers for Disease Control and Prevention. (2021, March 8). *How to Protect Yourself & Others*. Centers for Disease Control and Prevention. https://www.cdc.gov/coronavirus/2019-ncov / prevent-getting-sick/prevention.html

Centers for Disease Control and Prevention. (n.d.). Retrieved from https://www.cdc.gov/

Chawla, N., & Tom, A. (2021). Psychological Impact of Covid-19 on Children and Adolescents: A Systematic Review. *Indian Journal of Psychological Medicine*, *43*(4), 294–299.

Chun, J. Y., Kim, S. I., Park, E. Y., Park, S. Y., Koh, S. J., Cha, Y., Yoo, H. J., Joung, J. Y., Yoon, H. M., Eom, B. W., Park, C. M., Han, J.-Y., Kim, M., Lee, D.-W., Kim, J.-W., Keam, B., Lee, M., Kim, T. M., Choi, Y. J., ... Lim, M. C. (2021). Cancer Patients' Willingness to Take COVID-19 Vaccination: A Nationwide Multicenter Survey in Korea. *Cancers (Basel)*, *13*(15), 3883. doi:10.3390/cancers13153883 PMID:34359783

Cielo, F., Ulberg, R., & Giacomo, D. D. (2021). Psychological Impact of the Covid-19 Outbreak on Mental Health Outcomes among Youth: A Rapid Narrative Review. *International Journal of Environmental Research and Public Health*, *18*(6067), 1–15. doi:10.3390/ijerph18116067

Cleveland Clinic. (2019, September 25). *ADHD inattentive type in adults: Symptoms, diagnosis & treatment*. Cleveland Clinic. https://my.clevelandclinic .org/health/diseases/15253-attention-deficit-disorder-without-hyperactivity-add-in-adults

Conners, C. K., Erhardt, D., & Sparrow, E. (2002). *Conners' Adult ADHD Rating Scales–Self-Report: Long Version (CAARS–S: L)*. Toronto, Ontario, Canada: Multi-Health Systems. https://documents.acer.org/caars-self-l-int1.pdf

Correll, R. (2021). *Challenges that still exist for the Deaf Community*. Verywell Health. https://www.verywellhealth.com/what-challenges-still-exist-for-the-deaf-community-4153447

Cortese, S., Asherson, P., Sonuga-Barke, E., Banaschewski, T., Brandeis, D., Buitelaar, J., Coghill, D., Daley, D., Danckaerts, M., Dittmann, R. W., Doepfner, M., Ferrin, M., Hollis, C., Holtmann, M., Konofal, E., Lecendreux, M., Santosh, P., Rothenberger, A., Soutullo, C., ... Simonoff, E.European ADHD Guidelines Group. (2020). ADHD management during the COVID-19 pandemic: Guidance from the European ADHD Guidelines Group. *The Lancet. Child & Adolescent Health*, *4*(6), 412–414. doi:10.1016/S2352-4642(20)30110-3 PMID:32311314

COVID-19 (Coronavirus) Eye Health Care Guide for Patients. (n.d.). https://www.aoa.org/healthy-eyes/caring-for-your-eyes/covid-19-eye-health-care-guide-for-patients?sso=y

COVID-19: Medical Communication Access for Deaf and Hard of Hearing. (2020). *National Association of the Deaf.* https://www.nad.org/covid19-communication-medical-access-for-deaf-hard-of-hearing/

Cowden, R. G., Davis, E. B., Counted, V., Chen, Y., Rueger, S. Y., VanderWeele, T. J., Lemke, A. W., Glowiak, K. J., & Worthington, E. L. Jr. (2021). Suffering, mental health, and psychological well-being during the COVID-19 Pandemic: A longitudinal study of US adults with chronic health conditions. Wellbeing. *Space and Society*, *2*, 100048. doi:10.1016/j.wss.2021.100048 PMID:34746895

Cullen, W., Gulati, G., & Kelly, B. D. (2020). Mental health in the COVID-19 pandemic. *QJM: Monthly Journal of the Association of Physicians*, *113*(5), 311–312. doi:10.1093/qjmed/hcaa110 PMID:32227218

Cuncic, A. (2020, March 27). *Ways to Feel Less Lonely During the Coronavirus.* Verywell Mind. https://www.verywellmind.com/how-to-cope-with-loneliness-during-coronavirus4799661

D'Alessandro, A. (2020, May 8). *How Animated Pics Like 'Tom & Jerry', 'SpongeBob Movie', 'Sing 2', Skydance's 'Luck' & More Are Working Through The COVID-19 Crisis.* Deadline. https://deadline.com/2020/05/animated-movies-coronavirus-production-tom-and-jerry-spongebob-scoob-skydance-illumination-1202928961/

Damirchi, E. S., Mojarrad, A., Pireinaladin, S., & Grjibovski, A. M. (2020). The Role of Self-Talk in Predicting Death Anxiety, Obsessive-Compulsive Disorder, and Coping Strategies in the Face of Coronavirus Disease (COVID-19). *Iranian Journal of Psychiatry*, *15*(3), 182. doi:10.18502/ijps.v15i3.3810 PMID:33193766

Darvishi, E., Golestan, S., Demehri, F., & Jamalnia, S. (2020). A Cross-Sectional Study on Cognitive Errors and Obsessive-Compulsive Disorders among Young People During the Outbreak of Coronavirus Disease 2019. *Activitas Nervosa Superior*, *62*(4), 137–142. doi:10.100741470-020-00077-x PMID:33163111

Davico, C. (2021). Psychological Impact of the COVID-19 Pandemic on Adults and Their Children in Italy. *Frontiers in Psychiatry: Psychopathology*. doi:10.3389/fpsyt.2021.572997

Davide, P., Andrea, P., Martina, O., Andrea, E., Davide, D., & Mario, A. (2020). The impact of the COVID-19 pandemic on patients with OCD: Effects of contamination symptoms and remission state before the quarantine in a preliminary naturalistic study. *Psychiatry Research*, *291*, 113213. Advance online publication. doi:10.1016/j.psychres.2020.113213 PMID:32535508

De Benedictus, T., & Jaffe, J. (2004). Domestic violence and abuse: Types, signs, symptoms, causes, and effects. *Helpguide: Mental Health Issues.*

De Ridder, D., Geenen, R., Kuijer, R., & van Middendorp, H. (2008). Psychological adjustment to chronic disease. *Lancet, 372*(9634), 246–255. doi:10.1016/S0140-6736(08)61078-8 PMID:18640461

Demaria, F. & Vicari, S. (2021). Covid 19 Quarantine: Psychological Impact and Support for Children and Parents. *Italian Journal of Paediatrics, 14*(58).

Demmin, D., & Silverstein, S. (2020). *Visual Impairment and Mental Health: Unmet Needs and Treatment Options*. PubMed Central. https://www.ncbi.nlm.nih.gov/pmc/articles/PMC7721280/

Deschênes, S. S., Burns, R. J., Pouwer, F., & Schmitz, N. (2017). Diabetes complications and depressive symptoms: Prospective results from the montreal diabetes health and well-being study. *Psychosomatic Medicine, 79*(5), 603–612. doi:10.1097/PSY.0000000000000447 PMID:28060138

Donzé, C., Massot, C., Guenot, M., & Hautecoeur, P. (2021). CONFISEP: Impact of the COVID-19 pandemic lockdown on patients with multiple sclerosis in the north of France. *Revue Neurologique*. PMID:34538668

Dutton, M. A. (1993). Understanding women's responses to domestic violence: A redefinition of battered woman syndrome. *Hofstra Law Review, 21*(4), 2.

El Haj, M., Altintas, E., Chapelet, G., Kapogiannis, D., & Gallouj, K. (2020). High depression and anxiety in people with Alzheimer's disease living in retirement homes during the covid-19 crisis. *Psychiatry Research, 291*, 113294. doi:10.1016/j.psychres.2020.113294 PMID:32763552

Falk, G. (2021). *Unemployment rates during the COVID-19 pandemic: In brief*. Congressional Research Service. https://fas.org/sgp/crs/misc/R46554.pdf

Farhang, M., Miranda-Castillo, C., Behrens, M., Castillo, E., Mosquera, S., & Rojas, G. (2021) Impact of social isolation and coping strategies in older adults with mild cognitive impairment during the covid-19 pandemic: A qualitative study. *Aging & Mental Health*. https://www.tandfonline.com/doi/full/10.1080/13607863.2021.1958145 doi:10.1080/13607863.2021.1958145

Fegert, J. M., & Schulze, U. M. E. (2020). Covid-19 and Impact on Child and Adolescent Psychiatry – a German and Personal Perspective. *Irish Journal of Psychological Medicine, 37*(3), 234–245. doi:10.1017/ipm.2020.43 PMID:32404219

Fineberg, N. A., Van Ameringen, M., Drummond, L., Hollander, E., Stein, D. J., Geller, D., Walitza, S., Pallanti, S., Pellegrini, L., Zohar, J., Rodriguez, C. I., Menchon, J. M., Morgado, P., Mpavaenda, D., Fontenelle, L. F., Feusner, J. D., Grassi, G., Lochner, C., Veltman, D. J., ... Dell'Osso, B. (2020). How to manage obsessive-compulsive disorder (OCD) under COVID-19: A clinician's guide from the International College of Obsessive Compulsive Spectrum Disorders (ICOCS) and the Obsessive-Compulsive Research Network (OCRN) of the European College of Neuropsychopharmacology. *Comprehensive Psychiatry, 100*. Advance online publication. doi:10.1016/j.comppsych.2020.152174 PMID:32388123

Fisen, J. L., Sibrava, N. J., Boisseau, C. L., Mancebo, M. C., Stout, R. L., Pinto, A., & Rasmussen, S. A. (2013). Five-year course of obsessive-compulsive disorder: Predictors of remission and relapse. *The Journal of Clinical Psychiatry*, *74*(3), 233–239. doi:10.4088/JCP.12m07657 PMID:23561228

Flanagan, E. W., Beyl, R. A., Fearnbach, S. N., Altazan, A. D., Martin, C. K., & Redman, L. M. (2020). The impact of COVID-19 stay-at-home orders on health behaviors in adults. *Obesity (Silver Spring, Md.)*, *29*(2), 438–445. doi:10.1002/oby.23066 PMID:33043562

Flett, G. L., & Heisel, M. J. (2020, June 15). Aging and feeling valued versus expendable during the COVID-19 pandemic and beyond: A review and commentary of why mattering is fundamental to the health and well-being of older adults. *International Journal of Mental Health and Addiction*. https://link.springer.com/article/10.1007/s11469-020-00339-4

Foa, E. B. (2010). Cognitive behavioral therapy of obsessive-compulsive disorder. *Dialogues in Clinical Neuroscience*, *12*(2), 199–207. doi:10.31887/DCNS.2010.12.2/efoa PMID:20623924

Frenette, M., Frank, K., & Deng, Z. (2020). School Closures and the Online Preparedness of Children during the COVID-19 Pandemic. *Economic Insights*, 1–6. https://files.eric.ed.gov/fulltext/ED605398.pdf

Fullen, T., Galab, N., Abbott, K. A., & Adamou, M. (2020). Acceptance and Commitment therapy for adults with ADHD during COVID-19: An open trial. *Open Journal of Psychiatry*, *10*(04), 205–215. doi:10.4236/ojpsych.2020.104017

Galica, J., Liu, Z., Kain, D., Merchant, S., Booth, C., Koven, R., Brundage, M., & Haase, K. R. (2021). Coping during COVID-19: A mixed methods study of older cancer survivors. *Supportive Care in Cancer*, *29*(6), 3389–3398. doi:10.100700520-020-05929-5 PMID:33404813

Gallant, A. J., Flowers, P., Deakin, K., Cogan, N., Rasmussen, S., Young, D., & Williams, L. (2021). Barriers and enablers to influenza vaccination uptake in adults with chronic respiratory conditions: Applying the behaviour change wheel to specify multi-levelled tailored intervention content. *Psychology & Health*, •••, 1–20. doi:10.1080/08870446.2021.1957104 PMID:34328044

Gamble, A., Pham, Q., Goyal, S., & Cafazzo, J. A. (2020). The challenges of COVID-19 for people living with diabetes: Considerations for digital health. *JMIR Diabetes*, *5*(2), e19581. doi:10.2196/19581 PMID:32392473

Garbe, A., Ogurlu, U., Logan, N., & Cook, P. (2020). Parents' experiences with remote education during COVID-19 school closures. *American Journal of Qualitative Research*, *4*(3), 45–65.

Garza, A. (2020, August 24). *How Paramount Animation Shifted to Remote Work—and Made a "Beautiful" SpongeBob Movie in the Process.* Time. https://time.com/5882272/spongebob-movie-coronavirus/

Goldin-Meadow, S., & Mayberry, R. I. (2001). How do profoundly deaf children learn to read? *Learning Disabilities Research & Practice*, *16*(4), 222–229. https://doi.org/10.1111/0938-8982.00022

Goldschmidt, K. (2020). The COVID-19 Pandemic: Technology Use to Support the Wellbeing of Children. *Journal of Pediatric Nursing, 53,* 88–90. doi:10.1016/j.pedn.2020.04.013 PMID:32317129

Goodman-Casanova, J., Dura-Perez, E., Guzman-Parra, J., Cuesta-Vargas, A., & Mayoral-Cleries, F. (n.d.). *Telehealth Home Support During COVID-19 Confinement for Community-Dwelling Older Adults With Mild Cognitive Impairment or Mild Dementia: Survey Study*. Academic Press.

Goodman-Casanova, J. M., Dura-Perez, E., Guzman-Parra, J., Cuesta-Vargas, A., & Mayoral-Cleries, F. (2020). Telehealth Home Support During COVID-19 Confinement for Community-Dwelling Older Adults With Mild Cognitive Impairment or Mild Dementia: Survey Study. *Journal of Medical Internet Research, 22*(5), e19434. doi:10.2196/19434 PMID:32401215

Griffith, A. K. (2020). Parental burnout and child maltreatment during the COVID-19 pandemic. *Journal of Family Violence*, 1–7. doi:10.100710896-020-00172-2 PMID:32836736

Guo, M., Wu, C. F., Liu, W., Yang, J. Y., & Chen, D. (2004). Sex difference in psychological behavior changes induced by long-term social isolation in mice. *Progress in Neuro-Psychopharmacology & Biological Psychiatry, 28*(1), 115–121. doi:10.1016/j.pnpbp.2003.09.027

Hai, T., Swansburg, R., MacMaster, F. P., & Lemay, J. F. (2021). Impact of COVID-19 on Educational Services in Canadian Children With Attention-Deficit/Hyperactivity Disorder. In *Frontiers in Education* (Vol. 6, p. 32). Frontiers. doi:10.3389/feduc.2021.614181

Hallas, C. N., Howard, C., Theadom, A., & Wray, J. (2012). Negative beliefs about breathlessness increases panic for patients with chronic respiratory disease. *Psychology Health and Medicine, 17*(4), 467–477. doi:10.1080/13548506.2011.626434 PMID:22329594

Hamoda, H.M. (2021). Addressing the Consequences of the COVID-19 Lockdown for Children's Mental Health: Investing in School Mental Health Programs. *Psychiatric Services, 202*(1), 729-731. . doi:10.1176/appi.ps.202000597

Haring, B. (2020, March 27). *Nickelodeon & Disney Channel Address Kids' Coronavirus Concerns While Maintaining Quarantine*. Deadline. https://deadline.com/2020/03/kidstogether-the-nickelodeon-town-hall-addresses-kid-coronavirus-concerns-1202893877/

Hariyanto, T.I., Putri, C., & Situmeang, R.F.V. (2020). Dementia is a predictor for mortality outcome from coronavirus disease 2019 (COVID-19) infection. *Eur Arch Psychiatry Clin Neurosci, 271*, 393–395. doi:10.1007/s00406-020-01205-z

Hariyanto, T.I., Putri, C., Arisa, J., Fransisca, Situmeang, R.F., & Kurniawan, A. (2021). Dementia and outcomes from coronavirus disease 2019 (COVID-19) pneumonia: A systematic review and meta-analysis. *Archives of Gerontology and Geriatrics, 93*. https://www.sciencedirect.com/science/article/pii/S016749432030296X

Hayes, D. A. (1994). The Children's Hour Revisited: The Children's Television Act of 1990. *Federal Communications Law Journal, 46*(2), 294–311. https://www.repository.law.indiana.edu/cgi/viewcontent.cgi?referer=https://scholar.google.com/scholar?hl=en&as_sdt=0%2C33&q=children's+television+act&btnG=&httpsredir=1&referer=&httpredir=1&article=1016&context=fclj

Hinz, A., Krauss, O., Hauss, J. P., Höckel, M., Kortmann, R. D., Stolzenburg, J. U., & Schwarz, R. (2010). Anxiety and depression in cancer patients compared with the general population. *European Journal of Cancer Care, 19*(4), 522–529. doi:10.1111/j.1365-2354.2009.01088.x PMID:20030697

Holtmaat, K., Van der Spek, N., Lissenberg-Witte, B. I., Cuijpers, P., & Verdonck-de Leeuw, I. M. (2019). Positive mental health among cancer survivors: Overlap in psychological well-being, personal meaning, and posttraumatic growth. *Supportive Care in Cancer, 27*(2), 443–450. doi:10.100700520-018-4325-8 PMID:29959577

Hu, J., Fitzgerald, S. M., Owen, A. J., Ryan, J., Joyce, J., Chowdhury, E., Reid, C. M., Britt, C., Woods, R. L., McNeil, J. J., & Freak-Poli, R. (2021). Social isolation, social support, loneliness and cardiovascular disease risk factors: A cross-sectional study among older adults. *International Journal of Geriatric Psychiatry, 36*(11), 1795–1809. doi:10.1002/gps.5601 PMID:34231940

Humanitas University. (2021). *How technology could turn US into superheroes: The Future of Hearing*. Hunimed. https://www.hunimed.eu/news/how-technology-could-turn-us-into-superheroes-the-future-of-hearing/

Humphreys, K. L., Myint, M. T., & Zeanah, C. H. (2020). Increased risk for family violence during the COVID-19 pandemic. *Pediatrics, 146*(1). doi:10.1542/peds.2020-0982 PMID:32317306

Imran, N., Zeshan, M., & Pervaiz, Z. (2020). Mental health considerations for children & adolescents in COVID-19 Pandemic. *Pakistan Journal of Medical Sciences, 36*(S4), S67.

Imran, N., Aamer, I., Sharif, M., Bodla, Z., & Naveed, S. (2020). Psychological Burden of quarantine in children and adolescents: A rapid systematic review and proposed solutions. *Pakistan Journal of Medical Sciences, 36*(5). https://doi.org/10.12669/pjms.36.5.3088

Ingram, L. (2021). Integrating the visually impaired into the virtual future. In *Visually Impaired in the Digital Age*. IEEE Computer Society. https://www.computer.org/publications/tech-news/trends/integrating-the-visually-impaired-into-digital

Ismail, I. I., Kamel, W. A., & Al-Hashel, J. Y. (2021). Association of COVID-19 Pandemic and Rate of Cognitive Decline in Patients with Dementia and Mild Cognitive Impairment: A Cross-sectional Study. *Gerontology and Geriatric Medicine*. https://journals.sagepub.com/doi/full/10.1177/23337214211005223 doi:10.1177/23337214211005223

Jalloh, F. M., Li, W., Bunnell, R. E., Ethier, K. A., O'Leary, A., Hageman, K. M., Sengeh, P., Jalloh, M. B., Morgan, O., Hersey, S., Marston, B. J., Dafae, F., & Redd, J. T. (2018). Impact of Ebola Experiences and Risk Perceptions on Mental Health in Sierra Leone, July 2015. *BMJ Global Health, 3*(2), e000471. doi:10.1136/bmjgh-2017-000471 PMID:29607096

Jalongo, R. M. (2021). The Effects of COVID 19 on Early Childhood Education and Care: Research and Resources for Children, Families, Teachers and Teacher Educators. *Early Childhood Education Journal*, *49*(5), 763–774. doi:10.100710643-021-01208-y PMID:34054286

Jameson, J. (2019, December 5). *Pragmatic social communication: Activities to improve pragmatics*. Jewel Autism Centre Blog. http://jewelautismcentre.com/ jewel_blog/pragmatic-social-communication/

James, P. B., Wardle, J., Steel, A., & Adams, J. (2019). Post-Ebola Psychosocial Experiences and Coping Mechanism among Ebola Survivors: A Systematic Review. *Tropical Medicine & International Health*, *24*(6), 671–691. doi:10.1111/tmi.13226 PMID:30843627

Janssen, L.H.C. (2020). Does the Covid-19 Pandemic impact parents' and adolescents' well-being? An EMA-study on daily effect and parenting. *Plus One*. doi:10.1371/journal.pone.0240962

Jelinek, L., Moritz, S., Miegel, F., & Voderholzer, U. (2021). Obsessive-compulsive disorder during COVID-19: Turning a problem into an opportunity? *Journal of Anxiety Disorders*, *77*, 102329. Advance online publication. doi:10.1016/j.janxdis.2020.102329 PMID:33190017

Jeste, S., Hyde, C., Distefano, C., Halladay, A., Ray, S., Porath, M., Wilson, R. B., & Thurm, A. (2020). Changes in access to educational and healthcare services for individuals with intellectual and developmental disabilities during COVID-19 restrictions. *Journal of Intellectual Disability Research*, *64*(11), 825–833. doi:10.1111/jir.12776 PMID:32939917

Johnston, W. M., & Davey, G. C. L. (1997). The psychological impact of negative tv news bulletins: The catastrophizing of personal worries. *British Journal of Psychology*, *88*(1), 85–91. doi:10.1111/j.2044-8295.1997.tb02622.x PMID:9061893

Kakulla, B. N. (2020, January 1). *2020 tech trends of the 50+*. AARP. https://www.aarp.org/research/topics/technology/info-2019/2020-technology-trends-older-americans.html

Kang, C., Yang, S., Yuan, J., Xu, L., Zhao, X., & Yang, J. (2020). Patients with chronic illness urgently need integrated physical and psychological care during the COVID-19 outbreak. *Asian Journal of Psychiatry*, *51*, 102081. doi:10.1016/j.ajp.2020.102081 PMID:32289729

Kaputu-Kala-Malu, C. (2021). PTSD, Depression and Anxiety in Ebola Virus Disease Survivors in Beni Town, Democratic Republic of Congo. *BMC Psychiatry*, *21*(342). PMID:34238249

Karlsen, B., Idsoe, T., Hanestad, B. R., Murberg, T., & Bru, E. (2004). Perceptions of support, diabetes-related coping and psychological well-being in adults with type 1 and type 2 diabetes. *Psychology Health and Medicine*, *9*(1), 53–70. doi:10.1080/13548500310001637751

Khosravani, V., Aardema, F., Samimi Ardestani, S. M., & Sharifi Bastan, F. (2021). The impact of the coronavirus pandemic on specific symptom dimensions and severity in OCD: A comparison before and during COVID-19 in the context of stress responses. *Journal of Obsessive-Compulsive and Related Disorders*, *29*, 100626. Advance online publication. doi:10.1016/j.jocrd.2021.100626 PMID:33520614

Kladias, A. (2021). *Parent-Child Relationships and Student Outcomes in Children: A Comparison Before and During the COVID-19 Pandemic* (Doctoral dissertation). Otterbein University.

Kofman, Y. B., & Garfin, D. R. (2020). Home is not always a haven: The domestic violence crisis amid the COVID-19 pandemic. *Psychological Trauma: Theory, Research Practice and Policy.*

Kralik, D., van Loon, A., & Visentin, K. (2006). Resilience in the chronic illness experience. *Educational Action Research*, *14*(2), 187–201. doi:10.1080/09650790600718035

Kring, A. M., & Johnson, S. L. (2017). *Abnormal Psychology* (14th ed.). Wiley.

Kuhfeld, M., Soland, J., Tarasawa, B., Johnson, A., Ruzek, E., & Liu, J. (2020). Projecting the potential impact of COVID-19 school closures on academic achievement. *Educational Researcher*, *49*(8), 549–565. doi:10.3102/0013189X20965918

Lange, R. T. (2011). Full Scale IQ. In J. S. Kreutzer, J. DeLuca, & B. Caplan (Eds.), *Encyclopedia of Clinical Neuropsychology*. Springer. doi:10.1007/978-0-387-79948-3_1549

Larsen, L., Helland, M. S., & Holt, T. (2021, March 26). The impact of school closure and social isolation on children in vulnerable families during COVID-19: a focus on children's reactions. *European Child & Adolescent Psychiatry*. https://link.springer.com/article/10.1007/s00787-021-01758-x

Lawson, M., Piel, M. H., & Simon, M. (2020). Child maltreatment during the COVID-19 pandemic: Consequences of parental job loss on psychological and physical abuse towards children. *Child Abuse & Neglect*, *110*, 104709. doi:10.1016/j.chiabu.2020.104709 PMID:32893003

Lazarus, R. S., & Folkman, S. (1984). *Stress, Appraisal and Coping*. Springer.

Lee, K., Jeong, G.-C., & Yim, J. E. (2020, November 3). Consideration of the psychological and mental health of the elderly during COVID-19: A theoretical review. *International Journal of Environmental Research and Public Health*. https://www.ncbi.nlm.nih.gov/pmc/articles/PMC7663449/

Leese, J., Backman, C. L., Ma, J. K., Koehn, C., Hoens, A. M., English, K., ... Li, L. C. (2021). Experiences of self-care during the COVID-19 pandemic among individuals with rheumatoid arthritis: A qualitative study. *Health Expectations*. Advance online publication. doi:10.1111/hex.13341 PMID:34403189

Legg, T. J. (2018, September 17). *Parenting Tips for ADHD: Do's and Don'ts*. Healthline. https://www. healthline.com/health/adhd/parenting-tips

Leppänen, U. (2006). *Development of literacy in kindergarten and primary school* (No. 289). Jyväskylän yliopisto.

Leventhal, H., Diefenbach, M., & Leventhal, E. A. (1992). Illness cognition - using common-sense to understand treatment adherence and affect cognition interactions. *Cognitive Therapy and Research*, *16*(2), 143–163. doi:10.1007/BF01173486

Lévy-Weil, F. E., Jousse-Joulin, S., Tiffreau, V., Perez, R., Morisseau, V., & Bombezin, A. (2021). Physical activity and quality of life of patients with rheumatoid arthritis at the time of COVID-19 lockdown: Results from Carenity, an online patient community. *Joint, Bone, Spine*. Advance online publication. doi:10.1016/j.jbspin.2021.105212

Lexico. (n.d.a). *Comorbidity*. https://www.lexico. com/definition/comorbidity

Lexico. (n.d.b). *Neurotypical*. https://www.lexico. com/definition/neurotypical

Liao, K. Y. H., Yeung, N. C., Wong, C. C., Warmoth, K., & Lu, Q. (2017). Fear of cancer recurrence and physical well-being among Chinese cancer survivors: The role of conscientiousness, positive reappraisal and hopelessness. *Supportive Care in Cancer*, *25*(4), 1141–1149. doi:10.100700520-016-3504-8 PMID:27924358

Lindberg, L. (2020). The sexual and reproductive health of adolescents and young adults during the COVID-19 pandemic. *Perspectives on Sexual and Reproductive Health*. https://pubmed.ncbi.nlm.nih.gov/32537858/

Liu, J. J., Bao, Y., Huang, X., Shi, J., & Lu, L. (2020). Mental health considerations for children quarantined because of COVID-19. *The Lancet. Child & Adolescent Health*, *4*(5), 347–349. doi:10.1016/S2352-4642(20)30096-1 PMID:32224303

Liu, M., Xue, J., Zhao, N., Wang, X., Jiao, D., & Zhu, T. (2021). Using social media to explore the consequences of domestic violence on mental health. *Journal of Interpersonal Violence*, *36*(3-4). doi:10.1177/0886260518757756 PMID:29441804

Livneh, H. (2021). Psychosocial Adaptation to Chronic Illness and Disability: An Updated and Expanded Conceptual Framework. *Rehabilitation Counseling Bulletin*.

Livneh, H., & Antonak, R. F. (2005). Psychosocial adaptation to chronic illness and disability: A primer for counselors. *Journal of Counseling and Development*, *83*(1), 12–20. doi:10.1002/j.1556-6678.2005.tb00575.x

Livneh, H., Lott, S. M., & Antonak, R. F. (2004). Patterns of psychosocial adaptation to chronic illness and disability: A cluster analytic approach. *Psychology Health and Medicine*, *9*(4), 411–430. doi:10.1080/1354850042000267030

Lourens, H. (2021). The politics of touch-based help for visually impaired persons during the COVID-19 pandemic. *The COVID-19 Crisis: Social Perspectives*, 17.

Low, K. (2020, November 8). *Children With ADHD Need Structure in Their Lives to Stay Focused*. Verywell Mind. https://www.verywellmind.com/why-is-structure-important-for-kids-with-adhd-20747

Macchi, Z. A., Ayele, R., Dini, M., Lamira, J., Katz, M., Pantilat, S. Z., Jones, J., & Kluger, B. M. (2021). Lessons from the COVID-19 pandemic for improving outpatient neuropalliative care: A qualitative study of patient and caregiver perspectives. *Palliative Medicine*, *35*(7). doi:10.1177/02692163211017383 PMID:34006157

Manganello, J. (2020). Media use for children with disabilities in the United States during COVID-19. *Journal of Children and Media*, *15*(1), 29–32. doi:10.1080/17482798.2020.1857281

Manning, L. K., Carr, D. C., & Kail, B. L. (2016). Do higher levels of resilience buffer the deleterious impact of chronic illness on disability in later life? *The Gerontologist*, *56*(3), 514–524. doi:10.1093/geront/gnu068 PMID:25063353

Marques, E. S., Moraes, C. L. D., Hasselmann, M. H., Deslandes, S. F., & Reichenheim, M. E. (2020). Violence against women, children, and adolescents during the COVID-19 pandemic: Overview, contributing factors, and mitigating measures. *Cadernos de Saude Publica*, *36*, e00074420. doi:10.1590/0102-311x00074420 PMID:32374808

Masonbrink, A. R., & Hurley, E. (2020). Advocating for children during the COVID-19 school closures. *Pediatrics*, *146*(3), e20201440. doi:10.1542/peds.2020-1440 PMID:32554517

Matsunaga, H., Mukai, K., & Yamanishi, K. (2020). The acute impact of the pandemic of COVID -19 on the phenomenological features in the full or partial remitted patients with obsessive–compulsive disorder (OCD*). Psychiatry and Clinical Neurosciences*, *74*(10). Advance online publication. doi:10.1111/pcn.13119 PMID:32697002

Maynard, S. (2021, January 20). *Rule #2: Ban Negative Thoughts*. ADDitude. https://www.additudemag. com/anger-management-tips/

McLeod, S. A. (2019, August 3). *Likert scale*. Simply Psychology. https://www.simplypsychology.org/likert-scale.html

Megan, L., Evans, M. D., Margo, M. P. H., Lindauer, J. D., Maureen, E., & Farrell, M. D. (2020). A pandemic within a pandemic— Intimate partner violence during COVID-19. *The New England Journal of Medicine*, *383*(24), 2302–2304. doi:10.1056/NEJMp2024046 PMID:32937063

Merzon, E., Manor, I., Rotem, A., Schneider, T., Vinker, S., Golan Cohen, A., Lauden, A., Weizman, A., & Green, I. (2021). ADHD as a Risk Factor for Infection With Covid-19. *Journal of Attention Disorders*, *25*(13), 1783–1790. doi:10.1177/1087054720943271 PMID:32697120

Miller, S. (n.d.). *Ages and stages: Nurturing young children's independence*. Scholastic. https://www.scholastic.com/teachers/articles/teaching-content/ages-stages-nuturing-young-childrens-independence/

Miyashita, S., Yamada, T., Mikami, T., Miyashita, H., Chopra, N., & Rizk, D. (2020). Impact of dementia on clinical outcomes in elderly patients with coronavirus 2019 (COVID-19): An experience in New York. *Geriatrics & Gerontology International*, *20*(7), 732–734. doi:10.1111/ggi.13942 PMID:32691924

Monroe, S. M., & Slavich, G. M. (2016). Psychological stressors: overview. Academic Press.

Moore, S. A., Faulkner, G., Rhodes, R. E., Brussoni, M., Chulak-Bozzer, T., Ferguson, L. J., Mitra, R., O'Reilly, N., Spence, J. C., Vanderloo, L. M., & Tremblay, M. S. (2020, July 6). Impact of the COVID-19 virus outbreak on movement and play behaviours of Canadian children and youth: A national survey. *International Journal of Behavioral Nutrition and Physical Activity*. https://ijbnpa.biomedcentral.com/articles/10.1186/s12966-020-00987-8

Moreland, A., Herlihy, C., Tynan, M. A., Sunshine, G., McCord, R. F., Hilton, C. A., Poovey, J., Werner, A., Jones, C. D., Fulmer, E., Gundlapalli, A., Strosnider, H., Potvien, A., García, M. C., Honeycutt, S., Baldwin, G., Clodfelter, C., Howard-Williams, M., Jeong, G., ... Popoola, A. (2020). Timing of state and territorial COVID-19 stay-at-home orders and changes in population movement—United States, March 1–May 31, 2020. *Morbidity and Mortality Weekly Report*, *69*(35), 1198–1203. doi:10.15585/mmwr.mm6935a2 PMID:32881851

Morelli, M., Cattelino, E., Baiocco, R., Trumello, C., Babore, A., Candelori, C., & Chirumbolo, A. (2020). Parents and Children During the Covid-19 Lockdown: The Influence of Parenting Distress and Parenting Self Efficacy on Children's Emotional Well-Being. *Health Psychology*, *11*, 584645. Advance online publication. doi:10.3389/fpsyg.2020.584645 PMID:33123063

Morgül, E., Kallitsoglou, A. & Essau, A.C. (2020). Psychological Effects of Covid-19 lockdown on Children and Families in the UK. *Revista de Psicología Clínica con Niños y Adolescentes*, *7*(3), 42–48. doi:10.21134/rpcna.2020.mon.2049

Motolese, F., Rossi, M., Albergo, G., Stelitano, D., Villanova, M., Di Lazzaro, V., & Capone, F. (2020). The psychological impact of COVID-19 pandemic on people with multiple sclerosis. *Frontiers in Neurology*, *11*, 1255. doi:10.3389/fneur.2020.580507 PMID:33193033

Müller, L. M., & Goldenberg, G. (2020). *Education in times of crisis: The potential implications of school closures for teachers and students. A review of research evidence on school closures and international approaches to education during the COVID-19 pandemic*. Chartered College of Teaching.

Mustaţă, A. E. (2021). The relationships between coping mechanisms, depression, anxiety and sleep disorders in cardiovascular patients. *Journal of Evidence-Based Psychotherapies*, *21*(1), 37–55. doi:10.24193/jebp.2021.1.3

N., & González-Dambrauskas, S. (2021). Schools closures during the covid-19 pandemic: a catastrophic global situation. *The Pediatric Infectious Disease Journal, 40*(4), e146-e150.

Nanyang, L., Jiahui, S., Xiyuan, W., Ming, Z., Qianqian, H., & Hao, L. (2020). The Impact of Dementia on the Clinical Outcome of COVID-19: A Systematic review and Meta-Analysis. *Journal of Alzheimer's Disease*, *78*(4), 1775–1782. https://content.iospress.com/articles/journal-of-alzheimers-disease/jad201016

Nearchou, F., Flinn, C., Niland, R., Subramaniam, S. S., & Hennessy, E. (2020). Exploring the Impact of Covid-19 on Mental Health Outcomes in Children and Adolescents: A Systematic Review. *International Journal of Environmental Research and Public Health*, *17*(22), 1–19. doi:10.3390/ijerph17228479 PMID:33207689

Newton, R. U., Hart, N. H., & Clay, T. (2020). Keeping patients with cancer exercising in the age of COVID-19. *JCO Oncology Practice*, *16*(10), 656–664. doi:10.1200/OP.20.00210 PMID:32603253

Nikoladis, A., Paksarian, D., Alexander, L., DeRosa, J., Dunn, J., Nielson, D. M., Droney, I., Kang, M., Douka, I., Bromet, E., Milham, M. P., Stingaris, A., & Merikangas, K. R. (2020). The Coronavirus Health and Impact Survey (CRISIS) reveals reproducible correlates of pandemic-related mood states across the Atlantic. [Preprint]. medRxiv doi:10.1101/2020.08.24.20181123

Nonweiler, J., Rattray, F., Baulcomb, J., Happé, F., & Absoud, M. (2020). Prevalence and associated factors of emotional and behavioural difficulties during COVID-*19 pandemic in children with neurodevelopmental disorders. Children (Basel, Switzerland)*, *7*(9), 128. doi:10.3390/children7090128 PMID:32899799

Oberle, E., & Schonert-Reichl, K. A. (2016). Stress contagion in the classroom? The link between classroom teacher burnout and morning cortisol in elementary school students. *Social Science & Medicine*, *159*, 30–33. doi:10.1016/j.socscimed.2016.04.031 PMID:27156042

OECD. (2020). Combatting Covid-19's Effect on Children. *OECD Policy Responses to Coronavirus (COVID-19)*. https://www.oecd.org/coronavirus/policy-responses/combatting-covid-19-s-effect-on-children-2e1f3b2f/

Office For Civil Rights. (2021). *Education in a pandemic*. https://www2.ed.gov/about/offices/list/ocr/docs/20210608-impacts-of-covid19.pdf?tpcc=nlcapsule

Oliveira, V. C., Ferreira, M. L., Morso, L., Albert, H. B., Refshauge, K. M., & Ferreira, P. H. (2015). Patients' perceived level of social isolation affects the prognosis of low back pain. *European Journal of Pain (London, England)*, *19*(4), 538–545. doi:10.1002/ejp.578 PMID:25185789

Olivo, S., Cheli, M., Dinoto, A., Stokelj, D., Tomaselli, M., & Manganotti, P. (2021). Telemedicine during the SARS-Cov-2 pandemic lockdown: Monitoring stress and quality of sleep in patients with epilepsy. *Epilepsy & Behavior*, *118*, 107864. doi:10.1016/j.yebeh.2021.107864 PMID:33743345

OrCam Technologies Personal AI Solutions. (n.d.). https://www.orcam.com/en/article/orcam-technologies-personal-ai-solutions-ces-2022-innovation-award-and-2021-time-best-invention/

Orenstein, G. A., & Lewis, L. (2020). *Erikson's stages of psychosocial development*. StatPearls. https://www.ncbi.nlm.nih.gov/books/NBK556096/

Owen, N., Healy, G. N., Matthews, C. E., & Dunstan, D. W. (2010, July). *Too much sitting: the population health science of sedentary behavior*. Retrieved from https://www.ncbi.nlm.nih.gov/pmc/articles/PMC3404815/

Pagel, J. I., & Choukèr, A. (2016). Effects of isolation and confinement on humans-implications for manned space explorations. *Journal of Applied Physiology*, *120*(12), 1449–1457. doi:10.1152/japplphysiol.00928.2015

Parolin, Z., & Lee, E. K. (2021). Large socio-economic, geographic and demographic disparities exist in exposure to school closures. *Nature Human Behaviour*, *5*(4), 522–528. doi:10.103841562-021-01087-8 PMID:33737734

Paterson, C., Bacon, R., Dwyer, R., Morrison, K. S., Toohey, K., O'Dea, A., & Hayes, S. (2020, October). The role of telehealth during the COVID-19 pandemic across the interdisciplinary cancer team: implications for practice. In *Seminars in oncology nursing* (p. 151090). WB Saunders. doi:10.1016/j.soncn.2020.151090

Patton, R. M. (1963). *Behavioral Testing During a 7-day Confinement.* Academic Press.

Pecor, K. W., Barbyannis, G., Yang, M., Johnson, J., Materasso, S., Borda, M., ... Ming, X. (2021). Quality of Life Changes during the COVID-19 Pandemic for Caregivers of Children with ADHD and/or ASD. *International Journal of Environmental Research and Public Health, 18*(7), 3667. doi:10.3390/ijerph18073667 PMID:33915884

Pedrozo-Pupo, J. C., & Campo-Arias, A. (2020). Depression, perceived stress related to COVID, post-traumatic stress, and insomnia among asthma and COPD patients during the COVID-19 pandemic. *Chronic Respiratory Disease, 17*, 1479973120962800. doi:10.1177/1479973120962800 PMID:33000648

Phelps, C., & Sperry, L. L. (2020). Children and the COVID-19 pandemic. *Psychological Trauma: Theory, Research, Practice, and Policy, 12*(S1), S73–S75. doi:10.1037/tra0000861 PMID:32525366

Philippe, K., Chabanet, C., Issanchou, S., & Monnery-Patris, S. (2021, January 23). Child eating behaviors, parental feeding practices and food shopping motivations during the COVID-19 lockdown in France: (How) did they change? *Appetite.* https://www.sciencedirect.com/science/article/pii/S0195666321000404

Pizarro-Ruiz, J. P., & Ordóñez-Camblor, N. (2021). Effects of Covid-19 Confinement on the Mental Health of Children and Adolescents in Spain. *Scientific Reports, 11*(11713), 11713. Advance online publication. doi:10.103841598-021-91299-9 PMID:34083653

Podsada, J. (2020). *Masks, Social Distancing Challenge Interpreters for the Deaf.* www.heraldnet.com/business/masks-social-distancing-challenge-interpreters-for-the-deaf/

Polenick, C. A., Perbix, E. A., Salwi, S. M., Maust, D. T., Birditt, K. S., & Brooks, J. M. (2021). Loneliness during the COVID-19 Pandemic among older adults with chronic conditions. *Journal of Applied Gerontology, 40*(8), 0733464821996527. doi:10.1177/0733464821996527 PMID:33641513

Pollak, Y., Dayan, H., Shoham, R., & Berger, I. (2020). Predictors of non-adherence to public health instructions during the COVID-19 pandemic. *Psychiatry and Clinical Neurosciences, 74*(11), 602–604. doi:10.1111/pcn.13122 PMID:32729646

Rafanelli, A. (2021, July 22). *Growing up in a pandemic: How covid is affecting children's development.* Direct Relief. Retrieved March 29, 2022, from https://www.directrelief.org/2021/01/growing-up-in-the-midst-of-a-pandemic-how-covid-is-affecting-childrens-development/

Rainero, I., Bruni, A. C., Marra, C., Cagin, A., Bonanni, L., Cupidi, C., Laganà, V., Rubino, E., Vacca, A., Di Lorenzo, R., Provero, P., Isella, V., Vanacore, N., Agosta, F., Appollonio, I., Caffarra, P., Bussè, C., Sambati, R., Quaranta, D., Guglielmi, V., … Ferrarese, C. (2021). The Impact of COVID-19 Quarantine on Patients With Dementia and Family Caregivers: A Nation-Wide Survey. *Front. Aging Neurosci., 12*. https://www.frontiersin.org/articles/10.3389/fnagi.2020.625781/full

Ravens-Sieberer, U., Kaman, A., Erhart, M., Devine, J., Schlack, R., & Otto, C. (2021). Impact of the COVID-19 Pandemic on Quality of Life and Mental Health in Children and Adolescents in Germany. *European Child & Adolescent Psychiatry, 1*, 3. doi:10.100700787-021-01726-5 PMID:33492480

Rayburn, D. (2021, March 11). *6 Perils of Working from Home with ADHD*. Dana Rayburn ADHD Coach. https://danarayburn.com/5-perils-of-working-from-home-with-adhd/

Rege, M., Hanselman, P., Solli, I. F., Dweck, C. S., Ludvigsen, S., Bettinger, E., Crosnoe, R., Muller, C., Walton, G., Duckworth, A., & Yeager, D. S. (2020). How can we inspire nations of learners? An investigation of growth mindset and challenge-seeking in two countries. *American Psychologist*. https://slb.mmm.edu:2208/10.1037/amp0000647.supp

Rhodes, A., Martin, S., Guarna, J., Vowles, K., & Allen, T. (2020). A contextual-behavioral perspective on chronic pain during the COVID-19 pandemic and future times of mandated physical distancing. *Journal of Contextual Behavioral Science, 17*, 152–158. doi:10.1016/j.jcbs.2020.07.009

Riccardo, M., Matteo, D. M., & Annalena, V. (2020). The Impact of COVID-19 Infection and Enforced Prolonged Social Isolation on Neuropsychiatric Symptoms in Older Adults With and Without Dementia: A Review. *Frontiers in Psychiatry, 11*. https://www.frontiersin.org/article/10.3389/fpsyt.2020.585540 doi:10.3389/fpsyt.2020.585540

Rizzo, J. R., Beheshti, M., Fang, Y., Flanagan, S., & Giudice, N. A. (2020). COVID-19 and Visual Disability: Can't Look and Now Don't Touch. *PM & R*.

Roberta, B., Antonina, L., Alessandra, N., Maria, C., Edoardo, C. C., D'Agate, C., Lucia, D. G., Giuseppe, L. B., Tiziana, L. C., Mario, Z., & Roberto, M. (2020). Changes in Motor, Cognitive, and Behavioral Symptoms in Parkinson's Disease and Mild Cognitive Impairment During the COVID-19 Lockdown. *Frontiers in Psychiatry, 11*. https://www.frontiersin.org/article/10.3389/fpsyt.2020.590134

Rodrigues, J. V. S. & Lins, A.C.A. (2020). Possible Impacts Caused by the Covid-19 Pandemic on Children's Mental Health and the Role of Parents in this Scenario. *Research, Society & Development, 9*(8).

Rogers, M. M. (2020). Exploring the Domestic Abuse Narratives of Trans and Nonbinary People and the Role of Cisgenderism in Identity Abuse, Misgendering, and Pathologizing. *Violence Against Women*. PMID:34448660

Rohwerder, B. (2014). *Impact and Implications of the Ebola Crisis*. Applied Knowledge Services GSDRC Helpdesk Research Report 1177.

Rosa-Alcázar, Á., García-Hernández, M. D., Parada-Navas, J. L., Olivares-Olivares, P. J., Martínez-Murillo, S., & Rosa-Alcázar, A. I. (2021). Coping strategies in obsessive-compulsive patients during Covid-19 lockdown. *International Journal of Clinical and Health Psychology*, *21*(2), 100223. Advance online publication. doi:10.1016/j.ijchp.2021.100223 PMID:33519939

Roth, E. (2018, April 24). *What are the Three Types of ADHD?* Healthline. https://www.healthline.com/health/adhd/three-types-adhd

Rundle, A. G., Park, Y., Herbstman, J. B., Kinsey, E. W., & Wang, Y. C. (2020). COVID-19–related school closings and risk of weight gain among children. *Obesity (Silver Spring, Md.)*, *28*(6), 1008–1009. doi:10.1002/oby.22813 PMID:32227671

Ryoo, N., Pyun, J.-M., Baek, M. J., Suh, J., Kang, M.-J., Wang, M.-J., Youn, Y., Yang, D.-W., Kim, S.-Y., Park, Y.-H., & Kim, S.-Y. (2020). Coping With Dementia in the Middle of the COVID- 19 Pandemic. *Journal of Korean Medical Science*, *35*(42), e383.

Sabate, J. M., Deutsch, D., Melchior, C., Entremont, A., Mion, F., Bouchoucha, M., Façon, S., Raynaud, J.-J., Zerbib, F., & Jouët, P. (2021). COVID-19 pandemic and lockdown stress consequences in people with and without Irritable Bowel Syndrome. *Ethics, Medicine, and Public Health*, *18*, 100660. doi:10.1016/j.jemep.2021.100660 PMID:34150971

Saltzman, L. Y., Hansel, T. C., & Bordnick, P. S. (2020). Loneliness, isolation, and social support factors in post-COVID-19 mental health. *Psychological Trauma: Theory, Research, Practice, and Policy*, *12*(S1), S55–S57. doi:10.1037/tra0000703 PMID:32551762

Saxe, G., Chawla, N., Stoddard, F., Kassam-Adams, N., Courtney, D., Cunningham, K., Lopez, C., Hall, E., Sheridan, R., King, D., & King, L. (2003). Child stress disorders checklist: A measure of ASD and PTSD in children. *Journal of the American Academy of Child and Adolescent Psychiatry*, *42*(8), 972–978. doi:10.1097/01.CHI.0000046887.27264.F3 PMID:12874500

Saya Des Marais. (2020, December 4). *A Comprehensive History of OCD: From Religious Scruples to Modern Treatment*. Impulse Therapy. https://impulsetherapy.com/a-comprehensive-history-of-ocd-from-religious-scruples-to-modern-treatment/

Schmidt, S., Barblan, L. P., Lory, I., & Landolt, M. A. (2021). Age-related effects of the COVID-19 pandemic on mental health of child8ren and adolescents. *European Journal of Psychotraumatology*, *12*(1), 1–17. doi:10.1080/20008198.2021.1901407 PMID:34912501

Schnaiderman, D. (2021). Psychological impact of COVID-19 lockdown in children and adolescents from San Carlos de Bariloche, Argentina: Parents' perspective. *Archivos Argentinos de Pediatria*, *119*(3), 170–176. PMID:34033416

Schneiderman, N., Ironson, G., & Siegel, S. D. (2005). Stress and health: Psychological, behavioral, and biological determinants. *Annual Review of Clinical Psychology*, *1*(1), 607–628. doi:10.1146/annurev.clinpsy.1.102803.144141 PMID:17716101

Schuster, S. (2015, October 12). *17 Quotes That Prove OCD Is So Much More Than Being Neat*. The Mighty. https://themighty.com/2015/10/what-ocd-feels-like/

Sciberras, E., Patel, P., Stokes, M. A., Coghill, D., Middeldorp, C. M., Bellgrove, M. A., Becker, S. P., Efron, D., Stringaris, A., Faraone, S. V., Bellows, S. T., Quach, J., Banaschewski, T., McGillivray, J., Hutchinson, D., Silk, T. J., Melvin, G., Wood, A. G., Jackson, A., ... Westrupp, E. (2020). Physical health, media use, and mental health in children and adolescents with ADHD during the COVID-19 pandemic in Australia. *Journal of Attention Disorders*. Advance online publication. doi:10.1177/1087054720978549 PMID:33331195

Sedlak, A. J., Mettenburg, J., Basena, M., Peta, I., McPherson, K., & Greene, A. (2010). Fourth national incidence study of child abuse and neglect (NIS-4). Washington, DC: US Department of Health and Human Services.

Selye, H. (1976). *Stress in Health and Disease*. Butterworth.

Senjam, S. S. (2020). Impact of COVID-19 pandemic on people living with visual disability. *Indian Journal of Ophthalmology*, *68*(7), 1367.

Serge. (2021). Interviewing children: The impact of the COVID-19 quarantine on children's perceived Psychological distress and changes in routine. *BMC Pediatrics*, *21*(231), 1–11. doi:10.118612887-021-02704-1 PMID:33985448

Shah, R., Raju, V. V., Sharma, A., & Grover, S. (2021). Impact of COVID-19 and lockdown on children with ADHD and Their families-an online survey and a continuity care model. *Journal of Neurosciences in Rural Practice*, *12*(01), 71–79. doi:10.1055-0040-1718645 PMID:33531763

Shamblaw, A. L., Rumas, R. L., & Best, M. W. (2021). Coping during the COVID-19 pandemic: Relations with mental health and quality of life. *Canadian Psychology*, *62*(1), 92–100. doi:10.1037/cap0000263

Sharma, A., & Borah, S. B. (2020). Covid-19 and domestic violence: An indirect path to social and economic crisis. *Journal of Family Violence*, 1–7. doi:10.100710896-020-00188-8 PMID:32836737

Shen, J. (2020). *Impact of the Covid-19 Pandemic on Children, Youth and Families*. A brief produced by the Evidence-Based Policy Institute.

Shiloh, S., Peleg, S., & Nudelman, G. (2021). Making sense of COVID-19: A longitudinal investigation of the initial stages of developing illness representations. *Psychology & Health*, 1–17. doi:10.1080/08870446.2021.1925670 PMID:33998908

Shoham, R., Sonuga-Barke, E. J., Aloni, H., Yaniv, I., & Pollak, Y. (2016). ADHD-associated risk taking is linked to exaggerated views of the benefits of positive outcomes. *Scientific Reports*, *6*(1), 1–8. doi:10.1038rep34833 PMID:27725684

Sigmund Freud. (n.d.). *OCD History*. https://www.ocdhistory.net/20thcentury/freud.html

Silva, R. M., Shavitt, R. G., & Costa, D. L. (2020) Obsessive-compulsive disorder during the COVID-19 pandemic. *Brazilian Journal of Psychiatry*. doi:10.1590/1516-4446-2020-1189

Silva-Tinoco, R., González-Cantú, A., De La Torre-Saldaña, V., Guzmán-Olvera, E., Cuatecontzi-Xochitiotzi, T., Castillo-Martínez, L., ... Ochoa-Moreno, J. (2020). Effect in self-care behavior and difficulties in coping with diabetes during the COVID-19 pandemic. *Revista Mexicana de Endocrinología, Metabolismo y Nutrición*, 1-7.

Simonetti, A., Pais, C., Jones, M., Cipriani, M. C., Janiri, D., Monti, L., Landi, F., Bernabei, R., Liperoti, R., & Sani, G. (2020). Neuropsychiatric Symptoms in Elderly With Dementia During COVID-19 Pandemic: Definition, Treatment, and Future Directions. *Front. Psychiatry, 11*. https://www.frontiersin.org/articles/10.3389/fpsyt.2020.579842/full

Simon, J., Helter, T. M., White, R. G., van der Boor, C., & Łaszewska, A. (2021). Impacts of the Covid-19 Lockdown and Relevant Vulnerabilities on Capability Well- being, Mental Health and Social Support: An Austrian Survey Study. *BMC Public Health, 21*(314), 314. doi:10.118612889-021-10351-5 PMID:33557816

Sinfield, J. (2020, April 1). *How ADHD Combined Type Has Both Inattention and Hyperactivity*. Verywell Mind. https://www.verywellmind.com/what-is-adhd-combined-type-4135385

Singh, S. (2020). Impact of COVID-19 and lockdown on mental health of children and adolescents: A narrative review with recommendations. *Psychiatry Res, 293*. . doi:10.1016/j.psychres.2020.113429

Skene, I. P., & Pfeffer, P. E. (2021). Improved asthma control during the COVID-19 pandemic: Are there lessons to be learnt. *Thorax, 76*(9), 852–853. doi:10.1136/thoraxjnl-2021-216930 PMID:33837141

Slavin, R. E., & Storey, N. (2020). The US educational response to the COVID-19 pandemic. *Best Evid Chin Edu, 5*(2), 617–633. doi:10.15354/bece.20.or027

Solari-Twadell, P. A., Flinter, M., Rambur, B., Renda, S., Witwer, S., Vanhook, P., & Poghosyan, L. (2021). The Impact of the COVID-19 Pandemic on the future of telehealth in primary care. *Nursing Outlook*. Advance online publication. doi:10.1016/j.outlook.2021.09.004 PMID:34763897

Sorenson, M. (2020). *The Impact of the Coronavirus on the Deaf Community*. doorinternational.org/the-impact-of-the-coronavirus-on-the-deaf-community

Spiteri, J. (2021). The impact of the COVID-19 Pandemic on Children's Mental Health and Wellbeing, and Beyond: A Scoping Review. *Journal of Childhood, Education & Society, 2*(2), 126–138. doi:10.37291/2717638X.20212294

Sprang, G., & Silman, M. (2013, April 25). *Posttraumatic stress disorder in parents and youth after health-related disasters: Disaster Medicine and Public Health Preparedness*. Cambridge Core. Retrieved March 29, 2022, from https://www.cambridge.org/core/journals/disaster-medicine-and-public-health-preparedness/article/abs/posttraumatic-stress-disorder-in-parents-and-youth-after-healthrelated-disasters/4F3E4300F74CEEAFA8EE95E490944888

Stankovska, G., & Memedi, I. (2020). Stress, anxiety and depression in patients with cardiovascular diseases. *ACTA MEDICA BALKANICA, 5*(9-10), 46–52.

Stanton, A. L., Revenson, T. A., & Tennen, H. (2007). Health psychology: Psychological adjustment to chronic disease. *Annual Review of Psychology, 58*(1), 565–592. doi:10.1146/annurev.psych.58.110405.085615 PMID:16930096

Stroebe, M., Schut, H., & Boerner, K. (2017). Cautioning Health-Care Professionals. *Omega, 74*(4), 455–473. doi:10.1177/0030222817691870 PMID:28355991

Suárez-González, A., Rajagopalan, J., Livingston, G., & Alladi, S. (2021). The effect of COVID-19 isolation measures on the cognition and mental health of people living with dementia: A rapid systematic review of one year of quantitative evidence. *EClinicalMedicine, 39*. https://www.sciencedirect.com/science/article/pii/S2589537021003278

Sundarasen, S., Chinna, K., Kamaludin, K., Nurunnabi, M., Baloch, G. M., Khoshaim, H. B., Hossain, S. F. A., & Sukayt, A. (2020). Psychological Impact of COVID-19 and Lockdown among University Students in Malaysia: Implications and Policy Recommendation. *International Journal of Environmental Research and Public Health, 17*(6206), 1–13. doi:10.3390/ijerph17176206 PMID:32867024

Swick, S. D., & Jellinek, M. S. (2020, September 16). *Virtual school is especially difficult for children with ADHD*. MDedge Pediatrics. https://www.mdedge.com/pediatrics/article/ 228663/mental-health/virtual-school-especially-difficult-children-adhd

Tahira, A. C., Verjovski-Almeida, S., & Ferreira, S. T. (2021). Dementia is an age-independent risk factor for severity and death in COVID-19 inpatients. *Alzheimer's & Dementia, 17*, 1818–1831. https://doi.org/10.100TT2/alz.12352

Tanir, Y., Karayagmurlu, A., Kaya, İ., Kaynar, T. B., Türkmen, G., Dambasan, B. N., Meral, Y., & Coşkun, M. (2020). Exacerbation of obsessive compulsive disorder symptoms in children and adolescents during COVID-19 pandemic. *Psychiatry Research, 293*, 113363. Advance online publication. doi:10.1016/j.psychres.2020.113363 PMID:32798931

Tany, R. F., & Saha, A. K. (2017). A study on stress and anxiety in relation to asthma. *Journal of Psychosomatic Research, 12*(1), 117.

Tartakovsky, M. (2013, April 2). *9 Tips for Creating a Routine for Adults with ADHD*. Psych Central. https://psychcentral.com/blog/9-tips-for-creating-a-routine-for-adults-with- adhd#1

Taylor, D. B. (2020). For the Deaf, Social Distancing Can Mean Social Isolation. *The New York Times*. www.nytimes.com/2020/06/04/us/coronavirus-deaf-culture-challenges.html

Taylor, S. E., & Aspinwall, L. G. (1996). Psychosocial aspects of chronic illness. In P. T. Costa Jr & G. R. VandenBos (Eds.), *Psychological aspects of serious illness: Chronic conditions, fatal diseases, and clinical care* (pp. 3–60). American Psychological Association., doi:10.1037/10076-007

Taylor, S., Landry, C. A., Paluszek, M. M., Fergus, T. A., McKay, D., & Asmundson, G. J. (2020). COVID stress syndrome: Concept, structure, and correlates. *Depression and Anxiety, 37*(8), 706–714. doi:10.1002/da.23071 PMID:32627255

Thombs, B. D., Kwakkenbos, L., Levis, B., Bourgeault, A., Henry, R. S., Levis, A. W., Harb, S., Tao, L., Carrier, M.-E., Bustamante, L., Duchek, D., Dyas, L., El-Baalbaki, G., Ellis, K., Rice, D. B., Wurz, A., Nordlund, J., Gagarine, M., Turner, K. A., ... Benedetti, A.Scleroderma Patient-centered Intervention Network Investigators. (2021). Effects of a multi-faceted education and support programme on anxiety symptoms among people with systemic sclerosis and anxiety during COVID-19 (SPIN-CHAT): A two-arm parallel, partially nested, randomised, controlled trial. *The Lancet. Rheumatology*, *3*(6), e427–e437. doi:10.1016/S2665-9913(21)00060-6 PMID:33899008

Thorell, L. B., Skoglund, C., de la Peña, A. G., Baeyens, D., Fuermaier, A., Groom, M. J., Mammarella, I. C., van der Oord, S., van den Hoofdakker, B. J., Luman, M., de Miranda, D. M., Siu, A., Steinmayr, R., Idrees, I., Soares, L. S., Sörlin, M., Luque, J. L., Moscardino, U. M., Roch, M., ... Christiansen, H. (2021). Parental experiences of homeschooling during the COVID-19 pandemic: Differences between seven European countries and between children with and without mental health conditions. *European Child & Adolescent Psychiatry*, 1–13. Advance online publication. doi:10.100700787-020-01706-1 PMID:33415470

Tondo, G., Sarasso, B., Serra, P., Tesser, F., & Comi, C. (2021). The Impact of the COVID-19 Pandemic on the Cognition of People with Dementia. *International Journal of Environmental Research and Public Health*, *18*(8), 4285.

Tran, T. D., Hammarberg, K., Kirkman, M., Nguyen, H. T. M., & Fisher, J. (2020, December 1). Alcohol use and mental health status during the first months of COVID-19 pandemic in Australia. *Journal of Affective Disorders*. https://www.ncbi.nlm.nih.gov/pmc/articles/PMC7476559/

Tsapanou, A., Papatriantafyllou, J. D., Yiannopoulou, K., Sali, D., Kalligerou, F., Ntanasi, E., Zoi, P., Margioti, E., Kamtsadeli, V., Hatzopoulou, M., Koustimpi, M., Zagka, A., Papageorgiou, S. G., & Sakka, P. (2021). The impact of COVID-19 pandemic on people with mild cognitive impairment/dementia and on their caregivers. *International Journal of Geriatric Psychiatry*, *36*, 583–587. https://doi.org/10.1002/gps.5457

Tulchin-Francis, K., Stevens, W., Jr., Gu, X., Zhang, T., Roberts, H., Keller, J., Dempsey, D., Borchard, J., Jeans, K., & VanPelt, J. (2021). The impact of the coronavirus disease 2019 pandemic on physical activity in US children. *Journal of Sports and Health Science*, 1–10. https://reader.elsevier.com/reader/sd/pii/S2095254621000259?token=CA20D877B2AE88EDF759D7077742CCA3BAE816FCBBC709F360B40BC35A1049173DA8A15C17204192E366AAB188DA804A&originRegion=us-east-1&originCreation=20210406004449

Tyson, L., Hardeman, W., Stratton, G., Wilson, A. M., & Semlyen, J. (2021). The effects of social distancing and self-isolation during the COVID-19 pandemic on adults diagnosed with asthma: A qualitative study. *Journal of Health Psychology*. doi:10.1177/13591053211012766 PMID:33947267

U.S. Department of Health and Human Services. (2017, November). *Attention-Deficit/Hyperactivity Disorder (ADHD)*. National Institute of Mental Health. https://www.nimh.nih.gov/health/ statistics/attention-deficit-hyperactivity-disorder-adhd#:~:text=The%20overall%20prevalence%20of%20current,all%20other%20race%2Fethni city%20groups

Umucu, E., & Lee, B. (2020). Examining the impact of COVID-19 on stress and coping strategies in individuals with disabilities and chronic conditions. *Rehabilitation Psychology*, *65*(3), 193–198. Advance online publication. doi:10.1037/rep0000328 PMID:32406739

UN. (2020). *The Impact of Covid-19 on Children.* Policy Brief. United Nations. https://unsdg.un.org/sites/default/files/2020-04/160420_Covid_Children_Policy_Brief.pdf

UNIC Press. (2017). *Nigeria: Southern Leaders Insist on New Constitution.* UNIC Press. https://unicpress.com/2017/09/07/nigeria-southern-leaders-insist-new-constitution/

United States Environmental Protection Agency. (2015). America's children and the environment: Neurodevelopmental disorders (Excerpt from the third edition). In C. Croft (Ed.), Environmental hazards and neurodevelopment: Where ecology and well-being connect (pp. 3–39). CRC Press/Routledge/Taylor & Francis Group. doi:10.1201/b18030-3

Usher, K., Bhullar, N., Durkin, J., Gyamfi, N., & Jackson, D. (2020). *Family violence and COVID-19: Increased vulnerability and reduced options for support.* Academic Press.

Van Lancker, W., & Parolin, Z. (2020). COVID-19, school closures, and child poverty: A social crisis in the making. *The Lancet. Public Health*, *5*(5), e243–e244. doi:10.1016/S2468-2667(20)30084-0 PMID:32275858

Vanderloo, L., Carsley, S., Aglipay, M., Cost, K., Maguire, J., & Birken, C. (2020). Applying Harm Reduction Principles to Address Screen Time in Young Children Amidst the COVID-19 Pandemic. *Journal Of Development And Behavioral Pediatrics, 41*(5), 335–336. https://journals.lww.com/jrnldbp/Citation/2020/07000/Applying_Harm_Reduction_Principles_to_Address.1.aspx

Vardi, N. (2021). COVID-19 pandemic: Impacts on mothers' and infants' mental health during pregnancy and shortly thereafter. *Clinical Child Psychology and Psychiatry*. Advance online publication. doi:10.1177/13591045211009297 PMID:33855857

Viner, R. (2021). *Impacts of school closures on physical and mental health of children and young people: a systematic review*. MedReview., doi:10.1101/2021.02.10.21251526

Volavka, J., & Swanson, J. (2010). Violent behavior in mental illness: The role of substance abuse. *Journal of the American Medical Association*, *304*(5), 563–564. doi:10.1001/jama.2010.1097 PMID:20682936

Wagner, B. (2020). *Decline in marriage associated with the COVID-19 pandemic in the United States*. https://journals.sagepub.com/doi/full/10.1177/2378023120980328

Waite, P., Pearcey, S., Shum, A., Raw, J. A. L., Patalay, P., & Creswell, C. (2021). How did the mental health symptoms of children and adolescents change over early lockdown during the COVID-19 pandemic in the UK? *JCPP Advances: Child and Adolescent Mental Health*, *1*(1), 1–10. doi:10.1111/jcv2.12009 PMID:34485988

Walby, S. (2004). *The cost of domestic violence*. Academic Press.

Walker, L. E. A. (1992). Battered women syndrome and self-defense. *Notre Dame Journal of Law and Ethics*, *6*(2), 321–334.

Wang, Q. Q., Xu, R., & Volkow, N. D. (2021). Increased risk of COVID -19 infection and mortality in people with mental disorders: Analysis from electronic health records in the United States. *World Psychiatry; Official Journal of the World Psychiatric Association (WPA)*, *20*(1), 124–130. doi:10.1002/wps.20806 PMID:33026219

Wigg, C. D. M., Coutinho, I. M. F. A., Silva, I. C., & Lopes, L. B. (2020). The Mental Health of Children and Adolescents During the Covid-19 Pandemic: A Narrative Review. *Research, Society and Development*, *9*(9), 1–31. doi:10.33448/rsd-v9i9.7687

Wong, A. (2015, July 16). *The 1960s 'Sesame Street' Revolution and the Persistence of America's Educational Problems.* The Atlantic. https://www.theatlantic.com/education/archive/2015/07/the-1960s-experiment-childrens-tv/398681/

Wong, F. H., Liu, T., Leung, D. K., Zhang, A. Y., Au, W. S., Kwok, W. W., Shum, A. K., Wong, G. H., & Lum, T. Y.-S. (2021). Consuming information related to COVID-19 on social media among older adults and its association with anxiety, social trust in information, and COVID-safe behaviors: Cross-sectional telephone survey (preprint). doi:10.2196/preprints.26570

World Health Organization. (2020). Addressing violence against children, women and older people during the COVID-19 Pandemic: Key actions (No. WHO/2019-nCoV/ Violence_actions/2020.1). World Health Organization.

World Health Organization. (2020). *Constitution of the World Health Organization.* Available at https://www.who.int/about/governance/constitution

World Health Organization. (2020). https://www.who.int/health-topics/coronavirus#tab=tab_1

Wu, Y., Kwakkenbos, L., Henry, R. S., Carrier, M. E., Gagarine, M., Harb, S., Bourgeault, A., Tao, L., Carboni-Jiménez, A., Negeri, Z., Patten, S., Bartlett, S. J., Mouthon, L., Varga, J., Benedetti, A., Thombs, B. D., Fortuné, C., Gietzen, A., Guillot, G., ... Ellis, K. (2021). Factors associated with fears due to COVID-19: A Scleroderma Patient-centered Intervention Network (SPIN) COVID-19 cohort study. *Journal of Psychosomatic Research*, *140*, 110314. doi:10.1016/j.jpsychores.2020.110314 PMID:33271402

Wu, Y., Kwakkenbos, L., Henry, R. S., Tao, L., Harb, S., Bourgeault, A., Carrier, M.-E., Levis, B., Sun, Y., Bhandari, P. M., Carboni-Jiménez, A., Gagarine, M., He, C., Krishnan, A., Negeri, Z. F., Neupane, D., Mouthon, L., Bartlett, S. J., Benedetti, A., ... Welling, J. (2020). Validation of the COVID-19 Fears Questionnaires for Chronic Medical Conditions: A scleroderma patient-centered intervention network covid-19 cohort study. *Journal of Psychosomatic Research*, *139*, 110271. doi:10.1016/j.jpsychores.2020.110271 PMID:33096402

Ye, G., Baldwin, D. S., & Hou, R. (2021). Anxiety in asthma: A systematic review and meta-analysis. *Psychological Medicine*, *51*(1), 11–20. doi:10.1017/S0033291720005097 PMID:33431086

Yunier, B. P., Jiménez-Morales, R. M., Monasterio-Ramos, L. O., Vázquez-Gómez, L. A., & Fernández-Fleites, Z. (2021). Fear of COVID-19, problems accessing medical appointments, and subjective experience of disease progression, predict anxiety and depression reactions in patients with Multiple Sclerosis. *Multiple Sclerosis and Related Disorders*. PMID:34119745

Zambelli, Z., Fidalgo, A. R., Halstead, E. J., & Dimitriou, D. (2021). Acute impact of a national lockdown during the COVID-19 pandemic on wellbeing outcomes among individuals with chronic pain. *Journal of Health Psychology*. PMID:33601977

Zhai, Y., & Du, X. (2020). Loss and grief amidst COVID-19: A path to adaptation and resilience. *Brain, Behavior, and Immunity*, *87*, 80–81. doi:10.1016/j.bbi.2020.04.053

Zhang, J., Shuai, L., Yu, H., Wang, Z., Qiu, M., Lu, L., Cao, X., Xia, W., Wang, Y., & Chen, R. (2020). Acute stress, behavioural symptoms and mood states among school-age children with attention-deficit/hyperactive disorder during the COVID-19 outbreak. *Asian Journal of Psychiatry*, *51*, 102077. doi:10.1016/j.ajp.2020.102077 PMID:32315967

Zvolensky, M. J., Garey, L., Rogers, A. H., Schmidt, N. B., Vujanovic, A. A., Storch, E. A., Buckner, J. D., Paulus, D. J., Alfano, C., Smits, J. A. J., & O'Cleirigh, C. (2020). Psychological, addictive, and health behavior implications of the COVID-19 pandemic. *Behaviour Research and Therapy*, *134*, 103715. doi:10.1016/j.brat.2020.103715 PMID:32891956

Related References

To continue our tradition of advancing media and communications research, we have compiled a list of recommended IGI Global readings. These references will provide additional information and guidance to further enrich your knowledge and assist you with your own research and future publications.

Abashian, N., & Fisher, S. (2018). Intercultural Effectiveness in Libraries: Supporting Success Through Collaboration With Co-Curricular Programs. In B. Blummer, J. Kenton, & M. Wiatrowski (Eds.), *Promoting Ethnic Diversity and Multiculturalism in Higher Education* (pp. 219–236). Hershey, PA: IGI Global. doi:10.4018/978-1-5225-4097-7.ch012

Adebayo, O., Fagbohun, M. O., Esse, U. C., & Nwokeoma, N. M. (2018). Change Management in the Academic Library: Transition From Print to Digital Collections. In R. Bhardwaj (Ed.), *Digitizing the Modern Library and the Transition From Print to Electronic* (pp. 1–28). Hershey, PA: IGI Global. doi:10.4018/978-1-5225-2119-8.ch001

Adegbore, A. M., Quadri, M. O., & Oyewo, O. R. (2018). A Theoretical Approach to the Adoption of Electronic Resource Management Systems (ERMS) in Nigerian University Libraries. In A. Tella & T. Kwanya (Eds.), *Handbook of Research on Managing Intellectual Property in Digital Libraries* (pp. 292–311). Hershey, PA: IGI Global. doi:10.4018/978-1-5225-3093-0.ch015

Adesola, A. P., & Olla, G. O. (2018). Unlocking the Unlimited Potentials of Koha OSS/ILS for Library House-Keeping Functions: A Global View. In M. Khosrow-Pour (Ed.), *Optimizing Contemporary Application and Processes in Open Source Software* (pp. 124–163). Hershey, PA: IGI Global. doi:10.4018/978-1-5225-5314-4.ch006

Adesola, A. P., & Olla, G. O. (2019). Bridging the Digital Divide in Nigerian Information Landscape: The Role of the Library. *International Journal of Digital Literacy and Digital Competence*, *10*(3), 10–31. doi:10.4018/IJDLDC.2019070102

Adetayo, A. J. (2021). Fake News and Social Media Censorship: Examining the Librarian Role. In R. Blankenship (Ed.), *Deep Fakes, Fake News, and Misinformation in Online Teaching and Learning Technologies* (pp. 69–92). IGI Global. https://doi.org/10.4018/978-1-7998-6474-5.ch004

Adetayo, A. J. (2022). Building Civic Engagement in Smart Cities: Role of Smart Libraries. In M. Taher (Ed.), *Handbook of Research on the Role of Libraries, Archives, and Museums in Achieving Civic Engagement and Social Justice in Smart Cities* (pp. 314–333). IGI Global. https://doi.org/10.4018/978-1-7998-8363-0.ch017

Adigun, G. O., Sobalaje, A. J., & Salau, S. A. (2018). Social Media and Copyright in Digital Libraries. In A. Tella & T. Kwanya (Eds.), *Handbook of Research on Managing Intellectual Property in Digital Libraries* (pp. 19–36). Hershey, PA: IGI Global. doi:10.4018/978-1-5225-3093-0.ch002

Adriyana, L., & Fitrina Cahyaningtyas, D. (2022). The Importance of Rural Library Services Based on Social Inclusion in Indonesia. In M. Taher (Ed.), *Handbook of Research on the Role of Libraries, Archives, and Museums in Achieving Civic Engagement and Social Justice in Smart Cities* (pp. 201–218). IGI Global. https://doi.org/10.4018/978-1-7998-8363-0.ch010

Afolabi, O. A. (2018). Myths and Challenges of Building an Effective Digital Library in Developing Nations: An African Perspective. In A. Tella & T. Kwanya (Eds.), *Handbook of Research on Managing Intellectual Property in Digital Libraries* (pp. 51–79). Hershey, PA: IGI Global. doi:10.4018/978-1-5225-3093-0.ch004

Ahuja, Y., & Kumar, P. (2017). Web 2.0 Tools and Application: Knowledge Management and Sharing in Libraries. In B. Gunjal (Ed.), *Managing Knowledge and Scholarly Assets in Academic Libraries* (pp. 218–234). Hershey, PA: IGI Global. doi:10.4018/978-1-5225-1741-2.ch010

Ajmi, A. (2018). Developing In-House Digital Tools: Case Studies From the UMKC School of Law Library. In L. Costello & M. Powers (Eds.), *Developing In-House Digital Tools in Library Spaces* (pp. 117–139). Hershey, PA: IGI Global. doi:10.4018/978-1-5225-2676-6.ch006

Al-Kharousi, R., Al-Harrasi, N. H., Jabur, N. H., & Bouazza, A. (2018). Soft Systems Methodology (SSM) as an Interdisciplinary Approach: Reflection on the Use of SSM in Adoption of Web 2.0 Applications in Omani Academic Libraries. In M. Al-Suqri, A. Al-Kindi, S. AlKindi, & N. Saleem (Eds.), *Promoting Interdisciplinarity in Knowledge Generation and Problem Solving* (pp. 243–257). Hershey, PA: IGI Global. doi:10.4018/978-1-5225-3878-3.ch016

Alenzuela, R. (2017). Research, Leadership, and Resource-Sharing Initiatives: The Role of Local Library Consortia in Access to Medical Information. In S. Ram (Ed.), *Library and Information Services for Bioinformatics Education and Research* (pp. 199–211). Hershey, PA: IGI Global. doi:10.4018/978-1-5225-1871-6.ch012

Alenzuela, R., & Terry, M. A. (2020). Diversity, Indigenous Knowledge, and LIS Pedagogy: Conceptualizing Formal Education in Library and Information Studies in Vanuatu. In R. Alenzuela, H. Kim, & D. Baylen (Eds.), *Internationalization of Library and Information Science Education in the Asia-Pacific Region* (pp. 50–77). IGI Global. doi:10.4018/978-1-7998-2273-8.ch003

Allison, D. (2017). When Sales Talk Meets Reality: Implementing a Self-Checkout Kiosk. In E. Iglesias (Ed.), *Library Technology Funding, Planning, and Deployment* (pp. 36–54). Hershey, PA: IGI Global. doi:10.4018/978-1-5225-1735-1.ch003

Anglim, C. T., & Rusk, F. (2018). Empowering DC's Future Through Information Access. In A. Burtin, J. Fleming, & P. Hampton-Garland (Eds.), *Changing Urban Landscapes Through Public Higher Education* (pp. 57–77). Hershey, PA: IGI Global. doi:10.4018/978-1-5225-3454-9.ch003

Asmi, N. A. (2017). Social Media and Library Services. *International Journal of Library and Information Services*, *6*(2), 23–36. doi:10.4018/IJLIS.2017070103

Attademo, G., & Maccaro, A. (2022). Research Ethics in the Social Sciences. In G. Punziano & A. Delli Paoli (Eds.), *Handbook of Research on Advanced Research Methodologies for a Digital Society* (pp. 54–64). IGI Global. https://doi.org/10.4018/978-1-7998-8473-6.ch005

Awoyemi, R. A. (2018). Adoption and Use of Innovative Mobile Technologies in Nigerian Academic Libraries. In J. Keengwe (Ed.), *Handbook of Research on Digital Content, Mobile Learning, and Technology Integration Models in Teacher Education* (pp. 354–389). Hershey, PA: IGI Global. doi:10.4018/978-1-5225-2953-8.ch019

Awoyemi, R. A. (2018). Adoption and Use of Innovative Mobile Technologies in Nigerian Academic Libraries. In J. Keengwe (Ed.), *Handbook of Research on Digital Content, Mobile Learning, and Technology Integration Models in Teacher Education* (pp. 354–389). Hershey, PA: IGI Global. doi:10.4018/978-1-5225-2953-8.ch019

Awoyemi, R. A., & Awoyemi, R. O. (2021). Beyond the Physical Library Space: Creating a 21st Century Digitally-Oriented Library Environment. In C. Chisita, R. Enakrire, O. Durodolu, V. Tsabedze, & J. Ngoaketsi (Eds.), *Handbook of Research on Records and Information Management Strategies for Enhanced Knowledge Coordination* (pp. 189–203). IGI Global. https://doi.org/10.4018/978-1-7998-6618-3.ch012

Babatope, I. S. (2018). Social Media Applications as Effective Service Delivery Tools for Librarians. In M. Khosrow-Pour, D.B.A. (Ed.), Encyclopedia of Information Science and Technology, Fourth Edition (pp. 5252-5261). Hershey, PA: IGI Global. doi:10.4018/978-1-5225-2255-3.ch456

Bakare, A. A. (2018). Digital Libraries and Copyright of Intellectual Property: An Ethical Practice Management. In A. Tella & T. Kwanya (Eds.), *Handbook of Research on Managing Intellectual Property in Digital Libraries* (pp. 377–395). Hershey, PA: IGI Global. doi:10.4018/978-1-5225-3093-0.ch019

Baker, A. A. (2020). To Whose Benefit? At What Cost?: Consideration for Ethical Issues in Social Science Research. In M. Baran & J. Jones (Eds.), *Applied Social Science Approaches to Mixed Methods Research* (pp. 251–260). IGI Global. https://doi.org/10.4018/978-1-7998-1025-4.ch011

Baker-Gardner, R., & Smart, C. (2017). Ignorance or Intent?: A Case Study of Plagiarism in Higher Education among LIS Students in the Caribbean. In D. Velliaris (Ed.), *Handbook of Research on Academic Misconduct in Higher Education* (pp. 182–205). Hershey, PA: IGI Global. doi:10.4018/978-1-5225-1610-1.ch008

Baker-Gardner, R., & Stewart, P. (2018). Educating Caribbean Librarians to Provide Library Education in a Dynamic Information Environment. In S. Bhattacharyya & K. Patnaik (Eds.), *Changing the Scope of Library Instruction in the Digital Age* (pp. 187–226). Hershey, PA: IGI Global. doi:10.4018/978-1-5225-2802-9.ch008

Baran, M. L., & Jones, J. E. (2020). Developing the Research Study: A Step-by-Step Approach. In M. Baran & J. Jones (Eds.), *Applied Social Science Approaches to Mixed Methods Research* (pp. 262–274). IGI Global. https://doi.org/10.4018/978-1-7998-1025-4.ch012

Baskaran, C. (2020). Altmetircs Research: An Impact and Tools. In C. Baskaran (Ed.), *Measuring and Implementing Altmetrics in Library and Information Science Research* (pp. 1–10). IGI Global. https://doi.org/10.4018/978-1-7998-1309-5.ch001

Bengtson, J. (2017). Funding a Gamification Machine. In E. Iglesias (Ed.), *Library Technology Funding, Planning, and Deployment* (pp. 99–112). Hershey, PA: IGI Global. doi:10.4018/978-1-5225-1735-1.ch006

Bhuda, M., & Koitsiwe, M. (2022). The Importance of Underpinning Indigenous Research Using African Indigenous Philosophies: Perspectives From Indigenous Scholars. In R. Tshifhumulo & T. Makhanikhe (Eds.), *Handbook of Research on Protecting and Managing Global Indigenous Knowledge Systems* (pp. 223–248). IGI Global. https://doi.org/10.4018/978-1-7998-7492-8.ch013

Blummer, B., & Kenton, J. M. (2017). Access and Accessibility of Academic Libraries' Electronic Resources and Services: Identifying Themes in the Literature From 2000 to the Present. In H. Alphin Jr, J. Lavine, & R. Chan (Eds.), *Disability and Equity in Higher Education Accessibility* (pp. 242–267). Hershey, PA: IGI Global. doi:10.4018/978-1-5225-2665-0.ch011

Blummer, B., & Kenton, J. M. (2018). Academic and Research Libraries' Portals: A Literature Review From 2003 to the Present. In R. Bhardwaj (Ed.), *Digitizing the Modern Library and the Transition From Print to Electronic* (pp. 29–63). Hershey, PA: IGI Global. doi:10.4018/978-1-5225-2119-8.ch002

Blummer, B., & Kenton, J. M. (2018). International Students and Academic Libraries: Identifying Themes in the Literature From 2001 to the Present. In B. Blummer, J. Kenton, & M. Wiatrowski (Eds.), *Promoting Ethnic Diversity and Multiculturalism in Higher Education* (pp. 237–263). Hershey, PA: IGI Global. doi:10.4018/978-1-5225-4097-7.ch013

Bohuski, L. (2020). What If Your Library Can't Go Green?: Promoting Wellness in Libraries. In A. Kaushik, A. Kumar, & P. Biswas (Eds.), *Handbook of Research on Emerging Trends and Technologies in Library and Information Science* (pp. 13–26). IGI Global. doi:10.4018/978-1-5225-9825-1.ch002

Boom, D. (2017). The Embedded Librarian: Do More With less. In B. Gunjal (Ed.), *Managing Knowledge and Scholarly Assets in Academic Libraries* (pp. 76–97). Hershey, PA: IGI Global. doi:10.4018/978-1-5225-1741-2.ch004

Bosire-Ogechi, E. (2018). Social Media, Social Networking, Copyright, and Digital Libraries. In A. Tella & T. Kwanya (Eds.), *Handbook of Research on Managing Intellectual Property in Digital Libraries* (pp. 37–50). Hershey, PA: IGI Global. doi:10.4018/978-1-5225-3093-0.ch003

Bradley-Sanders, C., & Rudshteyn, A. (2018). MyLibrary at Brooklyn College: Developing a Suite of Digital Tools. In L. Costello & M. Powers (Eds.), *Developing In-House Digital Tools in Library Spaces* (pp. 140–167). Hershey, PA: IGI Global. doi:10.4018/978-1-5225-2676-6.ch007

Brown, V. (2018). Technology Access Gap for Postsecondary Education: A Statewide Case Study. In M. Yildiz, S. Funk, & B. De Abreu (Eds.), *Promoting Global Competencies Through Media Literacy* (pp. 20–40). Hershey, PA: IGI Global. doi:10.4018/978-1-5225-3082-4.ch002

Browne, N. (2021). The IHS Library and Its Response to the COVID-19 Pandemic. In B. Holland (Eds.), *Handbook of Research on Library Response to the COVID-19 Pandemic* (pp. 298-320). IGI Global. https://doi.org/10.4018/978-1-7998-6449-3.ch016

Chaiyasoonthorn, W., & Suksa-ngiam, W. (2018). Users' Acceptance of Online Literature Databases in a Thai University: A Test of UTAUT2. *International Journal of Information Systems in the Service Sector, 10*(1), 54–70. doi:10.4018/IJISSS.2018010104

Chaudron, G. (2018). Burst Pipes and Leaky Roofs: Small Emergencies Are a Challenge for Libraries. In K. Strang, M. Korstanje, & N. Vajjhala (Eds.), *Research, Practices, and Innovations in Global Risk and Contingency Management* (pp. 211–231). Hershey, PA: IGI Global. doi:10.4018/978-1-5225-4754-9.ch012

Chemulwo, M. J. (2018). Managing Intellectual Property in Digital Libraries and Copyright Challenges. In A. Tella & T. Kwanya (Eds.), *Handbook of Research on Managing Intellectual Property in Digital Libraries* (pp. 165–183). Hershey, PA: IGI Global. doi:10.4018/978-1-5225-3093-0.ch009

Chen, J., Lan, X., Huang, Q., Dong, J., & Chen, C. (2017). Scholarly Learning Commons. In L. Ruan, Q. Zhu, & Y. Ye (Eds.), *Academic Library Development and Administration in China* (pp. 90–109). Hershey, PA: IGI Global. doi:10.4018/978-1-5225-0550-1.ch006

Chigwada, J. P. (2018). Adoption of Open Source Software in Libraries in Developing Countries. *International Journal of Library and Information Services, 7*(1), 15–29. doi:10.4018/IJLIS.2018010102

Chigwada, J. P. (2020). Librarian Skillsets in the 21st Century: The Changing Role of Librarians in the Digital Era. In N. Osuigwe (Ed.), *Managing and Adapting Library Information Services for Future Users* (pp. 41–58). IGI Global. https://doi.org/10.4018/978-1-7998-1116-9.ch003

Chigwada, J. P. (2020). The Role of the Librarian in the Research Life Cycle: Research Collaboration Among the Library and Faculty. In C. Chisita (Ed.), *Cooperation and Collaboration Initiatives for Libraries and Related Institutions* (pp. 335–346). IGI Global. https://doi.org/10.4018/978-1-7998-0043-9.ch017

Chigwada, J. P. (2021). Research Data Management Services in Tertiary Institutions in Zimbabwe. In B. Holland (Eds.), *Handbook of Research on Knowledge and Organization Systems in Library and Information Science* (pp. 419-437). IGI Global. https://doi.org/10.4018/978-1-7998-7258-0.ch022

Chigwada, J. P., & Maturure, R. (2019). Advocating for Library and Information Services by National Library Associations of Africa in the Context of Sustainable Development Goals. In P. Ngulube (Ed.), *Handbook of Research on Advocacy, Promotion, and Public Programming for Memory Institutions* (pp. 219–237). IGI Global. doi:10.4018/978-1-5225-7429-3.ch012

Chiparausha, B., & Chigwada, J. P. (2019). Promoting Library Services in a Digital Environment in Zimbabwe. In P. Ngulube (Ed.), *Handbook of Research on Advocacy, Promotion, and Public Programming for Memory Institutions* (pp. 284–296). IGI Global. https://doi.org/10.4018/978-1-5225-7429-3.ch015

Chisita, C. T., & Chinyemba, F. (2017). Utilising ICTs for Resource Sharing Initiatives in Academic Institutions in Zimbabwe: Towards a New Trajectory. In B. Gunjal (Ed.), *Managing Knowledge and Scholarly Assets in Academic Libraries* (pp. 174–187). Hershey, PA: IGI Global. doi:10.4018/978-1-5225-1741-2.ch008

Chu, S., Tu, S., Wang, N., & Zhang, W. (2020). Information Equity and Cultural Sharing: The Service for Migrant Workers in Hangzhou Public Library. *International Journal of Library and Information Services*, *9*(1), 10–24. https://doi.org/10.4018/IJLIS.2020010102

Clarance, M. M., & Angeline, X. M. (2019). User Opinion on Library Collections and Services: A Case Study of Branch Library in Karaikudi. In S. Thanuskodi (Ed.), *Literacy Skill Development for Library Science Professionals* (pp. 343–375). IGI Global. https://doi.org/10.4018/978-1-5225-7125-4.ch015

Costello, L., & Fazal, S. (2018). Developing Unique Study Room Reservation Systems: Examples From Teachers College and Stony Brook University. In L. Costello & M. Powers (Eds.), *Developing In-House Digital Tools in Library Spaces* (pp. 168–176). Hershey, PA: IGI Global. doi:10.4018/978-1-5225-2676-6.ch008

Cui, Y. (2017). Research Data Management: Models, Challenges, and Actions. In L. Ruan, Q. Zhu, & Y. Ye (Eds.), *Academic Library Development and Administration in China* (pp. 184–195). Hershey, PA: IGI Global. doi:10.4018/978-1-5225-0550-1.ch011

Dhamdhere, S. N., De Smet, E., & Lihitkar, R. (2017). Web-Based Bibliographic Services Offered by Top World and Indian University Libraries: A Comparative Study. *International Journal of Library and Information Services*, *6*(1), 53–72. doi:10.4018/IJLIS.2017010104

Eiriemiokhale, K. A. (2018). Copyright Issues in a Digital Library Environment. In A. Tella & T. Kwanya (Eds.), *Handbook of Research on Managing Intellectual Property in Digital Libraries* (pp. 142–164). Hershey, PA: IGI Global. doi:10.4018/978-1-5225-3093-0.ch008

El Mimouni, H., Anderson, J., Tempelman-Kluit, N. F., & Dolan-Mescal, A. (2018). UX Work in Libraries: How (and Why) to Do It. In L. Costello & M. Powers (Eds.), *Developing In-House Digital Tools in Library Spaces* (pp. 1–36). Hershey, PA: IGI Global. doi:10.4018/978-1-5225-2676-6.ch001

Emiri, O. T. (2017). Digital Literacy Skills Among Librarians in University Libraries In the 21st Century in Edo And Delta States, Nigeria. *International Journal of Library and Information Services*, *6*(1), 37–52. doi:10.4018/IJLIS.2017010103

Emmelhainz, C. (2020). Educating the Central Asian Librarian: Considering the International MLIS in Kazakhstan. In R. Alenzuela, H. Kim, & D. Baylen (Eds.), *Internationalization of Library and Information Science Education in the Asia-Pacific Region* (pp. 1–32). IGI Global. https://doi.org/10.4018/978-1-7998-2273-8.ch001

Esguerra, A. C. (2020). Library Education and Librarianship in Japan and the Philippines. In R. Alenzuela, H. Kim, & D. Baylen (Eds.), *Internationalization of Library and Information Science Education in the Asia-Pacific Region* (pp. 131–157). IGI Global. https://doi.org/10.4018/978-1-7998-2273-8.ch006

Esposito, T. (2018). Exploring Opportunities in Health Science Information Instructional Outreach: A Case Study Highlighting One Academic Library's Experience. In S. Bhattacharyya & K. Patnaik (Eds.), *Changing the Scope of Library Instruction in the Digital Age* (pp. 118–135). Hershey, PA: IGI Global. doi:10.4018/978-1-5225-2802-9.ch005

Fagbola, O. O., Smart, A. E., & Oluwaseun, B. O. (2020). Application of Cloud Computing Technologies in Academic Library Management: The National Open University of Nigeria Library in Perspective. In A. Tella (Ed.), *Handbook of Research on Digital Devices for Inclusivity and Engagement in Libraries* (pp. 135–159). IGI Global. https://doi.org/10.4018/978-1-5225-9034-7.ch007

Fan, Y., Zhang, X., & Li, G. (2017). Research Initiatives and Projects in Academic Libraries. In L. Ruan, Q. Zhu, & Y. Ye (Eds.), *Academic Library Development and Administration in China* (pp. 230–252). Hershey, PA: IGI Global. doi:10.4018/978-1-5225-0550-1.ch014

Farmer, L. S. (2017). ICT Literacy Integration: Issues and Sample Efforts. In J. Keengwe & P. Bull (Eds.), *Handbook of Research on Transformative Digital Content and Learning Technologies* (pp. 59–80). Hershey, PA: IGI Global. doi:10.4018/978-1-5225-2000-9.ch004

Farmer, L. S. (2017). Data Analytics for Strategic Management: Getting the Right Data. In V. Wang (Ed.), *Encyclopedia of Strategic Leadership and Management* (pp. 810–822). Hershey, PA: IGI Global. doi:10.4018/978-1-5225-1049-9.ch056

Farmer, L. S. (2017). Managing Portable Technologies for Special Education. In V. Wang (Ed.), *Encyclopedia of Strategic Leadership and Management* (pp. 977–987). Hershey, PA: IGI Global. doi:10.4018/978-1-5225-1049-9.ch068

Fujishima, D., & Kamada, T. (2017). Collective Relocation for Associative Distributed Collections of Objects. *International Journal of Software Innovation*, *5*(2), 55–69. doi:10.4018/IJSI.2017040104

Ghani, S. R. (2017). Ontology: Advancing Flawless Library Services. In T. Ashraf & N. Kumar (Eds.), *Interdisciplinary Digital Preservation Tools and Technologies* (pp. 79–102). Hershey, PA: IGI Global. doi:10.4018/978-1-5225-1653-8.ch005

Gu, J. (2017). Library Buildings on New Campuses. In L. Ruan, Q. Zhu, & Y. Ye (Eds.), *Academic Library Development and Administration in China* (pp. 110–124). Hershey, PA: IGI Global. doi:10.4018/978-1-5225-0550-1.ch007

Guan, Z., & Wang, J. (2017). The China Academic Social Sciences and Humanities Library (CASHL). In L. Ruan, Q. Zhu, & Y. Ye (Eds.), *Academic Library Development and Administration in China* (pp. 31–54). Hershey, PA: IGI Global. doi:10.4018/978-1-5225-0550-1.ch003

Gul, S., & Shueb, S. (2018). Confronting/Managing the Crisis of Indian Libraries: E-Consortia Initiatives in India - A Way Forward. In R. Bhardwaj (Ed.), *Digitizing the Modern Library and the Transition From Print to Electronic* (pp. 129–163). Hershey, PA: IGI Global. doi:10.4018/978-1-5225-2119-8.ch006

Gunjal, B. (2017). Managing Knowledge and Scholarly Assets in Academic Libraries: Issues and Challenges. In B. Gunjal (Ed.), *Managing Knowledge and Scholarly Assets in Academic Libraries* (pp. 270–279). Hershey, PA: IGI Global. doi:10.4018/978-1-5225-1741-2.ch013

Guo, J., Zhang, H., & Zong, Y. (2017). Leadership Development and Career Planning. In L. Ruan, Q. Zhu, & Y. Ye (Eds.), *Academic Library Development and Administration in China* (pp. 264–279). Hershey, PA: IGI Global. doi:10.4018/978-1-5225-0550-1.ch016

Hahn, J. (2020). Student Engagement and Smart Spaces: Library Browsing and Internet of Things Technology. In B. Holland (Eds.), *Emerging Trends and Impacts of the Internet of Things in Libraries* (pp. 52-70). IGI Global. https://doi.org/10.4018/978-1-7998-4742-7.ch003

Halder, D. (2020). A Transitional Shift From Traditional Library to Digital Library. In A. Kaushik, A. Kumar, & P. Biswas (Eds.), *Handbook of Research on Emerging Trends and Technologies in Library and Information Science* (pp. 147–155). IGI Global. https://doi.org/10.4018/978-1-5225-9825-1.ch011

Hallis, R. (2018). Leveraging Library Instruction in a Digital Age. In S. Bhattacharyya & K. Patnaik (Eds.), *Changing the Scope of Library Instruction in the Digital Age* (pp. 1–23). Hershey, PA: IGI Global. doi:10.4018/978-1-5225-2802-9.ch001

Halupa, C. (2022). An Introduction to Survey Research. In A. Zimmerman (Ed.), *Methodological Innovations in Research and Academic Writing* (pp. 41–62). IGI Global. https://doi.org/10.4018/978-1-7998-8283-1.ch003

Hartsock, R., & Alemneh, D. G. (2018). Electronic Theses and Dissertations (ETDs). In M. Khosrow-Pour, D.B.A. (Ed.), Encyclopedia of Information Science and Technology, Fourth Edition (pp. 6748-6755). Hershey, PA: IGI Global. https://doi.org/ doi:10.4018/978-1-5225-2255-3.ch584

Haugh, D. (2018). Mobile Applications for Libraries. In L. Costello & M. Powers (Eds.), *Developing In-House Digital Tools in Library Spaces* (pp. 76–90). Hershey, PA: IGI Global. doi:10.4018/978-1-5225-2676-6.ch004

Hayes, C. (2022). Methodology and Method in Case Study Research: Framing Research Design in Practice. In S. Watson, S. Austin, & J. Bell (Eds.), *Conceptual Analyses of Curriculum Inquiry Methodologies* (pp. 138-154). IGI Global. https://doi.org/10.4018/978-1-7998-8848-2.ch007

Hayes, C., & Graham, Y. N. (2022). Phenomenology: Conceptually Framing Phenomenological Research Design and Methodology. In S. Watson, S. Austin, & J. Bell (Eds.), *Conceptual Analyses of Curriculum Inquiry Methodologies* (pp. 28-50). IGI Global. https://doi.org/10.4018/978-1-7998-8848-2.ch002

Hill, V. (2017). Digital Citizens as Writers: New Literacies and New Responsibilities. In E. Monske & K. Blair (Eds.), *Handbook of Research on Writing and Composing in the Age of MOOCs* (pp. 56–74). Hershey, PA: IGI Global. doi:10.4018/978-1-5225-1718-4.ch004

Hoh, A. (2019). Expanding the Awareness and Use of Library Collections Through Social Media: A Case Study of the Library of Congress International Collections Social Media Program. In J. Joe & E. Knight (Eds.), *Social Media for Communication and Instruction in Academic Libraries* (pp. 212–236). IGI Global. doi:10.4018/978-1-5225-8097-3.ch013

Holland, B. (2020). Emerging Technology and Today's Libraries. In B. Holland (Eds.), *Emerging Trends and Impacts of the Internet of Things in Libraries* (pp. 1-33). IGI Global. https://doi.org/10.4018/978-1-7998-4742-7.ch001

Homza, A., & Fontno, T. J. (2021). Supporting Teacher Candidates as Social Justice Change-Makers: A Faculty-Librarian Collaboration for Building and Using Diverse Youth Collections. In D. Hartsfield (Ed.), *Handbook of Research on Teaching Diverse Youth Literature to Pre-Service Professionals* (pp. 398–421). IGI Global. https://doi.org/10.4018/978-1-7998-7375-4.ch020

Horne-Popp, L. M., Tessone, E. B., & Welker, J. (2018). If You Build It, They Will Come: Creating a Library Statistics Dashboard for Decision-Making. In L. Costello & M. Powers (Eds.), *Developing In-House Digital Tools in Library Spaces* (pp. 177–203). Hershey, PA: IGI Global. doi:10.4018/978-1-5225-2676-6.ch009

Huang, C., & Xue, H. F. (2017). The China Academic Digital Associative Library (CADAL). In L. Ruan, Q. Zhu, & Y. Ye (Eds.), *Academic Library Development and Administration in China* (pp. 20–30). Hershey, PA: IGI Global. doi:10.4018/978-1-5225-0550-1.ch002

Huang, J., & Vedantham, A. (2019). Cabot Science Library: Creating Transformative Learning Environments in Library Spaces. In A. Darshan Singh, S. Raghunathan, E. Robeck, & B. Sharma (Eds.), *Cases on Smart Learning Environments* (pp. 284–298). IGI Global. doi:10.4018/978-1-5225-6136-1.ch016

Hunsaker, A. J., Majewski, N., & Rocke, L. E. (2018). Pulling Content out the Back Door: Creating an Interactive Digital Collections Experience. In L. Costello & M. Powers (Eds.), *Developing In-House Digital Tools in Library Spaces* (pp. 205–226). Hershey, PA: IGI Global. doi:10.4018/978-1-5225-2676-6.ch010

Hussain, A. (2020). Cutting Edge: Technology's Impact on Library Services. In J. Jesubright & P. Saravanan (Eds.), *Innovations in the Designing and Marketing of Information Services* (pp. 16–27). IGI Global. https://doi.org/10.4018/978-1-7998-1482-5.ch002

Idiegbeyan-ose, J., Owolabi, S. E., Ayooluwa, A., Foluke, O., Toluwani, E., & Sunday, O. (2019). Digital Library and Distance Learning in Developing Countries: Benefits and Challenges. In R. Bhardwaj & P. Banks (Eds.), *Research Data Access and Management in Modern Libraries* (pp. 220–245). IGI Global. https://doi.org/10.4018/978-1-5225-8437-7.ch011

Ifijeh, G., Adebayo, O., Izuagbe, R., & Olawoyin, O. (2018). Institutional Repositories and Libraries in Nigeria: Interrogating the Nexus. *Journal of Cases on Information Technology*, *20*(2), 16–29. doi:10.4018/JCIT.2018040102

Igbinovia, M. O., Solanke, E. O., & Obinyan, O. O. (2020). Building Influence: Strategising for Library Advocacy. In N. Osuigwe (Ed.), *Managing and Adapting Library Information Services for Future Users* (pp. 221–241). IGI Global. https://doi.org/10.4018/978-1-7998-1116-9.ch013

Iglesias, E. (2017). Insourcing and Outsourcing of Library Technology. In E. Iglesias (Ed.), *Library Technology Funding, Planning, and Deployment* (pp. 113–123). Hershey, PA: IGI Global. doi:10.4018/978-1-5225-1735-1.ch007

Ikolo, V. E. (2018). Transformational Leadership for Academic Libraries in Nigeria. In M. Khosrow-Pour, D.B.A. (Ed.), Encyclopedia of Information Science and Technology, Fourth Edition (pp. 5726-5735). Hershey, PA: IGI Global. doi:10.4018/978-1-5225-2255-3.ch497

Ikolo, V. E. (2020). Doctor's Awareness and Perception of Medical Library Resources and Services: A Case Study of Delta State University Teaching Hospital (Delsuth), Nigeria. *International Journal of Library and Information Services*, *9*(2), 58–71. https://doi.org/10.4018/IJLIS.2020070104

Joe, J. A. (2018). Changing Expectations of Academic Libraries. In M. Khosrow-Pour, D.B.A. (Ed.), Encyclopedia of Information Science and Technology, Fourth Edition (pp. 5204-5212). Hershey, PA: IGI Global. doi:10.4018/978-1-5225-2255-3.ch452

Juliana, I., Izuagbe, R., Itsekor, V., Fagbohun, M. O., Asaolu, A., & Nwokeoma, M. N. (2018). The Role of the School Library in Empowering Visually Impaired Children With Lifelong Information Literacy Skills. In P. Epler (Ed.), *Instructional Strategies in General Education and Putting the Individuals With Disabilities Act (IDEA) Into Practice* (pp. 245–271). Hershey, PA: IGI Global. doi:10.4018/978-1-5225-3111-1.ch009

Kalu, C. O., Chidi-Kalu, E. I., & Mafe, T. A. (2021). Research Data Management in an Academic Library. In J. Chigwada & G. Tsvuura (Eds.), *Handbook of Research on Information and Records Management in the Fourth Industrial Revolution* (pp. 38–55). IGI Global. https://doi.org/10.4018/978-1-7998-7740-0.ch003

Kalusopa, T. (2018). Preservation and Access to Digital Materials: Strategic Policy Options for Africa. In P. Ngulube (Ed.), *Handbook of Research on Heritage Management and Preservation* (pp. 150–174). Hershey, PA: IGI Global. doi:10.4018/978-1-5225-3137-1.ch008

Kamau, G. W. (2018). Copyright Challenges in Digital Libraries in Kenya From the Lens of a Librarian. In A. Tella & T. Kwanya (Eds.), *Handbook of Research on Managing Intellectual Property in Digital Libraries* (pp. 312–336). Hershey, PA: IGI Global. doi:10.4018/978-1-5225-3093-0.ch016

Karagöz, E., Güney, L. Ö., & Baran, B. (2022). The Collaborative Digital Content Library Fostering Faculty Members' Collaboratively Building Learning Sources. In G. Durak & S. Çankaya (Eds.), *Handbook of Research on Managing and Designing Online Courses in Synchronous and Asynchronous Environments* (pp. 196–213). IGI Global. doi:10.4018/978-1-7998-8701-0.ch010

Karmakar, R. (2018). Development and Management of Digital Libraries in the Regime of IPR Paradigm. *International Journal of Library and Information Services, 7*(1), 44–57. doi:10.4018/IJLIS.2018010104

Kasemsap, K. (2017). Mastering Knowledge Management in Academic Libraries. In B. Gunjal (Ed.), *Managing Knowledge and Scholarly Assets in Academic Libraries* (pp. 27–55). Hershey, PA: IGI Global. doi:10.4018/978-1-5225-1741-2.ch002

Kehinde, A. (2018). Digital Libraries and the Role of Digital Librarians. In A. Tella & T. Kwanya (Eds.), *Handbook of Research on Managing Intellectual Property in Digital Libraries* (pp. 98–119). Hershey, PA: IGI Global. doi:10.4018/978-1-5225-3093-0.ch006

Kenausis, V., & Herman, D. (2017). Don't Make Us Use the "Get Along Shirt": Communication and Consensus Building in an RFP Process. In E. Iglesias (Ed.), *Library Technology Funding, Planning, and Deployment* (pp. 1–22). Hershey, PA: IGI Global. doi:10.4018/978-1-5225-1735-1.ch001

Kohl, L. E., Lombardi, P., & Moroney, M. (2017). Moving from Local to Global via the Integrated Library System: Cost-Savings, ILS Management, Teams, and End-Users. In E. Iglesias (Ed.), *Library Technology Funding, Planning, and Deployment* (pp. 23–35). Hershey, PA: IGI Global. doi:10.4018/978-1-5225-1735-1.ch002

Kowalsky, M. (2020). School Librarian Experiences of Learning Management Implementation. In A. Tella (Ed.), *Handbook of Research on Digital Devices for Inclusivity and Engagement in Libraries* (pp. 160–184). IGI Global. https://doi.org/10.4018/978-1-5225-9034-7.ch008

Kumar, K. (2018). Library in Your Pocket Delivery of Instruction Service Through Library Mobile Apps: A World in Your Pocket. In S. Bhattacharyya & K. Patnaik (Eds.), *Changing the Scope of Library Instruction in the Digital Age* (pp. 228–249). Hershey, PA: IGI Global. doi:10.4018/978-1-5225-2802-9.ch009

Kwanya, T. (2018). Social Bookmarking in Digital Libraries: Intellectual Property Rights Implications. In A. Tella & T. Kwanya (Eds.), *Handbook of Research on Managing Intellectual Property in Digital Libraries* (pp. 1–18). Hershey, PA: IGI Global. doi:10.4018/978-1-5225-3093-0.ch001

Lapo, P., Makhmudov, G., & Rakhmatullaev, M. (2020). Internationalization of Library and Information Science Education in Tajikistan and Uzbekistan: Implications in Central Asia. In R. Alenzuela, H. Kim, & D. Baylen (Eds.), *Internationalization of Library and Information Science Education in the Asia-Pacific Region* (pp. 225–245). IGI Global. https://doi.org/10.4018/978-1-7998-2273-8.ch010

Lewis, J. K. (2018). Change Leadership Styles and Behaviors in Academic Libraries. In M. Khosrow-Pour, D.B.A. (Ed.), Encyclopedia of Information Science and Technology, Fourth Edition (pp. 5194-5203). Hershey, PA: IGI Global. doi:10.4018/978-1-5225-2255-3.ch451

Lillard, L. L. (2018). Is Interdisciplinary Collaboration in Academia an Elusive Dream?: Can the Institutional Barriers Be Broken Down? A Review of the Literature and the Case of Library Science. In M. Al-Suqri, A. Al-Kindi, S. AlKindi, & N. Saleem (Eds.), *Promoting Interdisciplinarity in Knowledge Generation and Problem Solving* (pp. 139–147). Hershey, PA: IGI Global. doi:10.4018/978-1-5225-3878-3.ch010

Liu, C., Dou, T., Zhou, H., Zhang, B., & Zhang, C. (2021). Library Service Innovation Based on New Information Technology: Taking the Interactive Experience Space "Tsinghua Impression" as an Example. *International Journal of Library and Information Services, 10*(1), 71–81. https://doi.org/10.4018/IJLIS.2021010106

Long, X., & Yao, B. (2017). The Construction and Development of the Academic Digital Library of Chinese Ancient Collections. In L. Ruan, Q. Zhu, & Y. Ye (Eds.), *Academic Library Development and Administration in China* (pp. 126–135). Hershey, PA: IGI Global. doi:10.4018/978-1-5225-0550-1.ch008

Long, X., & Yao, B. (2020). The Construction and Development of the Academic Digital Library of Chinese Ancient Collections. In I. Management Association (Ed.), *Digital Libraries and Institutional Repositories: Breakthroughs in Research and Practice* (pp. 78-87). IGI Global. https://doi.org/10.4018/978-1-7998-2463-3.ch006

Lowe, M., & Reno, L. M. (2018). Academic Librarianship and Burnout. In *Examining the Emotional Dimensions of Academic Librarianship: Emerging Research and Opportunities* (pp. 72–89). Hershey, PA: IGI Global. doi:10.4018/978-1-5225-3761-8.ch005

Lowe, M., & Reno, L. M. (2018). Emotional Dimensions of Academic Librarianship. In *Examining the Emotional Dimensions of Academic Librarianship: Emerging Research and Opportunities* (pp. 54–71). Hershey, PA: IGI Global. doi:10.4018/978-1-5225-3761-8.ch004

Lowe, M., & Reno, L. M. (2018). Why Isn't This Being Studied? In *Examining the Emotional Dimensions of Academic Librarianship: Emerging Research and Opportunities* (pp. 90–108). Hershey, PA: IGI Global. doi:10.4018/978-1-5225-3761-8.ch006

Lowe, M., & Reno, L. M. (2018). Research Agenda: Research Ideas and Recommendations. In *Examining the Emotional Dimensions of Academic Librarianship: Emerging Research and Opportunities* (pp. 109–125). Hershey, PA: IGI Global. doi:10.4018/978-1-5225-3761-8.ch007

Luyombya, D., Kiyingi, G. W., & Naluwooza, M. (2018). The Nature and Utilisation of Archival Records Deposited in Makerere University Library, Uganda. In P. Ngulube (Ed.), *Handbook of Research on Heritage Management and Preservation* (pp. 96–113). Hershey, PA: IGI Global. doi:10.4018/978-1-5225-3137-1.ch005

Ma, W. Y. (2022). Supporting Indigenous Education From a Distance: Adjusting Strategies to Maintain Access to a Rare Library Collection During a Global Crisis. In P. Pangelinan & T. McVey (Eds.), *Learning and Reconciliation Through Indigenous Education in Oceania* (pp. 197–209). IGI Global. https://doi.org/10.4018/978-1-7998-7736-3.ch012

Mabe, M., & Ashley, E. A. (2017). The Natural Role of the Public Library. In *The Developing Role of Public Libraries in Emergency Management: Emerging Research and Opportunities* (pp. 25–43). Hershey, PA: IGI Global. doi:10.4018/978-1-5225-2196-9.ch003

Mabe, M., & Ashley, E. A. (2017). I'm Trained, Now What? In *The Developing Role of Public Libraries in Emergency Management: Emerging Research and Opportunities* (pp. 87–95). Hershey, PA: IGI Global. doi:10.4018/978-1-5225-2196-9.ch007

Mabe, M., & Ashley, E. A. (2017). Emergency Preparation for the Library and Librarian. In *The Developing Role of Public Libraries in Emergency Management: Emerging Research and Opportunities* (pp. 61–78). Hershey, PA: IGI Global. doi:10.4018/978-1-5225-2196-9.ch005

Mabe, M., & Ashley, E. A. (2017). The CCPL Model. In *The Developing Role of Public Libraries in Emergency Management: Emerging Research and Opportunities* (pp. 15–24). Hershey, PA: IGI Global. doi:10.4018/978-1-5225-2196-9.ch002

Mabe, M., & Ashley, E. A. (2017). The Local Command Structure and How the Library Fits. In *In The Developing Role of Public Libraries in Emergency Management: Emerging Research and Opportunities* (pp. 44–60). Hershey, PA: IGI Global. doi:10.4018/978-1-5225-2196-9.ch004

Mafube, M. A., & Keakopa, S. M. (2019). Customer Services at the Library Archives of the National University of Lesotho. In P. Ngulube (Ed.), *Handbook of Research on Advocacy, Promotion, and Public Programming for Memory Institutions* (pp. 62–76). IGI Global. doi:10.4018/978-1-5225-7429-3.ch004

Majumdar, S. (2022). Community Engagement Through Extension and Outreach Activities: Scope of a College Library. In M. Taher (Ed.), *Handbook of Research on the Role of Libraries, Archives, and Museums in Achieving Civic Engagement and Social Justice in Smart Cities* (pp. 121–138). IGI Global. https://doi.org/10.4018/978-1-7998-8363-0.ch006

Mangone, E. (2022). The Difficult Joining of Theory and Empirical Research: Strengths and Weaknesses of Digital Research Methods. In G. Punziano & A. Delli Paoli (Eds.), *Handbook of Research on Advanced Research Methodologies for a Digital Society* (pp. 11–23). IGI Global. https://doi.org/10.4018/978-1-7998-8473-6.ch002

Manzoor, A. (2018). Social Media: A Librarian's Tool for Instant and Direct Interaction With Library Users. In R. Bhardwaj (Ed.), *Digitizing the Modern Library and the Transition From Print to Electronic* (pp. 112–128). Hershey, PA: IGI Global. doi:10.4018/978-1-5225-2119-8.ch005

Maringanti, H. (2018). A Decision Making Paradigm for Software Development in Libraries. In L. Costello & M. Powers (Eds.), *Developing In-House Digital Tools in Library Spaces* (pp. 59–75). Hershey, PA: IGI Global. doi:10.4018/978-1-5225-2676-6.ch003

Markman, K. M., Ferrarini, M., & Deschenes, A. H. (2018). User Testing and Iterative Design in the Academic Library: A Case Study. In R. Roscoe, S. Craig, & I. Douglas (Eds.), *End-User Considerations in Educational Technology Design* (pp. 160–183). Hershey, PA: IGI Global. doi:10.4018/978-1-5225-2639-1.ch008

Marrazzo, F. (2022). Doing Research With Online Platforms: An Emerging Issue Network. In G. Punziano & A. Delli Paoli (Eds.), *Handbook of Research on Advanced Research Methodologies for a Digital Society* (pp. 65–86). IGI Global. https://doi.org/10.4018/978-1-7998-8473-6.ch006

Mertens, D. (2022). Designing Mixed Methods Studies to Contribute to Social, Economic, and Environmental Justice: Implications for Library and Information Sciences. In P. Ngulube (Ed.), *Handbook of Research on Mixed Methods Research in Information Science* (pp. 173–189). IGI Global. https://doi.org/10.4018/978-1-7998-8844-4.ch009

Moahi, K. H. (2020). The Research Process and Indigenous Epistemologies. In P. Ngulube (Ed.), *Handbook of Research on Connecting Research Methods for Information Science Research* (pp. 245–265). IGI Global. https://doi.org/10.4018/978-1-7998-1471-9.ch013

Mohapatra, N. (2021). Webrarian: A Librarian on the Web. In C. Chisita, R. Enakrire, O. Durodolu, V. Tsabedze, & J. Ngoaketsi (Eds.), *Handbook of Research on Records and Information Management Strategies for Enhanced Knowledge Coordination* (pp. 458–470). IGI Global. https://doi.org/10.4018/978-1-7998-6618-3.ch027

Munatsi, R. (2020). National Research and Knowledge Systems: Role of Libraries. In C. Chisita (Ed.), *Cooperation and Collaboration Initiatives for Libraries and Related Institutions* (pp. 273–293). IGI Global. https://doi.org/10.4018/978-1-7998-0043-9.ch014

Musimbi, W. L., & Mutuku, P. K. (2019). The Future of LIS and Media Training in the Global Era: Challenges and Prospects. In C. Chisita & A. Rusero (Eds.), *Exploring the Relationship Between Media, Libraries, and Archives* (pp. 82–101). IGI Global. doi:10.4018/978-1-5225-5840-8.ch006

Mwanzu, A. (2019). Economics of Resource Sharing via Library Consortia. In C. Chisita & A. Rusero (Eds.), *Exploring the Relationship Between Media, Libraries, and Archives* (pp. 19–34). IGI Global. https://doi.org/10.4018/978-1-5225-5840-8.ch002

Na, L. (2017). Library and Information Science Education and Graduate Programs in Academic Libraries. In L. Ruan, Q. Zhu, & Y. Ye (Eds.), *Academic Library Development and Administration in China* (pp. 218–229). Hershey, PA: IGI Global. doi:10.4018/978-1-5225-0550-1.ch013

Nagarkar, S. P. (2017). Biomedical Librarianship in the Post-Genomic Era. In S. Ram (Ed.), *Library and Information Services for Bioinformatics Education and Research* (pp. 1–17). Hershey, PA: IGI Global. doi:10.4018/978-1-5225-1871-6.ch001

Natarajan, M. (2017). Exploring Knowledge Sharing over Social Media. In R. Chugh (Ed.), *Harnessing Social Media as a Knowledge Management Tool* (pp. 55–73). Hershey, PA: IGI Global. doi:10.4018/978-1-5225-0495-5.ch003

Nazir, T. (2017). Preservation Initiatives in E-Environment to Protect Information Assets. In T. Ashraf & N. Kumar (Eds.), *Interdisciplinary Digital Preservation Tools and Technologies* (pp. 193–208). Hershey, PA: IGI Global. doi:10.4018/978-1-5225-1653-8.ch010

Ngulube, P. (2017). Embedding Indigenous Knowledge in Library and Information Science Education in Anglophone Eastern and Southern Africa. In P. Ngulube (Ed.), *Handbook of Research on Social, Cultural, and Educational Considerations of Indigenous Knowledge in Developing Countries* (pp. 92–115). Hershey, PA: IGI Global. doi:10.4018/978-1-5225-0838-0.ch006

Ngulube, P. (2022). Using Simple and Complex Mixed Methods Research Designs to Understand Research in Information Science. In P. Ngulube (Ed.), *Handbook of Research on Mixed Methods Research in Information Science* (pp. 20–46). IGI Global. doi:10.4018/978-1-7998-8844-4.ch002

Nicolajsen, H. W., Sorensen, F., & Scupola, A. (2018). User Involvement in Service Innovation Processes. In M. Khosrow-Pour (Ed.), *Optimizing Current Practices in E-Services and Mobile Applications* (pp. 42–61). Hershey, PA: IGI Global. doi:10.4018/978-1-5225-5026-6.ch003

Ocholla, D. N. (2022). A Research Dashboard for Aligning Research Components in Research Proposals, Theses, and Dissertations in Library and Information Science. In P. Ngulube (Ed.), *Handbook of Research on Mixed Methods Research in Information Science* (pp. 629–640). IGI Global. https://doi.org/10.4018/978-1-7998-8844-4.ch029

Ochonogor, W. C., & Okite-Amughoro, F. A. (2018). Building an Effective Digital Library in a University Teaching Hospital (UTH) in Nigeria. In A. Tella & T. Kwanya (Eds.), *Handbook of Research on Managing Intellectual Property in Digital Libraries* (pp. 184–204). Hershey, PA: IGI Global. doi:10.4018/978-1-5225-3093-0.ch010

Okada, D. (2020). 10,000 Newly Certified Librarians, 100 Secure Jobs. In R. Alenzuela, H. Kim, & D. Baylen (Eds.), *Internationalization of Library and Information Science Education in the Asia-Pacific Region* (pp. 78–101). IGI Global. https://doi.org/10.4018/978-1-7998-2273-8.ch004

Oladapo, Y. O. (2018). Open Access to Knowledge and Challenges in Digital Libraries. In A. Tella & T. Kwanya (Eds.), *Handbook of Research on Managing Intellectual Property in Digital Libraries* (pp. 260–291). Hershey, PA: IGI Global. doi:10.4018/978-1-5225-3093-0.ch014

Oladokun, O., & Zulu, S. F. (2017). Document Description and Coding as Key Elements in Knowledge, Records, and Information Management. In P. Jain & N. Mnjama (Eds.), *Managing Knowledge Resources and Records in Modern Organizations* (pp. 179–197). Hershey, PA: IGI Global. doi:10.4018/978-1-5225-1965-2.ch011

Olubodun, O. J., & Oye, P. O. (2019). Library: A Tool for Information Dissemination and Creating Awareness in Conflict-Induced Situations. In E. Nyam & F. Idoko (Eds.), *Examining the Social and Economic Impacts of Conflict-Induced Migration* (pp. 55–63). IGI Global. https://doi.org/10.4018/978-1-5225-7615-0.ch003

Omeluzor, S. U., Abayomi, I., & Gbemi-Ogunleye, P. (2018). Contemporary Media for Library Users' Instruction in Academic Libraries in South-West Nigeria: Contemporary Library Instruction in the Digital Age. In S. Bhattacharyya & K. Patnaik (Eds.), *Changing the Scope of Library Instruction in the Digital Age* (pp. 162–185). Hershey, PA: IGI Global. doi:10.4018/978-1-5225-2802-9.ch007

Onwuchekwa, E. O. (2020). Library Signage and Information Graphics: A Communication Tool for Library Users. In A. Tella (Ed.), *Handbook of Research on Digital Devices for Inclusivity and Engagement in Libraries* (pp. 231–237). IGI Global. https://doi.org/10.4018/978-1-5225-9034-7.ch011

Onyancha, O. B. (2020). Informetrics Research Methods Outlined. In P. Ngulube (Ed.), *Handbook of Research on Connecting Research Methods for Information Science Research* (pp. 320–348). IGI Global. https://doi.org/10.4018/978-1-7998-1471-9.ch017

Oshilalu, A. H., & Ogochukwu, E. T. (2017). Modeling a Software for Library and Information Centers. *International Journal of Library and Information Services, 6*(2), 1–10. doi:10.4018/IJLIS.2017070101

Oswal, S. K. (2017). Institutional, Legal, and Attitudinal Barriers to the Accessibility of University Digital Libraries: Implications for Retention of Disabled Students. In H. Alphin Jr, J. Lavine, & R. Chan (Eds.), *Disability and Equity in Higher Education Accessibility* (pp. 223–241). Hershey, PA: IGI Global. doi:10.4018/978-1-5225-2665-0.ch010

Oukrich, J., & Bouikhalene, B. (2017). A Survey of Users' Satisfaction in the University Library by Using a Pareto Analysis and the Automatic Classification Methods. *International Journal of Library and Information Services, 6*(1), 17–36. doi:10.4018/IJLIS.2017010102

Oyelude, A. A., & Oluwaniyi, S. A. (2020). Managing Future Library Services for the Medical Sciences: A Pharmacy Library Experience. In N. Osuigwe (Ed.), *Managing and Adapting Library Information Services for Future Users* (pp. 200–220). IGI Global. https://doi.org/10.4018/978-1-7998-1116-9.ch012

Özel, N. (2018). Developing Visual Literacy Skills Through Library Instructions. In V. Osinska & G. Osinski (Eds.), *Information Visualization Techniques in the Social Sciences and Humanities* (pp. 32–48). Hershey, PA: IGI Global. doi:10.4018/978-1-5225-4990-1.ch003

Paganelli, A. L., & Paganelli, A. L. (2021). Blockchain and the Research Libraries: Expanding Interlibrary Loan and Protecting Privacy. In D. Gunter (Ed.), *Transforming Scholarly Publishing With Blockchain Technologies and AI* (pp. 232–250). IGI Global. https://doi.org/10.4018/978-1-7998-5589-7.ch012

Patel, D., & Thakur, D. (2017). Managing Open Access (OA) Scholarly Information Resources in a University. In A. Munigal (Ed.), *Scholarly Communication and the Publish or Perish Pressures of Academia* (pp. 224–255). Hershey, PA: IGI Global. doi:10.4018/978-1-5225-1697-2.ch011

Patnaik, K. R. (2018). Crafting a Framework for Copyright Literacy and Licensed Content: A Case Study at an Advanced Management Education and Research Library. In S. Bhattacharyya & K. Patnaik (Eds.), *Changing the Scope of Library Instruction in the Digital Age* (pp. 136–160). Hershey, PA: IGI Global. doi:10.4018/978-1-5225-2802-9.ch006

Paynter, K. (2017). Elementary Library Media Specialists' Roles in the Implementation of the Common Core State Standards. In M. Grassetti & S. Brookby (Eds.), *Advancing Next-Generation Teacher Education through Digital Tools and Applications* (pp. 262–283). Hershey, PA: IGI Global. doi:10.4018/978-1-5225-0965-3.ch014

Perry, S. C., & Waggoner, J. (2018). Processes for User-Centered Design and Development: The Omeka Curator Dashboard Project. In L. Costello & M. Powers (Eds.), *Developing In-House Digital Tools in Library Spaces* (pp. 37–58). Hershey, PA: IGI Global. doi:10.4018/978-1-5225-2676-6.ch002

Perumalsamy, R., & Kannan, S. P. (2019). User Information Needs in the Public Libraries in India. In S. Thanuskodi (Ed.), *Literacy Skill Development for Library Science Professionals* (pp. 25–53). IGI Global. https://doi.org/10.4018/978-1-5225-7125-4.ch002

Phuritsabam, B., & Devi, A. B. (2017). Information Seeking Behavior of Medical Scientists at Jawaharlal Nehru Institute of Medical Science: A Study. In S. Ram (Ed.), *Library and Information Services for Bioinformatics Education and Research* (pp. 177–187). Hershey, PA: IGI Global. doi:10.4018/978-1-5225-1871-6.ch010

Quadri, R. F., & Sodiq, O. A. (2018). Managing Intellectual Property in Digital Libraries: The Roles of Digital Librarians. In A. Tella & T. Kwanya (Eds.), *Handbook of Research on Managing Intellectual Property in Digital Libraries* (pp. 337–355). Hershey, PA: IGI Global. doi:10.4018/978-1-5225-3093-0.ch017

Quintana, A. J. (2021). Ensuring Research Integrity. In K. Elufiede & C. Barker Stucky (Eds.), *Strategies and Tactics for Multidisciplinary Writing* (pp. 192–201). IGI Global. https://doi.org/10.4018/978-1-7998-4477-8.ch015

Qutab, S., Adil, S. A., Gardner, L. A., & Ullah, F. S. (2022). The Role of Libraries, Archives, and Museums for Metaliteracy in Smart Cities: Implications, Challenges, and Opportunities. In M. Taher (Ed.), *Handbook of Research on the Role of Libraries, Archives, and Museums in Achieving Civic Engagement and Social Justice in Smart Cities* (pp. 355–375). IGI Global. https://doi.org/10.4018/978-1-7998-8363-0.ch019

Raj, S. K., & De, K. (2020). Electronic Resource Management and Digitisation: Library System of the University of Calcutta. In A. Kaushik, A. Kumar, & P. Biswas (Eds.), *Handbook of Research on Emerging Trends and Technologies in Library and Information Science* (pp. 231–265). IGI Global. https://doi.org/10.4018/978-1-5225-9825-1.ch017

Ram, S. (2017). Library Services for Bioinformatics: Establishing Synergy Data Information and Knowledge. In S. Ram (Ed.), *Library and Information Services for Bioinformatics Education and Research* (pp. 18–33). Hershey, PA: IGI Global. doi:10.4018/978-1-5225-1871-6.ch002

Rao, M. (2017). Use of Institutional Repository for Information Dissemination and Knowledge Management. In B. Gunjal (Ed.), *Managing Knowledge and Scholarly Assets in Academic Libraries* (pp. 156–173). Hershey, PA: IGI Global. doi:10.4018/978-1-5225-1741-2.ch007

Rao, Y., & Zhang, Y. (2017). The Construction and Development of Academic Library Digital Special Subject Databases. In L. Ruan, Q. Zhu, & Y. Ye (Eds.), *Academic Library Development and Administration in China* (pp. 163–183). Hershey, PA: IGI Global. doi:10.4018/978-1-5225-0550-1.ch010

Rao, Y., & Zhang, Y. (2020). The Construction and Development of Academic Library Digital Special Subject Databases. In I. Management Association (Ed.), *Digital Libraries and Institutional Repositories: Breakthroughs in Research and Practice* (pp. 24-44). IGI Global. https://doi.org/10.4018/978-1-7998-2463-3.ch002

Razip, S. N., Kadir, S. F., Saim, S. N., Dolhan, F. N., Jarmil, N., Salleh, N. H., & Rajin, G. (2017). Predicting Users' Intention towards Using Library Self-Issue and Return Systems. In N. Suki (Ed.), *Handbook of Research on Leveraging Consumer Psychology for Effective Customer Engagement* (pp. 102–115). Hershey, PA: IGI Global. doi:10.4018/978-1-5225-0746-8.ch007

Rothwell, S. L. (2018). Librarians and Instructional Design Challenges: Concepts, Examples, and a Flexible Design Framework. In S. Bhattacharyya & K. Patnaik (Eds.), *Changing the Scope of Library Instruction in the Digital Age* (pp. 24–59). Hershey, PA: IGI Global. doi:10.4018/978-1-5225-2802-9.ch002

Roy, L., & Frydman, A. (2018). Community Outreach. In M. Khosrow-Pour, D.B.A. (Ed.), Encyclopedia of Information Science and Technology, Fourth Edition (pp. 6685-6694). Hershey, PA: IGI Global. doi:10.4018/978-1-5225-2255-3.ch579

Rutto, D., & Yudah, O. (2018). E-Books in University Libraries in Kenya: Trends, Usage, and Intellectual Property Issues. In A. Tella & T. Kwanya (Eds.), *Handbook of Research on Managing Intellectual Property in Digital Libraries* (pp. 120–141). Hershey, PA: IGI Global. doi:10.4018/978-1-5225-3093-0.ch007

Sabharwal, A. (2017). The Transformative Role of Institutional Repositories in Academic Knowledge Management. In B. Gunjal (Ed.), *Managing Knowledge and Scholarly Assets in Academic Libraries* (pp. 127–155). Hershey, PA: IGI Global. doi:10.4018/978-1-5225-1741-2.ch006

Sadiku, S. A., Kpakiko, M. M., & Tsafe, A. G. (2018). Institutional Digital Repository and the Challenges of Global Visibility in Nigeria. In A. Tella & T. Kwanya (Eds.), *Handbook of Research on Managing Intellectual Property in Digital Libraries* (pp. 356–376). Hershey, PA: IGI Global. doi:10.4018/978-1-5225-3093-0.ch018

Sahu, M. K. (2018). Web-Scale Discovery Service in Academic Library Environment: A Birds Eye View. *International Journal of Library and Information Services*, *7*(1), 1–14. doi:10.4018/IJLIS.2018010101

Salim, F., Saigar, B., Armoham, P. K., Gobalakrishnan, S., Jap, M. Y., & Lim, N. A. (2017). Students' Information-Seeking Intention in Academic Digital Libraries. In N. Suki (Ed.), *Handbook of Research on Leveraging Consumer Psychology for Effective Customer Engagement* (pp. 259–273). Hershey, PA: IGI Global. doi:10.4018/978-1-5225-0746-8.ch017

Saroja, G. (2017). Changing Face of Scholarly Communication and Its Impact on Library and Information Centres. In A. Munigal (Ed.), *Scholarly Communication and the Publish or Perish Pressures of Academia* (pp. 100–117). Hershey, PA: IGI Global. doi:10.4018/978-1-5225-1697-2.ch006

Sauti, L. (2020). Social Media and Library Collaboration: Analysis of Government Libraries (Kaguvi Building). In C. Chisita (Ed.), *Cooperation and Collaboration Initiatives for Libraries and Related Institutions* (pp. 312–334). IGI Global. https://doi.org/10.4018/978-1-7998-0043-9.ch016

Schuster, D. W. (2017). Selection Process for Free Open Source Software. In E. Iglesias (Ed.), *Library Technology Funding, Planning, and Deployment* (pp. 55–71). Hershey, PA: IGI Global. doi:10.4018/978-1-5225-1735-1.ch004

Seagraves, K., & Weyand, L. (2021). From Bake-Alongs to Tech Talks: How One Public Library System Pivoted to Virtual Programming. In B. Holland (Ed.), *Handbook of Research on Library Response to the COVID-19 Pandemic* (pp. 447-480). IGI Global. https://doi.org/10.4018/978-1-7998-6449-3.ch023

Segaetsho, T. (2018). Environmental Consideration in the Preservation of Paper Materials in Heritage Institutions in the East and Southern African Region. In P. Ngulube (Ed.), *Handbook of Research on Heritage Management and Preservation* (pp. 183–212). Hershey, PA: IGI Global. doi:10.4018/978-1-5225-3137-1.ch010

Shakhsi, L. (2017). Cataloging Images in Library, Archive, and Museum. In T. Ashraf & N. Kumar (Eds.), *Interdisciplinary Digital Preservation Tools and Technologies* (pp. 119–141). Hershey, PA: IGI Global. doi:10.4018/978-1-5225-1653-8.ch007

Sharma, C. (2017). Digital Initiatives of the Indian Council of World Affairs' Library. In T. Ashraf & N. Kumar (Eds.), *Interdisciplinary Digital Preservation Tools and Technologies* (pp. 231–241). Hershey, PA: IGI Global. doi:10.4018/978-1-5225-1653-8.ch012

Shook, R. (2022). Achieving Balance Through Fundamentals of Digital Librarianship. In P. Pangelinan & T. McVey (Eds.), *Learning and Reconciliation Through Indigenous Education in Oceania* (pp. 185–196). IGI Global. https://doi.org/10.4018/978-1-7998-7736-3.ch011

Shukla, P., & Das, C. (2020). Plagiarism: The Role of Librarian and Teachers in Combating It. In J. Jesubright & P. Saravanan (Eds.), *Innovations in the Designing and Marketing of Information Services* (pp. 148–158). IGI Global. https://doi.org/10.4018/978-1-7998-1482-5.ch011

Siddaiah, D. K. (2018). Commonwealth Professional Fellowship: A Gateway for the Strategic Development of Libraries in India. In R. Bhardwaj (Ed.), *Digitizing the Modern Library and the Transition From Print to Electronic* (pp. 270–286). Hershey, PA: IGI Global. doi:10.4018/978-1-5225-2119-8.ch012

Silvana de Rosa, A. (2018). Mission, Tools, and Ongoing Developments in the So.Re. Com. "A.S. de Rosa" @-library. In M. Khosrow-Pour, D.B.A. (Ed.), Encyclopedia of Information Science and Technology, Fourth Edition (pp. 5237-5251). Hershey, PA: IGI Global. https://doi.org/ doi:10.4018/978-1-5225-2255-3.ch455

Smolenski, N., Kostic, M., & Sofronijevic, A. M. (2018). Intrapreneurship and Enterprise 2.0 as Grounds for Developing In-House Digital Tools for Handling METS/ALTO Files at the University Library Belgrade. In L. Costello & M. Powers (Eds.), *Developing In-House Digital Tools in Library Spaces* (pp. 92–116). Hershey, PA: IGI Global. doi:10.4018/978-1-5225-2676-6.ch005

Sochay, L., & Junus, R. (2017). From Summon to SearchPlus: The RFP Process for a Discovery Tool at the MSU Libraries. In E. Iglesias (Ed.), *Library Technology Funding, Planning, and Deployment* (pp. 72–98). Hershey, PA: IGI Global. doi:10.4018/978-1-5225-1735-1.ch005

Soliudeen, M. J. (2021). The Relevance of Feedback Mechanisms to Library Databases in Academic Libraries. In A. Maake, B. Maake, & F. Awuor (Eds.), *Digital Solutions and the Case for Africa's Sustainable Development* (pp. 116–130). IGI Global. doi:10.4018/978-1-7998-2967-6.ch008

Sonawane, C. S. (2018). Library Catalogue in the Internet Age. In R. Bhardwaj (Ed.), *Digitizing the Modern Library and the Transition From Print to Electronic* (pp. 204–223). Hershey, PA: IGI Global. doi:10.4018/978-1-5225-2119-8.ch009

Sorokhaibam, S. D., & Mathabela, N. N. (2017). Information Needs and Assessment of Bioinformatics Students at the University of Swaziland: Librarian View. In S. Ram (Ed.), *Library and Information Services for Bioinformatics Education and Research* (pp. 188–198). IGI Global. https://doi.org/10.4018/978-1-5225-1871-6.ch011

Staley, C., Kenyon, R. S., & Marcovitz, D. M. (2018). Embedded Services: Going Beyond the Field of Dreams Model for Online Programs. In D. Polly, M. Putman, T. Petty, & A. Good (Eds.), *Innovative Practices in Teacher Preparation and Graduate-Level Teacher Education Programs* (pp. 368–381). Hershey, PA: IGI Global. doi:10.4018/978-1-5225-3068-8.ch020

Stevenson, C. N. (2020). Data Speaks: Use of Poems and Photography in Qualitative Research. In M. Baran & J. Jones (Eds.), *Applied Social Science Approaches to Mixed Methods Research* (pp. 119–144). IGI Global. doi:10.4018/978-1-7998-1025-4.ch006

Stewart, M. C., Atilano, M., & Arnold, C. L. (2017). Improving Customer Relations with Social Listening: A Case Study of an American Academic Library. *International Journal of Customer Relationship Marketing and Management, 8*(1), 49–63. doi:10.4018/IJCRMM.2017010104

Sukula, S. K., & Bhardwaj, R. K. (2018). An Extensive Discussion on Transition of Libraries: The Panoramic View of Library Resources, Services, and Evolved Librarianship. In R. Bhardwaj (Ed.), *Digitizing the Modern Library and the Transition From Print to Electronic* (pp. 255–269). Hershey, PA: IGI Global. doi:10.4018/978-1-5225-2119-8.ch011

Surendran, B., & Kumar, K. (2020). Implementing Information Literacy Skills and Soft Skills for Better Use of Library Resources and Services. In S. Thanuskodi (Ed.), *Handbook of Research on Digital Content Management and Development in Modern Libraries* (pp. 214–224). IGI Global. doi:10.4018/978-1-7998-2201-1.ch012

Suresh, M., & Ravi, S. (2020). Online Database Use by Science Research Scholars of Alagappa University, Karaikudi: A Study. In S. Thanuskodi (Ed.), *Handbook of Research on Digital Content Management and Development in Modern Libraries* (pp. 86-102). IGI Global. https://doi.org/10.4018/978-1-7998-2201-1.ch006

Tella, A., & Babatunde, B. J. (2017). Determinants of Continuance Intention of Facebook Usage Among Library and Information Science Female Undergraduates in Selected Nigerian Universities. *International Journal of E-Adoption, 9*(2), 59–76. doi:10.4018/IJEA.2017070104

Tella, A., Okojie, V., & Olaniyi, O. T. (2018). Social Bookmarking Tools and Digital Libraries. In A. Tella & T. Kwanya (Eds.), *Handbook of Research on Managing Intellectual Property in Digital Libraries* (pp. 396–409). Hershey, PA: IGI Global. doi:10.4018/978-1-5225-3093-0.ch020

Thobane, M. S., & Jansen van Rensburg, S. K. (2022). Transforming Methods for Research With Indigenous Communities: An African Social Sciences Perspective. In P. Ngulube (Ed.), *Handbook of Research on Mixed Methods Research in Information Science* (pp. 190–203). IGI Global. doi:10.4018/978-1-7998-8844-4.ch010

Thull, J. J. (2018). Librarians and the Evolving Research Needs of Distance Students. In I. Oncioiu (Ed.), *Ethics and Decision-Making for Sustainable Business Practices* (pp. 203–216). Hershey, PA: IGI Global. doi:10.4018/978-1-5225-3773-1.ch012

Titilope, A. O. (2017). Ethical Issues in Library and Information Science Profession in Nigeria: An Appraisal. *International Journal of Library and Information Services, 6*(2), 11–22. doi:10.4018/IJLIS.2017070102

Tutu, J. M. (2018). Intellectual Property Challenges in Digital Library Environments. In A. Tella & T. Kwanya (Eds.), *Handbook of Research on Managing Intellectual Property in Digital Libraries* (pp. 225–240). Hershey, PA: IGI Global. doi:10.4018/978-1-5225-3093-0.ch012

Udo-Anyanwu, A. J., & Alor, A. R. (2020). Library Associations, Leadership, and Programmes: IFLA, AfLIA, and NLA. In N. Osuigwe (Ed.), *Managing and Adapting Library Information Services for Future Users* (pp. 89–102). IGI Global. https://doi.org/10.4018/978-1-7998-1116-9.ch006

Wallace, D., & Hemment, M. (2018). Enabling Scholarship in the Digital Age: A Case for Libraries Creating Value at HBS. In S. Bhattacharyya & K. Patnaik (Eds.), *Changing the Scope of Library Instruction in the Digital Age* (pp. 86–117). Hershey, PA: IGI Global. doi:10.4018/978-1-5225-2802-9.ch004

Wang, W., & Wei, Z. (2021). Tongwei County Library: Practices of Social Cooperation in Grassroots Libraries in Western China. *International Journal of Library and Information Services, 10*(1), 48–60. https://doi.org/10.4018/IJLIS.2021010104

Wani, Z. A., Zainab, T., & Hussain, S. (2018). Web 2.0 From Evolution to Revolutionary Impact in Library and Information Centers. In M. Khosrow-Pour, D.B.A. (Ed.), Encyclopedia of Information Science and Technology, Fourth Edition (pp. 5262-5271). Hershey, PA: IGI Global. https://doi.org/ doi:10.4018/978-1-5225-2255-3.ch457

Watkins, K. E., Nicolaides, A., & Marsick, V. J. (2021). Action Research Approaches. In V. Wang (Ed.), *Promoting Qualitative Research Methods for Critical Reflection and Change* (pp. 119–139). IGI Global. https://doi.org/10.4018/978-1-7998-7600-7.ch007

Weiss, A. P. (2018). Massive Digital Libraries (MDLs). In M. Khosrow-Pour, D.B.A. (Ed.), Encyclopedia of Information Science and Technology, Fourth Edition (pp. 5226-5236). Hershey, PA: IGI Global. https://doi.org/ doi:10.4018/978-1-5225-2255-3.ch454

Wu, S. K., Bess, M., & Price, B. R. (2018). Digitizing Library Outreach: Leveraging Bluetooth Beacons and Mobile Applications to Expand Library Outreach. In R. Bhardwaj (Ed.), *Digitizing the Modern Library and the Transition From Print to Electronic* (pp. 193–203). Hershey, PA: IGI Global. doi:10.4018/978-1-5225-2119-8.ch008

Wulff, E. (2018). Evaluation of Digital Collections and Political Visibility of the Library. In R. Bhardwaj (Ed.), *Digitizing the Modern Library and the Transition From Print to Electronic* (pp. 64–89). Hershey, PA: IGI Global. doi:10.4018/978-1-5225-2119-8.ch003

Wulff, E. (2019). Research Data Access and Management in National Libraries. In R. Bhardwaj & P. Banks (Eds.), *Research Data Access and Management in Modern Libraries* (pp. 1–28). IGI Global. https://doi.org/10.4018/978-1-5225-8437-7.ch001

Xiao, L., & Liu, Y. (2017). Development of Innovative User Services. In L. Ruan, Q. Zhu, & Y. Ye (Eds.), *Academic Library Development and Administration in China* (pp. 56–73). Hershey, PA: IGI Global. doi:10.4018/978-1-5225-0550-1.ch004

Xin, X., & Wu, X. (2017). The Practice of Outreach Services in Chinese Special Libraries. In L. Ruan, Q. Zhu, & Y. Ye (Eds.), *Academic Library Development and Administration in China* (pp. 74–89). Hershey, PA: IGI Global. doi:10.4018/978-1-5225-0550-1.ch005

Yao, X., Zhu, Q., & Liu, J. (2017). The China Academic Library and Information System (CALIS). In L. Ruan, Q. Zhu, & Y. Ye (Eds.), *Academic Library Development and Administration in China* (pp. 1–19). Hershey, PA: IGI Global. doi:10.4018/978-1-5225-0550-1.ch001

Yin, Q., Yingying, W., Yan, Z., & Xiaojia, M. (2017). Resource Sharing and Mutually Beneficial Cooperation: A Look at the New United Model in Public and College Libraries. In L. Ruan, Q. Zhu, & Y. Ye (Eds.), *Academic Library Development and Administration in China* (pp. 334–352). Hershey, PA: IGI Global. doi:10.4018/978-1-5225-0550-1.ch019

Yuhua, F. (2018). Computer Information Library Clusters. In M. Khosrow-Pour, D.B.A. (Ed.), Encyclopedia of Information Science and Technology, Fourth Edition (pp. 4399-4403). Hershey, PA: IGI Global. doi:10.4018/978-1-5225-2255-3.ch382

Yusuf, F., & Owolabi, S. E. (2018). Open Access to Knowledge and Challenges in Digital Libraries: Nigeria's Peculiarity. In A. Tella & T. Kwanya (Eds.), *Handbook of Research on Managing Intellectual Property in Digital Libraries* (pp. 241–259). Hershey, PA: IGI Global. doi:10.4018/978-1-5225-3093-0.ch013

Zhang, Q., Zhang, C., & Zhang, Z. (2021). Open Data Services in the Library: Case Study of the Shanghai Library. *International Journal of Library and Information Services*, *10*(1), 1–17. https://doi.org/10.4018/IJLIS.2021010101

Zhang, W., Zou, W., & Qiu, X. (2019). A Unique Development Road of Urban Public Libraries of China: Practice and Exploration of Pudong Library. *International Journal of Library and Information Services*, *8*(2), 51–71. https://doi.org/10.4018/IJLIS.2019070104

Zhu, S., & Shi, W. (2017). A Bibliometric Analysis of Research and Services in Chinese Academic Libraries. In L. Ruan, Q. Zhu, & Y. Ye (Eds.), *Academic Library Development and Administration in China* (pp. 253–262). Hershey, PA: IGI Global. doi:10.4018/978-1-5225-0550-1.ch015

About the Contributors

Nava R. Silton, a Developmental Psychologist, received her B.S. from Cornell University in 2002 and her M.A. and Ph.D. from Fordham University in 2009. Silton has worked at Nickelodeon, Sesame Workshop, and Mediakidz, and has consulted for Netflix, Apple, Blue's Clues & You, 9Story Media, and The Autism Seaver Center. She appears regularly on Fox 5 News as a Psychological Correspondent, and has appeared on Good Day New York, Good Day Street Talk and NBC. Nava is currently a Professor of Psychology at Marymount Manhattan College. She has written over three dozen peer-reviewed journal articles, over twenty chapters, book reviews and encyclopedia entries and has edited six full textbooks, with this being her seventh. Her first two books discuss innovative technologies for individuals with autism and other disabilities, her third delves into creativity, her fourth into family dynamics and romantic relationships, her fifth explores the constructs of happiness, gratitude, kindness, empathy and well-being, her sixth text discusses best parenting and child development practices for the 21st century and this seventh book discusses the impact of COVID-19 on children, adolescents and adults. Silton has also produced a variety of creative works, including an Award-Winning children's comic book series, entitled *Realabilities*, an off-Broadway Alliance nominated Musical, *Addy & Uno*, which played off-Broadway at Theater Row for over 18 months and a soon-to-be TV show with The Jim Henson Company. Silton also created the podcast, *A Cup of Java with Dr. Nava, The Bashert Card Game,* and recently penned three full feature screenplays, *Pure, The Prof* and *Jackpot*, which are now being recognized in over a dozen screenplay contests. Silton is married and has five children, three boys and two little girls.

* * *

Vincent Agulonye obtained a BA from the Usmanu Danfodiyo University, Sokoto, (UDUS) Nigeria in 2007, a National Diploma in French (UDUS) 2005, a Postgraduate Diploma in Education from The National Teachers Institute and UDUS and a Postgraduate Diploma in Mass Communication from the Bayero University,

Kano, in 2011. He obtained a Masters in International Affairs and Diplomacy from the Ahmadu Bello University, Zaria and a Ph.D. in Development Studies from the Lisbon School of Economics and Management (ISEG), University of Lisbon in 2020. He is a Researcher with the Centre for Africa and Development (CEsA), ISEG. He has authored a few books, articles, and a book chapter.

Emily Angelillo is currently a senior at Marymount Manhattan College. She is majoring in Psychology and double minoring in Biology and Neuroscience. Her interest in the hypothesized correlation between college students' adjustment to remote learning and their mindset derived from her passion for education and her concern for her peers' mental health during the pandemic. With the results, she hopes to influence early education programs to implement lessons on how to sharpen adjustment skills. She also includes techniques on how to frame one's thinking more positively to cause smoother transitions throughout education, work, development, and life overall.

Samuel Bahago is a staff member of the Veritas University, Abuja and a serving priest of the Catholic Diocese of Minna, Niger State. He has decades of experience in the education sector from primary schools under his care. He was a Catholic Secondary School Principal and later a Polytechnic Registrar and Rector. His experience in education ranges from teaching to administration.

Brianna Blackwell received her Bachelor of Arts in Psychology from Marymount Manhattan College in 2021. Blackwell interned at the United Nations, where she demonstrated her ability to utilize psychology in different communities and is currently working as an Assistant Teacher at a Montessori preschool. Her motivation for writing this chapter is to spread awareness of the unique risk factors of domestic violence and child abuse during the COVID-19 pandemic. She also wanted to highlight the potentially severe effects of domestic violence, abuse, and child abuse for those enduring these circumstances that can interfere with overall development.

Ingrid Brussier is a French Psychology M.A. candidate with a concentration in Mental Health and Substance Abuse at the New School for Social Research. She is currently working as a research assistant investigating emotional regulation and support in a cross-cultural study. Ingrid is particularly interested in the influence culture has on child development.

Regina Colie is a graduate student, who is attaining her Master's in Clinical Mental Health Counseling at The School of Health Sciences at Touro College. She is an Alumna of Marymount Manhattan College, where she received her BA in

Psychology. She hopes to become a mental health counselor specializing in eating disorders and postpartum depression. She hopes to earn her doctoral degree in the near future.

Dilek Demirtepe-Saygili received her Ph.D. degree in Clinical Psychology from Middle East Technical University and currently works in the Department of Psychology at Atilim University, Turkey. Her recent interests include stress, coping, emotions, psychological well-being, chronic illnesses, and caregivers.

Amanda Hall graduated from Marymount Manhattan College with a Bachelor of Arts Degree in Psychology. She was motivated to write about the Deaf and Visually-Impaired communities due to her own personal experience with these communities. Her family has a history with visual-impairment and a number of her peers do, as well. She took an American Sign Language (ASL) Course at Marymount Manhattan College, where she also studied Deaf Culture. It opened her eyes to their worlds and she was able to make connections because of it, with the wish to help them and learn from them.

Manuella Hounton was born and raised in Benin, West Africa. She moved to New York City where she not only had to adapt to the culture but also had to learn a new language. She has since graduated with her Bachelor of Arts in Psychology from Marymount Manhattan College and will be applying to graduate schools in the fall for Occupational Therapy. Classes taken throughout her degree have helped to mold her interest in public and mental health.

Ariana Lopez was born and raised in the lower Hudson Valley, right outside of New York, New York. She attended Marymount Manhattan College where she graduated Cum Laude with a Bachelors of Art degree in Psychology. On her way to pursuing a Master's in Mental Health Counseling and Developmental Psychology, she had the outstanding opportunity to prepare this chapter. Her interest was piqued due to the nature of living through such a historical time and such a non-normative life event for the developing child and adult. She relishes the opportunity to educate people on the importance of taking their environment into account when examining various relevant developmental trajectories.

Ali McClellan is a senior at Marymount Manhattan College in New York City and is a double-major in Psychology and Dance. Fueled by a passion for understanding, the complexities of the mind and body, Ali is deeply interested in exploring their interconnectedness. While working on an independent study with Dr. Nava Silton in Fall of 2021, she began to explore the realm of psychological research and its many possibilities. This publication was of interest to Ali, since she wanted to learn more about how the Covid-19 pandemic affected various populations.

Justin Vrana received his B.A. in Psychology and Theatre Arts from Marymount Manhattan College in 2021. While at Marymount Manhattan College, Vrana spent much of his time conducting research centered on Attention Deficit Hyperactivity Disorder (ADHD). Having ADHD himself, Vrana wrote this chapter in the hopes of improving the lives of individuals with the disorder, who contracted COVID-19, as well as those who may encounter similar stressors in the future. He hopes to continue his work in ADHD research as he progresses towards the next stage of his life and pursues a career in the field of Psychology.

Index

F

G

H

I

L

M

N

O

P

www.ingramcontent.com/pod-product-compliance
Lightning Source LLC
LaVergne TN
LVHW081327300926
849161LV00008B/1902